W.B. SAUNDERS COMPANY
A Division of Elsevier Inc.

1600 John F. Kennedy Boulevard • Suite 1800 • Philadelphia, Pennsylvania 19103-2899

http://www.theclinics.com

ENDOCRINOLOGY AND METABOLISM CLINICS OF NORTH AMERICA Volume 38, Number 1
March 2009 ISSN 0889-8529, ISBN-13: 978-1-4377-0472-3, ISBN-10: 1-4377-0472-7

Editor: Rachel Glover
Developmental Editor: Theresa Collier

Endocrinology and Metabolism Clinics of North America (ISSN 0889-8529) is published quarterly by Elsevier Inc., 360 Park Avenue South, New York, NY 10010-1710. Months of issue are March, June, September, and December. Business and Editorial Offices: 1600 John F. Kennedy Boulevard, Suite 1800, Philadelphia, PA 19103-2899. Customer Service Office: 11830 Westline Industrial Drive, St. Louis, MO 63146. Periodicals postage paid at New York, NY and additional mailing offices. Subscription prices are USD 242.00 per year for US individuals, USD 408.00 per year for US institutions, USD 124.00 per year for US students and residents, USD 304.00 per year for Canadian individuals, USD 500.00 per year for Canadian institutions, USD 352.00 per year for international individuals, USD 500.00 per year for international institutions, and USD 184.00 per year for international and Canadian and foreign students/residents. To receive student/resident rate, orders must be accompanied by name of affiliated institution, date of term, and the signature of program/residency coordinator on institution letterhead. Orders will be billed at individual rate until proof of status is received. Foreign air speed delivery is included in all *Clinics* subscription prices. All prices are subject to change without notice. **POSTMASTER:** Send address changes to *Endocrinology and Metabolism Clinics of North America*, Elsevier Periodicals Customer Service, 11830 Westline Industrial Drive, St. Louis, MO 63146. **Customer Service: 1-800-654-2452 (U.S. and Canada). From outside of the US and Canada: 1-314-453-7041. Fax: 1-314-453-5170. For print support, e-mail: journalscustomerservice-usa@elsevier.com. For online support, e-mail: journals onlinesupport-usa@elsevier.com.**

Reprints. For copies of 100 or more, of articles in this publication, please contact the Commercial Rights Department, Elsevier Inc., 360 Park Avenue South, New York, NY 10010-1710; phone: (+1) 212-633-3813; fax: (+1) 212-462-1935; e-mail: reprints@elsevier.com.

Endocrinology and Metabolism Clinics of North America is covered in *MEDLINE/PubMed (Index Medicus), EMBASE/Excerpta Medica, Current Contents/Clinical Medicine, Current Contents/Life Sciences, Science Citation Index, ISI/BIOMED, BIOSIS,* and *Chemical Abstracts.*

Printed in the United States of America.

Contributors

CONSULTING EDITOR

DEREK LEROITH, MD, PhD
Chief, Division of Endocrinology, Metabolism, and Bone Diseases, Mount Sinai School of Medicine, New York, New York

GUEST EDITOR

DONALD A. SMITH, MD, MPH
Associate Professor of Medicine, Community and Preventive Medicine; and Director, Lipids and Metabolism, Zena and Michael A.Wiener Cardiovascular Institute, Marie-Josee and Henry R. Kravis Center for Cardiovascular Health, Mount Sinai School of Medicine, New York, New York

AUTHORS

JUDITH A. ABERG, MD
Director of Virology and Director of the AIDS Clinical Trials Unit, Bellevue Hospital Center; and Associate Professor of Medicine, New York University School of Medicine, New York, New York

BRUCE DARROW, MD, PhD
Assistant Professor of Medicine, Cardiovascular Institute, Mount Sinai Medical Center, New York, New York

SAMUEL S. GIDDING, MD
Nemours Cardiac Center, A. I. DuPont Hospital for Children, Wilmington, Delaware

ANNE CAROL GOLDBERG, MD, FACP
Associate Professor of Medicine, Division of Endocrinology, Metabolism, and Lipid Research, Washington University School of Medicine, St. Louis, Missouri

IRA J. GOLDBERG, MD
Dickinson Richards Professor of Medicine, Division of Preventive Medicine and Nutrition, Department of Medicine, Columbia University College of Physicians and Surgeons, New York, New York

ALISON M. HILL, PhD
Postdoctoral Research Scholar, Department of Nutritional Sciences, Pennsylvania State University, University Park, Pennsylvania

RUNHUA HOU, MD
Assistant Professor of Medicine, Endocrine Unit, University of Rochester, Rochester, New York

HEATHER I. KATCHER, PhD, RD
Postdoctoral Scholar, Department of Nutritional Sciences, Pennsylvania State University, University Park, Pennsylvania; and Clinical Research Coordinator, Washington Center for Clinical Research, Washington, District of Columbia

PENNY M. KRIS-ETHERTON, PhD, RD
Distinguished Professor of Nutrition, Department of Nutritional Sciences, Pennsylvania State University, University Park, Pennsylvania

JULIE L.G. LANFORD, MPH, RD
Wellness Director, Cancer Services, Inc., Winston-Salem, North Carolina

JOE F. LAU, MD, PhD
Cardiology Fellow, Mount Sinai Medical Center, New York, New York

TERRI MONTAGUE, MD
Assistant Professor of Medicine, Division of Kidney Disease and Hypertension, Brown Medical School, Providence, Rhode Island

BARBARA MURPHY, MD
Professor of Medicine, Division of Nephrology, Mount Sinai School of Medicine, New York, New York

AJITH P. NAIR, MD
Fellow, Cardiovascular Institute, Mount Sinai Medical Center, New York, New York

DONALD A. SMITH, MD, MPH
Associate Professor of Medicine, Community and Preventive Medicine; and Director, Lipids and Metabolism, Zena and Michael A.Wiener Cardiovascular Institute, Marie-Josee and Henry R. Kravis Center for Cardiovascular Health, Mount Sinai School of Medicine, New York, New York

EVAN A. STEIN, MD, PhD
Metabolic and Atherosclerosis Research Center; and Voluntary Professor, Pathology and Laboratory Medicine, University of Cincinnati, Cincinnati, Ohio

PAUL D. THOMPSON, MD
Director of Cardiology, The Henry Low Heart Center, Hartford Hospital, Hartford, Connecticut; and Professor of Medicine, University of Connecticut School of Medicine, Farmington, Connecticut

PETER P. TOTH, MD, PhD
Director of Preventive Cardiology, Sterling Rock Falls Clinic, Ltd., Sterling, Illinois; and Clinical Associate Professor, Department of Family and Community Medicine, University of Illinois College of Medicine, Peoria, Illinois

CARMELO V. VENERO, MD
Preventive Cardiology Fellow, The Henry Low Heart Center, Hartford Hospital, Hartford, Connecticut

PETER W.F. WILSON, MD
Professor of Medicine, Division of Cardiology, Emory University School of Medicine,
EPICORE; and Professor of Public Health, Department of Epidemiology, Atlanta VAMC
Epidemiology and Genetics Section; and Department of Global Health, Rollins School of
Public Health, Emory University, Atlanta, Georgia

JANEY S. YOO, MS, RD
Clinical Dietitian, Children's Hospital, New Orleans, Louisiana

FRANCES R. ZAPPALLA, DO
Nemours Cardiac Center, A. I. DuPont Hospital for Children, Wilmington, Delaware

Contents

> Low-density lipoprotein cholesterol (LDL-C) level currently is used as the major determinant of lipid- and lipoprotein-associated risk for ischemic cardiovascular disease, and varying levels have become the standard goals of lipid-altering treatment. The predictive value of the LDL-C cholesterol level, however, often is less than that provided by other variables such as non–high-density lipoprotein cholesterol (non-HDL-C), apolipoprotein B (apoB), and the number of LDL particles measured by nuclear magnetic resonance spectroscopy. This article reviews studies that compare these different lipoprotein variables, describes advanced methodologies of lipoprotein testing, and suggests goals of treatment and clinical situations in which these tests might be ordered.

> Risk scores for the prediction of coronary heart disease (CHD) have greatly improved in the past 30 years. While standardized baseline measurements and modern technology aid in the development of increasingly accurate CHD risk algorithms, recent reports have shown that simple prediction tools using a basic set of variables, including age, systolic blood pressure, smoking, hypertension, exercise, body mass index, diabetes, and family history are predictive of CHD risk and can potentially be self-administered.

> This article discusses specific dietary factors as well as dietary patterns that affect the major coronary heart disease (CHD) lipid risk factors

(ie, LDL-C, HDL-C, and TG). Based on a very large evidence base, it is clear that diet and lifestyle practices can markedly affect these major CHD lipid risk factors, and consequently decrease CHD risk substantively.

Statins, ezetimibe, and bile acid-binding resins can be used individually or in combination for lowering low-density lipoprotein cholesterol (LDL-C) levels. Statins are the most potent drugs for lowering LDL-C and are well tolerated in most patients. The addition of a bile acid sequestrant or ezetimibe to a statin produces additional LDL-C reduction allowing many patients to reach LDL-C targets. This article discusses the efficacy and safety of available statins, bile acid sequestrants, and ezetimibe in the treatment of hyperlipidemia.

Although the past 30 years have been fruitful and productive in lipid research, from basic science to drug development to demonstration of clinical benefit, cardiovascular disease remains the major cause of mortality and morbidity in industrialized societies. With the rapid industrialization of countries, such as India and China, cardiovascular disease rapidly is becoming the leading cause of global death and disability. Although most of the effective lipid-lowering drugs, the statins, have become generic and inexpensive, there remains a need for effective and safe agents. Hopefully, some of those discussed in this article will fill that need.

Approximately 10% of patients treated with statins experience some form of muscle-related side effects in clinical practice. These can range from asymptomatic creatine kinase (CK) elevation, to muscle pain, weakness, and its most severe form, rhabdomyolysis. Higher risk patients for statin myopathy are those older than 80, with a small body frame, on higher statin doses, on other medications, or with other systemic diseases including hepatic or renal diseases, diabetes mellitus, or hypothyroidism. The cause of statin myopathy is presumed to be the same for its variable presentation but has not been defined. In patients with myopathic symptoms, their symptoms and CK levels determine whether statin therapy can be continued or must be stopped.

> The treatment of elevated levels of low-density lipoprotein cholesterol is standard medical practice supported by conclusive outcome data. Less definitive information exists for hypertriglyceridemia. Only in the setting of severe hyperchylomicronemia is the benefit of triglyceride lowering clear: it is a means to reduce the risk of pancreatitis. The relationship of triglycerides and cardiovascular disease is still unclear. Moreover, the cardiovascular benefits of reducing triglycerides and of using triglyceride-lowering medications remain unproved. Nonetheless it has become almost standard to reduce the levels of triglyceride-rich lipoproteins that are a major component of plasma non–high-density lipoprotein cholesterol.

> The protectiveness of elevated HDL-C against CHD and its long-term sequelae is a subject of intense investigation throughout the world. HDL has the capacity to modulate a large number of atherogenic mechanisms, such as inflammation, oxidation, thrombosis, and cell proliferation. Among lipoproteins, HDL is also unique, in that it promotes the mobilization and clearance of excess lipid via the series of reactions collectively termed "reverse cholesterol transport." Numerous therapeutic agents are being developed in an attempt to modulate serum levels of HDL-C as well as its functionality. This article discusses the development of newer treatments targeted at raising HDL-C and HDL particle numbers to reduce residual risk in patients at risk for CHD.

> Atherosclerosis begins in childhood, and early initiation of prevention through behavioral means may lower the risk of future cardiovascular disease. The obesity epidemic threatens the cardiovascular health of today's children. Genetic dyslipidemias such as familial hypercholesterolemia and the presence of multiple risk factors in the same child or adolescent may require pharmacologic therapy.

> Elderly individuals are at higher risk for cardiovascular events, and thus this population stands to gain a greater reduction in events from lipid therapy than younger individuals. Multiple primary and secondary prevention trials

have demonstrated that the benefits of statins in geriatric patients are equivalent to, or greater than, those seen in younger patients. Combination therapy with non-statin agents should be considered in patients who do not meet cholesterol goals or who have concomitant hypertriglyceridemia or low levels of high-density lipoprotein cholesterol. Although increased side effects may occur with high-dose statin therapy, careful vigilance of drug interactions and limiting polypharmacy can reduce these effects.

Dyslipidemia now is recognized as a significant potential adverse event in HIV-infected patients who are receiving antiretroviral therapy. HIV-infected persons who have hyperlipidemia should be managed similarly to those without HIV infection in accordance with the National Cholesterol Education Program. Providers must treat the HIV infection first; if dyslipidemia develops, patients should be prescribed lipid-lowering therapies or should consider modifying their current antiretroviral therapy, if indicated. Evidence for these two strategies is discussed.

Recent studies have shown the spectrum of dyslipidemia in patients who have chronic kidney disease (CKD) or end-stage renal disease to be different from that of the general population. This article discusses the pathophysiology of dyslipidemia in CKD, dialysis, and renal transplant patients, the therapeutic options, and their association with clinical outcomes. Whenever possible, comparisons are made to outcomes in the general population.

THE CLINICS ARE NOW AVAILABLE ONLINE!

Access your subscription at:
www.theclinics.com

Foreword

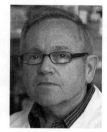

Derek LeRoith, MD, PhD
Consulting Editor

This issue, written by experts in the field of lipidology and compiled by Donald Smith, brings to the reader both basic aspects and clinical applicability.

An important question that often arises is the benefit of ordering more advanced lipoprotein profiles. The main reason for the quandary, as pointed out in the article by Lau and Smith, is that calculated low-density lipoprotein (LDL) cholesterol, measured by standard technologies, or non–high-density lipoprotein (non-HDL) cholesterol, are less predictive of ischemic cardiovascular risk than are apolipoprotein B (apoB) and nuclear magnetic resonance (NMR)–measured LDL particles in numerous studies. This is especially true in the presence of high triglycerides, or low-HDL cholesterol. Although apoB levels and the number of NMR-measured LDL particles may be more predictive, no clinical trials comparing the use of these goals versus LDL cholesterol or non-HDL cholesterol goals have been performed. For those who can interpret the results, their use may be justified occasionally to confirm lipid goal attainment in those with mixed dyslipidemias and particularly in patients already at standard lipid goals in the presence of progressive coronary heart disease.

Prediction of coronary heart disease is extremely important in clinical practice for primary and secondary prevention. Wilson emphasizes in his article the importance of standardizing baseline measurements of the factors involved, such as the lipid profile and diabetes status, to enable outcome studies to lead to definitive decisions. It has been established that the Framingham score is still very useful as a predictive index except in Japanese-Americans and in African Americans. In addition, investigators in certain European countries have found that, while Framingham is useful, it may overestimate cardiovascular disease in some groups, such as Italians. Future estimates will undoubtedly add other biomarkers and imaging techniques for atheromatous burden, and eventually may add genetic markers to aid in the predictions.

An important aspect of lipid management involves lifestyle changes. Katcher, Hill, Lanford, Yoo, and Kris-Etherton comprehensively discuss dietary components contributing to elevated LDL cholesterol, including saturated fat, trans fats, and cholesterol. They present descriptions and clinical trial evidence of various dietary manipulations that can significantly alter the lipoprotein profile, including weight reduction and diets that include more soluble fiber, plant sterols, and soy, all having variable

Endocrinol Metab Clin N Am 38 (2009) xiii–xv
doi:10.1016/j.ecl.2009.01.015
0889-8529/09/$ – see front matter © 2009 Published by Elsevier Inc.

quantitative effects. In a separate section, the effects of low-carbohydrate and Mediterranean diets, omega 3 fatty acids, mono-unsaturated fatty acids, and alcohol on triglycerides and HDL cholesterol are presented. Finally the lipid-altering effects of physical exercise are discussed as an important component of lifestyle change that should always complement these dietary manipulations.

The minimal goal for reductions in LDL cholesterol is 40 mg/dL (1 mM/L). This is often achieved by a single statin drug, though often the practitioner has to consider additional therapies. Hou and Goldberg discuss these options and describe the mechanisms of action and practical aspects of their usage. The major drugs discussed are statins, ezetimibe, and bile acid sequestrants, as well as niacin and fibrates. Combination therapies have indeed reduced LDL cholesterol levels further and studies are ongoing to quantify their preventive effects in the clinical environment.

Research progresses on other new medications and other methodologies to reduce LDL cholesterol. Evan Stein has been involved in many of these early-phase clinical trials. He describes in detail compounds being studied that not only provide possible new therapies, but also illustrate the biochemistry of lipid metabolism and the safety problems of interfering with it. Compounds discussed include squalene synthase inhibitors, apoB antisense oligonucleotides, small interfering RNAs of apoB, and proprotein convertase subtilism kexin 9.

Venero and Thompson in their article describe the etiology and management of statin-induced myopathy, an important clinical problem given the widespread use of statins. The incidence as reported in clinical trials of approximately 5% is lower than that found in surveys of patients in clinical practice, where incidence is around 10%. The symptoms range from tolerable myalgias to fatal rhabdomyolysis in extremely rare cases. Creatine kinase measurements may be important at baseline with repeat testing only necessary when the patient actually experiences myopathic symptoms. Stopping the agent, reintroducing a different statin, increasing the dosing interval, and even trying coenzyme Q10 are suggested therapeutic ways to handle this.

Ira Goldberg discusses the value of treating hypertriglyceridemia. While treatment of hypercholesterolemia with statins and other agents has shown clear-cut results in preventing cardiovascular events, and while the treatment of very elevated tryglycerides to prevent pancreatitis is important, the value of treating moderate hypertriglyceridemia to prevent such cardiovascular events is debatable. There are numerous dietary regimens and drugs that can effectively lower triglycerides and they are effective both for very high levels (>500 mg/dL) as well as for levels below 500 mg/dL. Despite inconsistent evidence in preventive clinical trials, lowering triglycerides to below 150 mg/dL in patients at risk is considered a secondary lipid-altering goal, which often also provides the additional benefit of raising HDL cholesterol.

An important risk factor for the development of atheromatous cardiovascular disease is reduced HDL cholesterol, and a few trials have shown that raising HDL cholesterol reduces cardiovascular risk. While statins are extremely effective in reducing LDL cholesterol, they are only mildly effective in raising HDL cholesterol. Drugs, such as niacin, and fibrates in the presence of hypertriglyceridemia are more effective. Peter Toth describes efforts to find agents that will raise HDL cholesterol. Investigators have looked into therapies involving apolipoprotein A1 (apoA1) itself, apoA1-mimetics, novel peroxisome proliferator-activated receptor alpha agonists, liver X receptor alpha agonists, cholesterol ester transfer protein inhibitors, and farnesoid X receptor antagonists. To date these agents, while demonstrating effectiveness in preclinical studies and in some clinical studies, are not yet adequately developed for use in patients.

Atherosclerosis can clearly begin in childhood and adolescence. Initially it was thought to be purely the consequence of genetic causes, such as familial hypercholesterolemia. However, with the epidemic of obesity that is affecting youth, environmental factors normally involved in atherosclerosis in adults are clearly in play. Dietary intervention and lifestyle changes are clearly indicated to reverse these processes. On the other hand, in cases of familial hyperlipidemia and in those adolescents that fail lifestyle intervention and are at high risk, pharmacological intervention is clearly indicated. Zappalla and Gidding develop these issues in their article.

Nair and Darrow address the important topic of lipid management in the geriatric patient. As the population ages, more patients are at risk for cardiovascular disease. Such patients require lipid-lowering agents for primary and secondary prevention, a strategy that has been shown to work quite effectively in a number of well-known trials. Statins are particularly useful. However, when statins are inadequate as solo agents, combinations with other lipid-altering therapies should be considered, as in the nongeriatric age group. Judicious usage is essential, especially when considering high doses, as the elderly are more prone to the known side effects. However, this caution should not result in avoidance of prescribing these agents to the elderly with dyslipidemia.

Use of anti-retroviral agents in treating HIV-infected individuals commonly results in dyslipidemia. Once dyslipidemia appears, there are two therapeutic approaches: altering the anti-retroviral therapy or initiating therapy for the dyslipidemia. These therapies, however, may interfere with each other, as outlined in the article by Judith Aberg. If changes in anti-retrovirals is undertaken to affect the lipid profile, it should be done under supervision to maintain virologic suppression. Nutritional alternatives to lipid therapy should undoubtedly be considered first.

Chronic kidney disease is associated with increased cardiovascular morbidity and mortality. Montague and Murphy discuss the notion that, while numerous factors may account for this effect, the role of lipid abnormalities is unclear. This arises from two important aspects. One is the fact that, in end-stage renal disease with patients on dialysis, the profile of lipid abnormalities changes from that seen in the general population. Total cholesterol, LDL cholesterol, and HDL cholesterol may all be lower, whereas small dense LDL particles and lipoprotein (a) may increase. Furthermore, only a few clinical trials using lipid-lowering drugs have been completed, while others are ongoing. All in all, the clinical-trial preventive evidence is not yet clear-cut.

I believe that this up-to-date presentation will be of tremendous value and will be most appreciated by all of us involved in an important area of endocrinology.

Derek LeRoith, MD, PhD
Division of Endocrinology, Metabolism, and Bone Diseases
Mount Sinai School of Medicine
One Gustave L. Levy Place
Box 1055, Altran 4-36
New York, NY 10029, USA

E-mail address:
derek.leroith@mssm.edu (D. LeRoith)

Preface

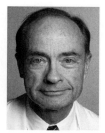

Donald A. Smith, MD, MPH
Guest Editor

The field of clinical lipidology has rapidly progressed beyond the simple lipid profile and the highly useful and simple paradigm of the National Cholesterol Education's Adult Treatment Panel III and its more recent modifications. More advanced measures of lipoprotein testing are being heavily marketed, newer risk-factor prediction models are being tested, more data are being accumulated on the benefits of lifestyle and pharmacologic therapies and the risks of the latter, and the use of lipid-lowering therapies are extending to younger and older patients, and to patients with renal disease or HIV where lipid-lowering therapy becomes more complex. In addition, newer medications to further lower low-density lipoprotein cholesterol and raise high-density lipoprotein cholesterol help us better understand lipoprotein biochemistry and the enormous creativity and difficulty required to develop a new safe and effective pharmaceutical compound. I have been extremely privileged in this issue of *Endocrinology and Metabolism Clinics of North America* to have worked and written with an extraordinarily gifted and informed group of experts in all these areas with the hope of helping clinicians responsible for lipid-altering therapy become more knowledgeable and thus in the end more effective in managing their patients.

Donald A. Smith, MD, MPH
Associate Professor of Medicine, Community and Preventive Medicine
Zena and Michael A. Wiener Cardiovascular Institute
Marie-Josee and Henry R. Kravis Center for Cardiovascular Health
Mount Sinai School of Medicine
Box 1014, 1 Gustave Levy Place
New York, NY 10029-6574, USA

E-mail address:
donald.smith@mssm.edu (D.A. Smith)

Endocrinol Metab Clin N Am 38 (2009) xvii
doi:10.1016/j.ecl.2009.01.014
0889-8529/09/$ – see front matter © 2009 Published by Elsevier Inc.

endo.theclinics.com

Advanced Lipoprotein Testing: Recommendations Based on Current Evidence

Joe F. Lau, MD, PhD[a], Donald A. Smith, MD, MPH[b],*

KEYWORDS

- Advanced lipoprotein testing • Non-HDL cholesterol
- Apolipoprotein B • LDL particle number • LDL particle size
- Vertical density gradient ultracentrifugation
- Segmented gradient gel electrophoresis
- Nuclear magnetic resonance spectroscopy (NMR)

As information has emerged from recent clinical trials, it has become clear that the incidence of ischemic atherosclerotic events is related to low-density lipoprotein (LDL) cholesterol concentration as measured using the Friedewald equation.[1] Up to 50% of secondary cardiovascular events can be prevented simply by lowering the LDL cholesterol level to 70 to 80 mg/dL by using high-dose statin drugs.[2] Because there may be a discrepancy between the LDL cholesterol concentration and the number of LDL particles, and because the size of LDL particles may modify the risk associated with LDL cholesterol at any concentration, it has become important to understand better the more advanced methods of lipoprotein testing for all potential atherogenic lipoproteins—very-low-density lipoproteins (VLDL), intermediate-density lipoproteins (IDL), lipoprotein (a), and LDL. This article briefly describes these methods and possible therapeutic target values, with special attention to target values for patients who have coronary heart disease (CHD).

National guidelines have been based predominantly on LDL cholesterol levels.[3–5] By examining these goals, it is possible to determine at what percentiles these LDL cholesterol values lie within the Framingham Offspring population. One then can look at advanced lipoprotein measures of apolipoprotein B (apoB) and the number of LDL particles within the same population or within other populations representative

[a] Mount Sinai Medical Center, Box 1030, 1 Gustave Levy Place, New York, NY 10029-6574, USA
[b] Zena and Michael A. Wiener Cardiovascular Institute, Marie-Josee and Henry R. Kravis Center for Cardiovascular Health, Mount Sinai School of Medicine, Box 1014, 1 Gustave Levy Place, New York, NY 10029-6574, USA
* Corresponding author.
E-mail address: donald.smith@mssm.edu (D.A. Smith).

Endocrinol Metab Clin N Am 38 (2009) 1–31
doi:10.1016/j.ecl.2008.11.008
0889-8529/08/$ – see front matter © 2009 Elsevier Inc. All rights reserved.

of the United States such as the National Health and Nutrition Examination Survey III (NHANES III)[6] or the Multi-Ethnic Study of Atherosclerosis (MESA) populations[7] and determine where equivalent percentile goals for these parameters might lie. Lacking results from clinical trials to set target goals for these newer parameters, one only can hypothesize that in certain subgroups of the population attaining such population percentile–based goals may reduce risk more effectively than simply attaining the more evidence-based LDL cholesterol goals.

MEASURES OF LIPID TESTING

Some of the tests available to clinicians for measuring atherogenic lipoproteins are

1. Non–high-density lipoprotein (non-HDL) cholesterol (from a standard lipid profile)
2. ApoB
3. Vertical density gradient ultracentrifugation (Vertical Auto Profile [VAP]; Atherotech)
4. Segmented gradient gel electrophoresis (S-GGE; Berkeley HeartLab)
5. Nuclear magnetic resonance (NMR; Lipoprofile; Liposcience)

Refer to **Table 1** for a partial list of laboratories that offer advanced lipid tests with their associated costs.

LOW-DENSITY LIPOPROTEIN CHOLESTEROL LEVELS FROM THE STANDARD LIPID PROFILE

In the standard lipid profile, the LDL cholesterol level is calculated from the Friedewald equation,[8] which, in the fasting state and thus without chylomicrons, is as follows:

$$Total\ cholesterol\ level\ =\ LDL\ cholesterol\ level\ +\ HDL\ cholesterol\ level$$
$$+\ VLDL\ cholesterol\ level$$

Thus

$$LDL\ cholesterol\ level\ =\ total\ cholesterol\ level\ -\ HDL\ cholesterol\ level$$
$$-\ VLDL\ cholesterol\ level$$

Because

$$VLDL\ cholesterol\ level\ =\ triglyceride\ level/5$$

(a good approximation when fasting triglycerides levels are < 400 mg/dL and in the absence of type III, or dysbetalipoproteinemia), then

$$LDL\ cholesterol\ level\ =\ total\ cholesterol\ level\ -\ HDL\ cholesterol\ level$$
$$-\ triglycerides\ level/5$$

This calculation allows the total cholesterol and total triglyceride levels to be measured enzymatically and rapidly in serum, followed by precipitation of all apoB lipoproteins and enzymatic measurement of cholesterol in the supernate to give the HDL cholesterol level. The LDL cholesterol level then is calculated by the Friedewald equation.

NON–HIGH-DENSITY LIPOPROTEIN CHOLESTEROL

The non-HDL cholesterol level, the difference between the HDL cholesterol concentration and the total cholesterol concentration, is a measure of cholesterol in all potential atherogenic lipoproteins including IDL, VLDL, lipoprotein (a), and LDL. It was suggested by the National Cholesterol Education Program (NCEP) as a secondary target

Table 1
Prices of lipid and lipoprotein tests by various laboratories as of September 2008

Laboratory	Cost ($)
Quest Diagnostics (800-631-1390 – New York City)	
Lipid profile (standard)	75
ApoB	59
Vertical Auto Profile (VAP)	154
Berkeley HeartLab (800-432-7889)	
Lipid profile	27
LDL gradient gel electrophoresis (S_3-GGE)	51
ApoB	28
LipoScience (877-547-6837)	
Lipoprotein subparticles by nuclear magnetic resonance (NMR)	80
With standard lipid profile	99

in patients who have triglycerides levels of 200 mg/dL or higher, with goal levels being 30 mg/dL greater than those for LDL cholesterol.[3] This target assumes triglyceride levels of 150 mg/dL or lower, and thus a calculated VLDL cholesterol level of 30 mg/dL or less (ie, a triglyceride level of 150 divided by 5) is a reasonable goal. For patients who have CHD, especially those at highest risk,[4] the non-HDL cholesterol goal is less than 100 mg/dL. The Framingham Offspring population percentiles for NCEP III LDL cholesterol and calculated non-HDL cholesterol goals are listed in **Table 2**.

Table 2
Suggested LDL and non-HDL cholesterol and apoB goals based on three different populations

Population Percentile	LDL-C (mg/dL)	Non-HDL-C (mg/dL)	ApoB (mg/dL)	LDL Particle Number (nmol/L)	Risk Category
5th percentile	70	100	65	700	High risk of coronary heart disease
			80 (ADA/ACC)[51]		
20th percentile	100	130	85	1000	Coronary heart disease equivalent, diabetes mellitus
			90 (ADA/ACC)[51]		
50th percentile	130	160	105	1300	>2 cardiovascular risk factors
80th percentile	160	190	125	1600	0, 1 cardiovascular risk factors

Data from Refs. [6,7,55]

APOLIPOPROTEIN B

ApoB, a measure of all non-HDL lipoproteins (LDL, IDL, VLDL, lipoprotein (a), and chylomicrons [< 1% of all non-HDLlipoproteins])[9] but largely determined by the number of LDL particles, can be used as a surrogate measure of LDL or the number of atherogenic particles and may be a better measure of lipoprotein-associated atherosclerotic risk than the LDL cholesterol concentration.[10] There are many standardized immunochemical techniques for measuring ApoB levels in clinical laboratories, but in 1994 the World Health Organization, the International Federation for Clinical Chemistry, and the Centers for Disease Control and Prevention developed an international reference standard, SP3-07, that reduced the among-method coefficient of variation to 6% or less, imprecision to 5% or less, and bias compared with the reference to 6% or less.[11] Certified laboratories should have this level of accuracy and precision when using this reference standard.

Approximate percentile levels in the NHANES III study are shown in **Table 2**.[6] Thus, apoB goals corresponding to less than 70 mg/dL, less than 100 mg/dL, less than 130 mg/dL, and less than 160 mg/dL of LDL cholesterol in NHANES III population percentiles according to this inspection of the population data would be less than 65 mg/dL, less than 85 mg/dL, less than 105 mg/dL, and less than 125 mg/dL, respectively. However, one authority has recommended the preference for a 5 mg/dL higher goal for ApoB than the values established by population percentiles (ie, a goal of <90 mg/dL for LDL-C of <100 mg/dL; apoB goal of <110 mg/dL for LDL-C <130 mg/dL; apoB goal of <130 mg/dL for LDL-C <160 mg/dL; see **Table 2**).[12]

VERTICAL DENSITY GRADIENT ULTRACENTRIFUGATION

Based on ultracentrifugation studies at the Berkeley National Laboratories of the University of California in 1954, HDL, VLDL, LDL, and IDL particles were defined by a range of migration rates measured in Svedberg units.[13] The original Framingham lipid distributions associated with this technology required 20 hours of sequential ultracentrifugation, thus precluding the use of centrifugation in mass lipoprotein screening of individuals. A more practical approach, vertical density gradient ultracentrifugation, is marketed as the VAP test.[14] With this method, the major lipoprotein groups can be sorted by density into subcomponents, including four levels of LDL and at least three levels of each of the other major lipoprotein groups. The VAP evaluation includes measures of non-HDL cholesterol, total LDL cholesterol, and its three components: lipoprotein (a) cholesterol, IDL cholesterol, and "real" LDL cholesterol. The position of the most prominent peak of real LDL cholesterol is shown along a linear scale defining LDL particle size from large to small as patterns A, A/B, and B. The concentrations of each of the four LDL subfractions allow determination of the relative percentages of small, less-preferable LDL_{3+4} and large LDL_{1+2} particles, but the clinical use of this information has not been determined. Lipoprotein (a), measured as the cholesterol content in the lipoprotein (a) density peak, has elevated values higher than 10 mg/dL, rather than higher than 30 mg/dL (or higher than 75 nmol/L using the more common antibody assays of lipoprotein (a) mass).[15]

Goals for LDL cholesterol and non-HDL cholesterol levels in VAP reports are the same as the goals in the NCEP ATP III. Practically speaking, this test yields very accurate measures of LDL cholesterol, even in a nonfasting state or in the presence of hypertriglyceridemia. It also provides a determination of LDL size. For instance, a patient who has pattern B (small) or pattern A/B (intermediate) LDL may require an even lower LDL cholesterol goal, because the number of such small LDL particles generally is higher than the LDL cholesterol concentration might suggest. To obtain a measure of the number of LDL particles, one could use non-HDL cholesterol or order an immuno-chemical assay of apoB, using population percentiles from **Table 2** to obtain a comparative population-based estimate of LDL-associated risk.

Using non-HDL cholesterol and subclass lipoprotein data from fresh serum speci-mens with triglycerides lower than 500 mg/dL sent to Atherotech for vertical ultracen-trifugation, VAP reports provide a calculated apoB level that correlates with an immunochemical apoB assay calibrated to the international apoB standard with a correlation coefficient of 0.961; the mean bias of the calculated value is 3.8% higher than the measured value.[16] Thus this free calculated apoB value may be sufficiently accurate to avoid the extra expense of an immunochemical assay for apoB in addition to the VAP test itself.

SEGMENTED GRADIENT GEL ELECTROPHORESIS

Another way to separate lipoproteins involves electrophoresis in non-denaturing poly-acrylamide gels, available from Berkeley HeartLab. Such gels form cross-linked matrices that trap lipoproteins and proteins as they travel toward the anode. The original linear gel had only one concentration of polyacrylamide, limiting its separation power; large lipoproteins could not enter the gel, and smaller lipoproteins traversed the gel without entrapment in the matrix. The latest segmented-gradient gels consist of three gradients in sequence, providing greater lipoprotein separation of seven subclasses of LDL (LDL-S_3 GGE) and 10 subclasses of HDL (HDL-S_{10} GGE). The LDL diameter is given for the two predominant LDL peaks (in Angstrom units), determined by migration distances calibrated using proteins and latex beads of known sizes. The percentage goals given on the reports for fraction for small LDL particles (III a + b < 15% and IV b < 5%) are based on the values for the lowest coronary plaque progression rates measured by quantitative coronary angiography in the Stanford Coronary Risk Inter-vention Project.[17] Below-median versus above-median apoB levels of 116 mg/dL added to the efficacy of GGE-measured LDL particle size in predicting risk for angina, myocardial infarction (MI), and CHD death in the Quebec Cardiovascular Study.[18] Thus both information about the size of LDL particles obtained from GGE and information about the number of LDL particles from apoB, which can be ordered through the same laboratory, are important for maximizing preventive information using GGE-measured LDL particle sizing. This laboratory also can provide other advanced lipopro-tein information including HDL subclasses, lipoprotein (a), and apoE subtypes.

NUCLEAR MAGNETIC RESONANCE SPECTROSCOPY

Among the latest technological developments is proton nuclear magnetic resonance (NMR) spectroscopy.[19] A plasma sample is subjected to a microsecond radiofre-quency NMR pulse, and the emitted spectrum of interest reflects the terminal methyl groups of the cholesterol, cholesterol esters, triglycerides, and phospholipid mole-cules. Pure lipoprotein fractions obtained by GGE have specific NMR profiles based on size. These profiles are combined to give three size measurements for VLDL and HDL (large, intermediate, and small), two for LDL (large and small), and one for IDL. The clinical report contains the number of LDL particles and levels of risk based on percentiles in the MESA populations.[7] The lowest risk category (< 1000 nmol/L) corre-sponds to an LDL cholesterol level lower than 100 mg/dL, which defines the lowest 20% of the population. Conveniently, dividing the number of LDL particles by 10 gives the equivalent population percentile in the MESA population. Thus, one can determine easily whether the standard Friedewald LDL cholesterol concentration (eg, LDL cholesterol = 100 mg/dL) severely underestimates the percentile risk provided by the number of LDL particles (eg, if it is significantly higher than 1000 nmol/L). At a constant LDL cholesterol concentration, small increases in particle diameter correspond to large increases in LDL volume (ie, for a sphere, volume = 4/3 π radius^3) and thus large decreases in the number of LDL particles. Clinically, knowing the number of particles may be helpful when a patient's LDL cholesterol concentration meets the goal set by the newer NCEP criteria for highest-risk populations (eg, < 70 mg/dL)[4] and yet the patient's atherosclerosis has progressed angiographically or clinically in terms of CHD events. Often such patients have small LDL particles whose number may exceed the population percentile represented by the LDL cholesterol concentration, suggesting the need for further lowering of the LDL cholesterol concentration or the use of agents that increase LDL particle size to attain lower numbers of LDL particles. Although suggestive, the value of such an approach has not yet been proven.

EVIDENCE FOR ADVANCED LIPID TESTING

Before ordering advanced lipoprotein tests, the clinician should have a fundamental understanding of the emerging body of evidence that supports their clinical applicability. Several key studies performed during the past decade have sought to determine whether individual or combined ratio measures of lipid and lipoprotein constituents (ie, non-HDL cholesterol, apoB, the number of LDL particles, LDL particle size, the ratio of total cholesterol to HDL cholesterol, and the ratio of apoB to apolipoprotein A-1 [apoA-1]) are better predictors of atherogenic lipoprotein risk than LDL cholesterol level. The totality of results thus far suggests that all surrogate measures of LDL can provide additive information beyond that provided by LDL cholesterol concentration, with the non-HDL cholesterol level having slightly better predictive power and with the number of LDL particles and apoB levels offering the greatest (and seemingly equivalent) predictive value.

Whether the non-HDL cholesterol level can predict atherogenic risk and the progression of coronary artery disease better than the LDL cholesterol level has been the subject of earlier investigations. In 2001 the NCEP ATP III recommended using non-HDL cholesterol levels as a secondary target in patients who have triglyceride levels of 200 mg/dL or higher, with target levels being 30 mg/dL higher than those for LDL cholesterol.[3] Deriving a patient's non-HDL cholesterol level is simple and cost effective; it relies only on subtracting the HDL cholesterol level from the total cholesterol level, with both attainable from a standard lipid profile. Because total cholesterol and HDL cholesterol levels are not affected by eating, blood for non-HDL cholesterol evaluations can be drawn in the nonfasting state.[20]

Many epidemiologic studies have demonstrated that the HDL cholesterol level has greater predictive power than the LDL cholesterol level, and generally these studies increase the study hazard ratio (HR), relative risk (RR), or odds ratio (OR) predicted by the LDL cholesterol level by some absolute value, generally at least more than 0.5. In spite of the apparent increase in HR for non-HDL cholesterol over LDL cholesterol, the confidence intervals of the two variables still overlap, thus rendering the apparent increase in HR only a chance finding. In many studies, however, the LDL cholesterol level is not a significant univariate predictor, whereas the non-HDL cholesterol level or apoB level is. In other studies, when non-HDL cholesterol is added to LDL cholesterol in a multivariate model, LDL cholesterol becomes insignificant, but non-HDL cholesterol retains its significance.

The following sections discuss the details of the studies comparing the strength of the association of various lipid and lipoprotein variables with cardiovascular outcomes. For ease in comprehension, the reader should consult **Tables 3–6** before continuing with the text.

The Non–High-Density Lipoprotein Cholesterol Level Versus the Low-Density Lipoprotein Cholesterol Level as a Predictor of the Risk for Coronary Heart Disease

A combined Framingham and Framingham Cohort Study followed 5800 subjects (46% male), age 30 to 79 years (mean age, 48 years), for 15 years. The end points were incidents of fatal and nonfatal MI, coronary insufficiency, and sudden cardiovascular death (**Table 3**).[21] Adjusted for the presence of diabetes, systolic blood pressure, and other risk factors, the RR of an LDL cholesterol level of 160 mg/dL or higher, versus a level lower than 130 mg/dL, was 2.04 (95% confidence interval [CI], 1.44–2.90), and the RR for a non-HDL cholesterol level of 190 mg/dL or higher, versus a level lower than 160 mg/dL, was 2.21 (95% CI, 1.57–3.11). Although the numerical difference is small, at every stratum of LDL cholesterol, the RR of the highest versus the lowest stratum of non-HDL cholesterol was 2.3 (95% CI, 1.90–2.69), whereas increasing strata of LDL cholesterol within each stratum of non-HDL cholesterol added no increased RR, suggesting that the non-HDL cholesterol level adds information to the LDL cholesterol level.

The Boston Area Health Study matched 303 persons (77% male) with a mean age of 57 years who had survived a first MI with 297 age-, gender-, and community-matched controls.[22] After adjustment for age and gender, ORs for first nonfatal MI of the highest versus the lowest quartile for non-HDL cholesterol level and LDL cholesterol level were 2.27 (95% CI, 1.41–3.66) and 1.38 (not significant), respectively. The area under the receiving-operative curve (AUROC) also was larger for the non-HDL cholesterol level than for the LDL cholesterol: 0.582 and 0.537, respectively.

A study from Greece matched 100 individuals (88% male, and 9 of whom had familial heterozygous hypercholesterolemia) who had experienced MI under the age of 36 years with 100 age- and sex-matched healthy controls.[23] When conditional logistic regression analysis was used, after controlling for body mass index (BMI), history of diabetes, hypertension, and smoking, the significant OR for MI per 1 mg/dL increase in non-HDL cholesterol was 1.03, and was 1.02 for total cholesterol, for LDL cholesterol, for triglycerides, and for apoB. The OR for being in the highest versus the lowest tertile of non-HDL cholesterol level was 28 (95% CI, 7.5–104); no comparative values were given for other lipid parameters. When discriminant analysis was used to determine which lipid variables had the strongest ability to predict outcome, the non-HDL cholesterol level was the strongest (λ-Wilks = 0.68).

The Bypass Angioplasty Revascularization Investigation trial was an intervention trial of coronary artery bypass grafting versus percutaneous transluminal coronary angioplasty in 1514 individuals (73% male) with a mean age 61 years who had multivessel coronary disease on angiography. They were followed for 5 years with end points being nonfatal MI, all-cause death, nonfatal MI or death combined, angina, and coronary revascularization.[24] The baseline lipid values used were those drawn 4 to 14 weeks after randomization. For nonfatal MI, the RR, adjusted in a multivariate model for baseline risk factors including diabetes, was 1.049 per 10 mg/dL increase in non-HDL cholesterol, 1.43 for total cholesterol, 1.016 for triglycerides, and 1.033 (not significant) for LDL cholesterol. Although the non-HDL cholesterol level was a better predictor for nonfatal MI and angina at 5 years, it was not significantly better than the LDL cholesterol level in predicting the combined end point of MI or cardiovascular death or for revascularization.

Table 3
Predictive comparisons of LDL and non-HDL cholesterol and apoB in cardiovascular trials

Trial/Study Population	Events	Trial Type	Years Follow-up	Comparison Groups	Lipid or Lipoprotein Measure	HR, RR, OR, or AUROC
Framingham[21] n = 5800, Mean age, 48 y	MI, angina, coronary insufficiency, CHD death	Prospective cohort	15	≥ 160: < 130 mg/dL, RF adj ≤190: < 160 mg/dL, RF adj	LDL-C Non–HDL-C	2.04 2.21 but three strata of non–HDL-C add risk within each of three strata of LDL-C
Boston Area Health Study[22] n = 300 post-MI cases, 300 controls, Mean age, 57 y	Nonfatal MI	Case-control	NA	Q4:Q1	LDL-C Non–HDL-C	1.38 AUROC 0.537 2.27 AUROC 0.582
MI in young individuals[23] n = 100 MI < 36 y, 100 controls, Mean age, 32 y	Nonfatal MI	Case-control	NA	OR per 1 mg/dL increase, RF adj	LDL-C Non–HDL-C	1.02 1.03
Bypass Angioplasty Revascularization Investigation (BARI)[24] n = 1514 with multivessel CHD, Mean age, 61 y	Nonfatal MI	Randomized PTCA versus CABG	5	RR per 10 mg/dL increase, RF adj	LDL-C Non–HDL-C	1.033 (NS) 1.049
Rancho Bernardo Study[25] n = 2227, Mean age, 69 y	CHD death CVD death	Prospective cohort	10	RR per 1 SD, m/f	LDL-C Non–HDL-C TC:HDL-C ratio LDL-C Non–HDL-C TC:HDL-C ratio	NS/NS (male/female) NS/NS 1.32/1.43 NS/NS 1.18/NS 1.19/1.38

Study/Population	Outcome	Design	Follow-up (y)	Measure	Marker	Result
Nurses' Health Study[26] 33,000 women n = 234 cases, Mean age, 61 y	Non-fatal MI, fatal CHD	Prospective cohort Nested case-control	8	RR Q5:Q1/RR with RF adj	LDL-C Non–HDL-C ApoB TC:HDL-C ApoB:HDL-C	2.7/3.1 (RR/RR with RF adj) 5.0/4.4 4.7/4.1 6.3/4.1 6.5/4.6
AMORIS[27] n = 172,000 Swedish adults, Mean age, 48 y	MI death or sudden death	Prospective cohort	5.5	RR per 1 SD, m/f; both LDL-C and apoB simultaneously in model AUROC m/f in group LDL-C < 145 mg/dL	LDL-C ApoB LDL-C ApoB	1.14/0.85 (NS) (male/female) 1.33/1.53 0.60/0.60 0.65/0.69
Copenhagen Study[28] n = 9231 adults equal numbers by decade, Age 20–80+ y	Any ischemic cardiovascular event (MI, angina, TIA, stroke, amaurosis fugax)	Prospective cohort	8	HR:T3:T1, m/f AUROC, m/f	LDL-C non–HDL-C ApoB ApoB RF adj LDL-C non–HDL-C ApoB	1.4/1.4 (male/female) 1.7/1.4 1.6/1.8 1.4/1.5 0.58/0.64 0.60/0.66 0.60/0.66
Health Professionals Study[29] 18,225 men n = 266 cases, Mean age, 66 y	MI, CHD death	Prospective cohort nested case-control	6	RR:Q6:Q:1	LDLC non–HDL-C ApoB	1.81 2.16 3.01
Long-Term Intervention with Pravastatin in Ischemic Disease (LIPID)[30] n = 9014 adults who had CHD, Median age, 62 y	MI, CHD death	Interventional: pravastatin 40 mg versus placebo	6.1	HR per mmol/L LDL-C placebo group baseline values HR per g/L apo B HR per 1 unit TC:HDL-C HR per mmol/L-C pravastatin group, 1-y values HR per g/L apo B HR per 1 unit TCHDL-C	LDL-C ApoB TCHDL-C LDL-C ApoB TC:HDL-C	1.15 1.64 1.14 1.08 (NS) 1.49 1.03

(continued on next page)

Table 3
(continued)

Trial/Study Population	Events	Trial Type	Years Follow-up	Comparison Groups	Lipid or Lipoprotein Measure	HR, RR, OR, or AUROC
Air Force/Texas Coronary Atherosclerosis Prevention Study (AFCAPS/ TEXCAPS)[31] n = 6505 adults without CHD, low HDL-C, Mean age, 58 y	MI, CHD death, unstable angina	Interventional: lovastatin 10–20 mg versus placebo	5.2	RR T3:T1; lovastatin / placebo baseline values Logistic regression RF adj baseline values	LDL-C ApoB ApoB/A-I TC, LDL-C ApoB, apoB/A-I, HDL-C, TC:HDL-C, apoA-I	1.29/1.46 1.60/1.55 1.72/2.00 NS All significant
Treating to New Targets and Incremental Decrease in End Points through Aggressive Lipid Lowering (TNT+ IDEAL) trials[32] n = 18,018 individuals who had CHD, Mean age, 61 y	MI, CHD death, resuscitated cardiac arrest, CVA	Interventional: TNT: atorvastatin 80 mg versus 10 mg IDEAL: atorvastatin 80 mg versus simvastatin 40 mg	4.8	Cox proportional hazard model HR per 1 SD 1-year values Two lipids in same model Lipid/apoprotein in same model Apoprotein/lipid ratio in same model Two ratios in same model	LDL-C Non–HDL-C ApoB TC:HDL-C ApoB/A-I LDL-C Non–HDL-C LDL-C ApoB ApoB TC:HDL-C TC:HDL-C ApoB/A-1	1.15 1.19 1.19 1.21 1.24 NS 1.31 NS 1.24 NS 1.17 NS 1.24
National Health and Nutrition Examination Survey III (NHANES III)[33] American adults	MI, CVA, angina, intermittent claudication, CHF	Cross-sectional	NA	OR:T3:T1	LDL-C, non– HDL-C, apoB, LDL-C:HDL-C Non–HDL-C: HDL-C ApoB:HDL-C	all NS 1.24 1.37

Atherosclerosis Risk in Communities Study (ARIC)[34] n = 12,300 multiethnic American adults Ages, 45–64 y	MI, CHD death, coronary revascularization	Prospective cohort	10	RR per 1 SD, m/f	LDL-C	1.42/1.37 (male/female)
					ApoB	1.31/1.32
				RR per 1 SD, LDL-C, TG, HDL-C, apoB, apoA-1 in model	LDL-C	1.27
					ApoB	0.96 (NS)

All results are adjusted for age and gender. All results are significant (P < 0.05) unless indicated.

Abbreviations: AUROC, area under the receiver operating curve; CABG, coronary artery bypass grafting; CHD coronary heart disease; CVA, stroke; HDL-C, high-density lipoprotein cholesterol; HR, hazard ratio; LDL-C, low-density lipoprotein cholesterol; m/f, male/female; MI, myocardial infarction; NS, not significant; OR, odds ratio; PTCA, percutaneous transluminal coronary angioplasty; RF adj, adjusted for risk factors (smoking, body mass index, and diabetes); RR, relative risk; TC, total cholesterol; TIA, transient ischemic attack.

Less Favorable Results of the Non–High-Density Lipoprotein Cholesterol Level Versus the Low-Density Lipoprotein Cholesterol Level as a Predictor for the Risk of Coronary Heart Disease

Mixed results occurred in the Rancho Bernardo Study of an elderly cohort of white, middle- to upper-middle class persons in California consisting of 2227 coronary disease–free individuals (41% male; mean age, 69 years) who were not taking statins (see **Table 3**).[25] The subjects were followed for 10 years. The end points were death from coronary or cardiovascular disease (CVD). In this study LDL cholesterol had no association with the outcomes, and only a few lipid parameters did. In men non-HDL cholesterol level was not associated significantly with coronary death. It was associated with cardiovascular death, but only after the first 5 years (RR, 1.18 per SD). The ratio of total cholesterol to HDL cholesterol was associated with both coronary and cardiovascular death, but again only after the first 5 years (RR, 1.32 and 1.19, respectively). Neither association was significant when smoking, systolic blood pressure, fasting plasma glucose, BMI, and physical activity were added to the model. In women only the ratio of total cholesterol to HDL cholesterol, but not the non-HDL cholesterol level, was associated significantly with coronary and cardio-vascular death (RR, 1.43 and 1.38, respectively); the association remained significant after risk-factor adjustment but only in the first 3 to 5 years of the study.

Positive Results of the Apolipoprotein B Versus the Low-Density Lipoprotein Cholesterol Level as a Predictor of the Risk for Coronary Heart Disease

The Nurses Health Study followed 33,000 postmenopausal women (average age, 61 years) for 8 years; 234 of these women experienced a nonfatal MI or fatal CHD (see **Table 3**).[26] These cases, in this nested case-control study, were matched to two controls for age, smoking, and fasting status, and persons taking lipid-lowering medi-cations at baseline were excluded. In the matched analysis, the highest versus lowest quintile RRs for LDL cholesterol level, non-HDL cholesterol level, and apoB level were 2.7, 5.0, and 4.7, respectively; the values for the lipid ratios of total cholesterol to HDL cholesterol and of apoB to HDL cholesterol were higher, at 6.3 and 6.5, respectively. When a multivariate model was used that included weight, history of diabetes, hyper-tension, ultra-sensitive C-reactive protein, and physical activity, the RR for the LDL cholesterol level increased to 3.1, but the RRs for the non-HDL cholesterol and apoB levels were reduced to 4.4 and 4.1, respectively.

In the Apolipoprotein-related Mortality Risk (AMORIS) study,[27] 172,000 Swedish adults (56% male; mean age, 48 years) who had blood drawn as part of a check-up or in an outpatient setting, with no historical medical information, were followed through the national death registry for an average of 5.5 years. The end points were death recorded as MI or sudden death. Total cholesterol, triglyceride, apoB, and apoA-1 levels were measured on fresh serum, and the LDL cholesterol and HDL cholesterol levels were calculated by a formula using total cholesterol, triglycerides, and apoA-1. Correlation coefficients between the Friedewald-calculated LDL choles-terol levels and AMORIS-calculated LDL cholesterol levels were 0.97 to 0.99 in four different populations (15,000 total) in which both variables had been calculated. Nevertheless, interpreting this study as a comparison between the apoB level and the Friedewald-calculated LDL cholesterol level should be done with some caution. When both the AMORIS-calculated LDL cholesterol level and the apoB level were used in the same multivariate analysis, the RRs for MI death or sudden death for the LDL cholesterol level and the apoB level in men were 1.14 and 1.33, respectively, and in women were 0.85 (nonsignificant) and 1.53, respectively. The apoB level was a stronger predictor of risk in those who had LDL cholesterol levels lower than 145 mg/dL; the AUROC for MI death or sudden death for LDL cholesterol and apoB were 0.60 and 0.65, respectively, in men and were significantly different, 0.60 and 0.69, respectively, in women.

In the Copenhagen Study[28] 9231 asymptomatic adults, drawn in equal numbers from each decade from age 20 to more than 80 years, who were not taking lipid-altering agents at recruitment between 1991 and 1994, were followed for 8 years. There were 807 episodes of ischemic coronary heart disease or stroke. The HRs for myocardial ischemia in the highest and lowest tertiles of LDL cholesterol level, non-HDL cholesterol level, and apoB level were significant in men (1.8, 2.2, and 2.4, respectively) and women (2.2, 2.0, and 2.6, respectively); the HRs for apoB levels were higher than those for LDL cholesterol levels. For any ischemic cardiovascular event (including stroke), the HRs for LDL cholesterol level, non-HDL cholesterol level, and apoB level were 1.4, 1.7, and 1.6, respectively, for men, and were 1.4, 1.4, and 1.8, respectively, for women. ApoB HRs for any ischemic cardiovascular event remained significant when adjusted for LDL cholesterol level. The AUROC for any ischemic cardiovascular event in men was 0.58 for LDL cholesterol level, 0.60 for non-HDL cholesterol level, and 0.60 for apoB level. Respective areas for women were 0.64, 0.66, and 0.66, suggesting that although the apoB level may predict risk slightly better than the LDL and non-HDL cholesterol levels, it is only minimally better.

In the 6-year nested, case-control male Health Professionals Study, with subjects aged 40 to 75 years (mean age, 66 years), there were 266 cases of MI or CHD death.[29] Comparing highest and lowest quintiles of risk for MI and fatal CHD, the RR was 3.01 for the apoB level, 2.76 for the non-HDL cholesterol level, and 1.81 for the LDL cholesterol level. When the non-HDL cholesterol level and the apoB level or the LDL cholesterol level and the apoB level were placed into the same quintile model and mutually adjusted, only the apoB level was predictive, with an RR of 4.18, compared with 0.70 (not significant) for the non-HDL cholesterol level and 0.55 (not significant) for the LDL cholesterol level.

The Long-Term Intervention with Pravastatin in Ischemic Disease trial recruited 9014 subjects who had CHD (83% male; median age 62 years) who had a total cholesterol level of 155 to 270 mg/dL and assigned them randomly to pravastatin, 40 mg/d, or placebo. After 6.1 years, the pravastatin-treated group experienced a 24% reduction in MI and CHD mortality ($P < .001$).[30] Unadjusted HRs for this end point in the placebo group were 1.15 for baseline LDL cholesterol, 1.64 for apoB, and 1.14 for the ratio of total cholesterol to HDL cholesterol, all of which were significant. In the pravastatin group, using lipid levels at 1 year, unadjusted HRs for the same end point were 1.08 for the LDL cholesterol level (not significant), 1.49 for apoB, and 1.03 for the ratio of total cholesterol to HDL cholesterol. Unfortunately HRs were given per unit change in units specific to each variable (eg, mmol/L for LDL cholesterol or g/L for apoB), not in standardized units such as HR per SD, and thus the ability of these lipid variables to predict risk could not be compared.

The Air Force/Texas Coronary Atherosclerosis Prevention Study randomly assigned 6505 coronary disease–free adults (85% male; mean age, 58 years) who had HDL cholesterol levels below the mean in NHANES III, to lovastatin, 10 to 20 mg/d, or placebo.[31] ApoB, apoA-1, and apoB/apoA-1 levels at both baseline and 1 year predicted coronary events at 5.2 years. Neither the LDL cholesterol level nor the non-HDL cholesterol level was a significant predictor at either time point. The baseline HDL cholesterol level and the ratio of total cholesterol to HDL cholesterol were significant predictors, but their values at year 1 were not.

The largest analysis in secondary prevention comparing standard lipid profile parameters, apoB, apoA-1, and ratios was one combining the Treating to New Targets (TNT) and Incremental Decrease in End Points through Aggressive Lipid Lowering (IDEAL) trials. Results from the 18,018 subjects were combined because the design, clinical end points, 4.8-year follow-up, and interventions were similar.[32] Both the TNT and IDEAL trials were multicenter, secondary intervention trials randomizing and comparing aggressive versus usual-dose statin therapy—atorvastatin, 80 mg versus 10 mg, in the TNT trial and atorvastatin, 80 mg, versus simvastatin, 40 mg, in the IDEAL trial—in a combined population (81% male) with average age of 61 years. The comparative LDL cholesterol levels in the treatment groups were the same: 101 mg/dL and 77 mg/dL in the TNT trial and 104 mg/dL and 81 mg/dL in the IDEAL trial. Major cardiovascular events included nonfatal MI, coronary death, fatal or nonfatal stroke, and resuscitation after cardiac arrest. The Cox proportional hazard model was used and included the effects of study, age, and gender; HRs were given per SD change in the variable.

In this large population, HRs were significant for the LDL cholesterol level (1.15), the non-HDL cholesterol level (1.19), apoB level (1.19), the ratio of total cholesterol to HDL cholesterol (1.21), and the apoB to apoA-1 ratio (1.24). In pairwise comparisons, the LDL cholesterol level lost its significant predictive value when combined with the apoB level or with the non-HDL cholesterol level, although each of them remained significant at values of 1.24 and 1.31, respectively. Even more powerful as predictors were the ratios: the apoB level and the non-HDL cholesterol level lost their predictive value when compared individually with the ratio of total cholesterol to HDL cholesterol or with the ratio of apoB to apoA-1, each of which retained a significant predictive value of 1.17 and 1.24, respectively. In a pairwise comparison, the ratio of apoB to apoA-1 remained a significant predictor (1.24), but the ratio of total cholesterol to HDL cholesterol (1.0) was no longer significant.

In terms of treatment goals, although LDL cholesterol lost significance as a risk predictor (1.08) in subjects whose LDL cholesterol level was 100 mg/dL or lower, the non-HDL cholesterol level (1.15), the apoB level (1.15), and the ratios of total cholesterol to HDL cholesterol (1.22) and of apoB to apoA-1 (1.31) remained significant risk predictors. These findings suggest that taking both atherogenic and antiatherogenic lipids into account simultaneously has more predictive value in those treated to low LDL cholesterol levels.

Less Favorable Results of Apolipoprotein B Versus the Low-Density Lipoprotein Cholesterol Level as a Predictor for the Risk of Coronary Heart Disease

The NHANES III database of American adults gathered between 1988 and 1994 was a cross-sectional analysis for the association of lipids and their ratios with end points including prevalent history of MI or stroke, angina on exertion, intermittent claudication, and congestive heart failure (see **Table 3**).[33] Comparisons of the highest versus the lowest tertile were not significant for apoB, non-HDL cholesterol, and LDL cholesterol levels. Although the OR for the ratio of LDL cholesterol to HDL cholesterol was not significant, the ORs for the ratios of non-HDL cholesterol to HDL cholesterol and apoB to HDL cholesterol were significant, at 1.24 and 1.37, respectively, suggesting that in such ratios non-HDL cholesterol and apoB performed better as risk predictors than the LDL cholesterol level.

In the 10-year prospective Atherosclerosis Risk in Communities Study of 12,300 middle-aged (45–64 years), mixed-ethnicity participants free of CHD, there were 725 incident cases of MI, CHD death, or coronary revascularization.[34] The age- and race-adjusted RRs per SD of LDL cholesterol were 1.42 and 1.37 in men and women, respectively, and were 1.31 and 1.32, respectively, for apoB. In a three-lipid model containing LDL cholesterol, triglycerides, and apoB, the first two values remained significant predictors, but the apoB level was no longer significant, with RRs of 1.05 in men and 0.97 in women. In stratified models where apoB was thought to be more predictive, the apoB level still remained nonsignificant in subjects who had an LDL cholesterol level lower than 160 mg/dL and in subjects who had above-median triglyceride levels. Coefficients of variation for repeated measurements of LDL cholesterol and apoB were 10% and 17%, respectively, suggesting that poorer precision in measuring apoB might have caused some of the loss of its predictive ability.

Low-Density Lipoprotein Particle Number is Better than Low-Density Cholesterol Level as a Predictor of the Risk for Coronary Heart Disease

Fewer studies have compared the predictive risk of the number of LDL particles measured by NMR spectroscopy with standard lipid profile variables that have been performed using apoB (**Table 4**).

In the cross-sectional MESA study, 5400 CVD-free adults (47% male), age 45 to 84 years (mean age, 61 years) had standard lipid profile measures and proton NMR spectroscopy determinations for the number and size of all lipoprotein particles. Increases in maximal carotid intima media thickness (IMT) measured at eight points in the common and internal carotid arteries were calculated per 1 SD of the lipid parameter.[7] The change in IMT thickness (in μm) per 1 SD of lipid variable was 40.2 for the number of LDL particles, 37.4 for LDL cholesterol, −23.2 for the number of HDL particles, and −22.4 for HDL cholesterol. When the model included five measures, the change in IMT was 30.3 for the number of large LDL particles, 34.8 for the number of small LDL particles, 11.8 (not significant) for LDL cholesterol level, −17.3 for HDL cholesterol level, and −1.6 (not significant) for triglycerides level. These data suggest that the number of LDL particles is a more potent measure of atherosclerotic vascular changes than the LDL cholesterol level and that both small and large LDL particles are associated with increased atherosclerotic risk. This study also clearly shows that when the number of small LDL particles increases, the number of large LDL particles falls. In univariate analysis this inverse relationship gives the impression that small LDL particles are atherogenic, but large ones are not. When multivariate analysis is used, the apparently benign effect of large LDL cholesterol disappears, and the numbers of both large and small LDL particles have atherogenic predictive value.

The Cardiovascular Health Study performed a nested case control study of men and women over the age of 65 years comparing those who had incident MI or angina over a 5-year period with a healthy sample group whose maximal carotid IMT was lower than the twenty-fifth percentile, whose ankle brachial index was greater than 1, and who had no brain infarcts of 3 mm or larger on MRI, no ultrasound abdominal aortic aneurysms 3 cm or larger, and no wall motion abnormalities on cardiac echocardiography.[35] In men, the OR for MI/angina in these two groups generally was not significant for any measure, but in women the ORs for the number of LDL particles in quartile 4 and quartile 1 of the Friedewald-calculated LDL cholesterol level were 3.34 and 2.59, respectively. In a multivariate model including LDL and HDL cholesterol, triglycerides, insulin, glucose, and C-reactive protein levels and waist circumference, the number of LDL particles still had a statistically significant OR for MI/angina of 1.11 (95% CI, 1.04–1.18/100 LDL particles), but LDL size was no longer significant.

Table 4
Predictive comparisons in cardiovascular trials

Trial/Study Population	Events	Trial Type	Years Follow-up	Comparison Groups	Lipid or Lipoprotein Measure	HR, RR, OR, or Change in IMT (μm)
Multi-Ethnic Study of Atherosclerosis (MESA)[7] n = 5400 Age 45–84 y	Maximum carotid IMT, combined eight measures	Cross-sectional	NA	Change in IMT per 1 SD lipid	LDL-C	37.4
					LDL particle #	40.2
				Change in IMT per 1 SD lipid, 5 variables in model	LDL-C	11.8 (NS)
					Large LDL particle #	30.3
					Small LDL particle #	34.8
					HDL-C	–17.3
					TG	–1.6 (NS)
Cardiovascular Health Study[35] 5201 CVD-free adults age ≥ 65 y 434 cases 249 healthy controls Mean age, 73 y	MI, angina	Prospective cohort Nested case-control	5	No significance in men, thus only data for women are shown. OR: Q4:Q1	LDL-C	2.59
					LDL particle #	3.34
				Females only OR: per 100 particles, RF adj	LDL-C	NS
PLAC-1[36] n = 241 subjects 408 subjects who had CHD Mean age, 57 y	Progression in quantitative coronary angiography	Interventional pravastatin 40 mg versus placebo	3	OR: above versus below median values	LDL cholesterol	1.4 (NS)
					Number of LDL particles	
					Number of small LDL particles	

Abbreviations: IMT, intima media thickness; HDL-C, high-density lipoprotein cholesterol; HR, hazard ratio; LDL-C, low-density lipoprotein cholesterol; MI, myocardial infarction; NS, not significant; OR, odds ratio; RF adj, adjusted for risk factors (smoking, body mass index, and diabetes); RR, relative risk; TG, triglycerides.

Pravastatin Limitation of Atherosclerosis in the Coronary Arteries was a randomized, placebo-controlled trial of pravastatin 40 versus placebo looking at the quantitative coronary angiographic changes in 408 subjects who had LDL cholesterol levels between 130 and 190 mg/dL.[36] Pravastatin slowed the progression of arthrosclerosis by 40% and decreased MI by 60% (P < .05). In a subanalysis, frozen baseline and 6-month samples from 241 subjects (75% male; mean age, 58 years) were analyzed using NMR spectroscopy. ORs comparing above- versus below-median values of lipids or lipoproteins for predicting progression were 1.4 (not significant) for LDL cholesterol, 2.1 (not significant) for the number of LDL particles by NMR, and 7.7 (95% CI, 2.1–27) for the number of small LDL particles.

All Variables Compared in One Population

In the 13-year follow-up of the Quebec Cardiovascular Study[37] of 2072 CHD-free men, age 35 to 64 years, the univariate RRs for nonfatal MI and CHD death for highest versus lowest tertile for apoB and LDL cholesterol levels were 1.91 and 1.80, respectively (**Table 5**). Neither value (1.89 and 2.02, respectively) was attenuated after adjusting for nonlipid and lipid risk factors (including triglycerides and HDL cholesterol levels). Both the LDL cholesterol level and the apoB level added to the AUROC when a model was used that contained the risk factors of age, BMI, systolic blood pressure, smoking, diabetes, HDL cholesterol level, and log-transformed triglycerides: 70.7% and 70.3%, respectively, compared with 68.9% without either variable (P < .001; there was no difference between two variables). In the highest LDL cholesterol tertile (> 170 mg/dL) in this study, however, apoB levels modified risk; lower levels of apoB (< 128 mg/dL) were not associated with increased risk of CHD, but higher levels of APOB were. Similarly, in the tertile with highest LDL cholesterol levels, apoB significantly improved the AUROC for predicting incident CHD: .535 without apoB and .580 with apoB (P = .04).

In the same study, when the end point was expanded to include unstable angina, MI, and CHD death, 2% to 16% polyacrylamide GGE divided LDL into particles less than 255 Å (small), and greater than 260 Å (large).[38] The RR for those in the highest versus those in the lowest tertile of small LDL particles was 3.6, unadjusted, for ischemic heart disease, was 3.4 when adjusted for the risk factors of age, BMI, systolic blood pressure, smoking, and diabetes, and was 2.5, still significant, when adjusted further for HDL cholesterol, triglycerides, and apoB levels.

This increased risk was seen in the first 7.3 years of the study and not thereafter. In addition, when stratified on above- and below-median values for small and large LDL cholesterol particles, the apoB level added significantly to the RR (eg, the RR of 2.1 for above-median small LDL cholesterol particles increased to 3.3 when above-median apoB was added). This finding suggests that using the apoB level as a measure of particle number enhances the value of the size of LDL particles as a risk predictor. Of interest, there was no increased risk among the three tertiles of larger LDL particles (P = .09).

The European Prospective Investigation into Cancer and Nutrition-Norfolk study prospectively followed 26,000 individuals between age 45 and 79 years (mean age, 65 years) from the general practices in Norfolk, United Kingdom, for an average 6 years through 2002.[39] Hospitalization and death registries identified 1003 participants free of CHD at baseline, not taking statin therapy, who were hospitalized with or died from CHD as an underlying cause. These subjects were matched with two controls by age, gender, and enrollment date. When univariate models were used comparing highest versus lowest quartile for CHD, the ORs (all significant) for non-HDL

Table 5
Predictive comparisons in cardiovascular trials: all lipid/lipoprotein variables in the same population

Trial/Study Population	Events	Trial Type	Years Follow-up	Comparison Groups	Lipid or Lipoprotein Measure	HR, RR, OR, or Change in IMT (um)
Quebec CV Study[37] n = 2072 CHD-free men, Mean age, 57 y	MI, CHD death	Prospective cohort	13	RR: T3:T1 RF adj/RF adj + adj for HDL-C, TG	LDL-C apo B	
				AUROC in highest tertile of LDL-C (>120 mg/dL)	Usual RF, HDL-C, TG	0.54
					Usual RF, HDL-C, TG, with apoB	0.58
Quebec CV Study[38]	MI, CHD death, unstable angina	Prospective cohort	13	RR: T3:T1	Number of small (< 255Å) LDL particles 2%–16%	3.6
					PAGE RF adj, RF adj, and adjusted for HDL-C, TG	3.4
						2.5
European Prospective Investigation into Cancer and Nutrition (EPIC)-Norfolk Study[39] 25,663 adults n= 869 cases, Mean age, 65 y	Hospitalization or death from CHD	Prospective, Nested case control	6	OR: Q4:Q1	LDL-C	1.68
					Non–HDL-C	2.15
					TC:HDL-C	2.57
					ApoB:apoA-I	2.64
					TC:HDL-C RF+TG adj	1.23 (NS)
					ApoB:apoA-I RF+TG adj	2.03
				AUROCRF adj	TC:HDL-C	0.670
					ApoB:apoA-1	0.673

Study	Outcome	Design	Follow-up (y)	Statistic	Marker	Value
EPIC-Norfolk Study[40] n = 1003 cases	Hospitalization or death from CHD	Prospective, Nested case control	6	OR: Q4:Q1 univariate RF adj (smoking)	LDL-C	1.73
					non–HDL-C	2.14
					Number of LDL particles	2.00
				OR: Q4:Q1 LDL-C and LDL number of particles in same model	LDL-C	1.22
					LDL particle #	1.78
				OR: Q4:Q1 Adj for Framingham risk score	LDL-C	1.24 (NS)
					Non–HDL-C	1.38
					Number of LDL particles	1.34
Framingham Offspring Study[41] n = 3322 Median age, 51 y	MI, angina, coronary insufficiency, CHD death	Prospective cohort	15	RR per 1 SD, m/f	LDL-C	1.12 (NS)/1.18 (NS)
					Non–HDL-C	1.22/1.28
					ApoB	1.37/1.38
					TC:HDL-C ratio	1.39/1.39
					ApoB:apoA-1	1.39/1.39
Framingham Offspring Study[42] n = 3066	MI, angina, coronary insufficiency, CHD death, CHF, CVA, TIA, claudication	Prospective cohort	15	RR per 1 SD	LDL-C	1.06 (NS)
					Non–HDL-C	1.17
					Number of LDL particles	1.24
Women's Health Study[43] n = 15,632 women aged ≥ 45 y Mean age, 54 y	MI, CVA, coronary revascularization, CV death	Prospective cohort	10	HR: Q5:Q1, RF adj	LDL-C	1.62
					Non–HDL-C	2.51
					ApoB	2.50
					TC:HDL-C	3.81
					ApoB:HDL-C	3.56

(continued on next page)

Table 5
(continued)

Trial/Study Population	Events	Trial Type	Years Follow-up	Comparison Groups	Lipid or Lipoprotein Measure	HR, RR, OR, or Change in IMT (um)
Women's Health Study[44] 15,632 women aged ≥ 45 y n = 130 cases, 130 controls Mean age, 60 y	MI, CVA, CV death	Prospective cohort, Nested case-control	3	OR: Q4:Q1	LDL-C	2.05
					Non–HDL-C	2.94
					ApoB	2.43
					TC:HDL-C	3.11
					Number of LDL particles	4.17
					Number of LDL particles	2.85
				OR: Q4:Q1 adj for TC:HDL-C OR: Q4:Q1, RF adj	Number of LDL particles	2.67
				RR per 1 quartile, 2 variables in model RR per 1 quartile, 2 variables in model	Number of LDL particles	1.57
					ApoB	1.02 (NS)
					Number of LDL particles	1.44
					TC:HDL-C	1.22 (NS)
					Number of LDL particles alone	1.44
				AUROC	TC:HDL-C	1.22 (NS)
Veterans Affairs High-Density Lipoprotein Intervention Trial (VA-HIT)[47] 2531 men who had HDL-C < 40 mg/dL 364 cases, 697 controls Mean age, 64 y	MI, CHD death	Interventional gemfibrozil 1200 versus placebo, Nested case-control	5.1	OR per 1 SD, RF adj	LDL-C	1.08 (NS)
					Non–HDL-C	1.09 (NS)
					ApoB	1.14 (NS)
					Number of LDL particles	1.28
					TC:HDL-C	1.14
					ApoB:apoA-1	1.14 (NS)

Abbreviations: CHD, coronary heart disease; CHF, congestive heart failure; CV, cardiovascular; CVA, stroke; HDL-C, high-density lipoprotein cholesterol; HR, hazard ratio; IMT, intima media thickness; LDL-C, low-density lipoprotein cholesterol; m/f, male/female; MI, myocardial infarction; NS, not significant; OR, odds ratio; RR, relative risk; TC, total cholesterol; TG, triglycerides; TIA, transient ischemic attack.

cholesterol levels and number of LDL particles were 2.14 and 2.00, respectively, greater than the OR for the LDL cholesterol level (1.73). When a conditional logistic regression model with both LDL cholesterol concentration and the number of LDL particles was used, the OR for highest versus lowest quartile of LDL cholesterol, 1.22, was no longer significant, whereas the OR for the number of LDL particles was still significant at 1.78. Similarly the number of LDL particles and non-HDL cholesterol level retained significant ORs of 1.34 and 1.38, respectively, after adjusting for the Framingham risk score, whereas the LDL cholesterol level did not.

In another nested case control analysis in the same population[40] looking at 869 subjects and 1511 controls, ORs for CHD comparing the highest versus the lowest quartiles for LDL cholesterol, non-HDL cholesterol, the ratio of total cholesterol to HDL cholesterol, and the ratio of apoB to apoA-1 were 1.68, 2.15, 2.57, and 2.64, respectively, showing that ratios incorporating both atherogenic and non-atherogenic values in combination are more powerful than either alone. In a model adjusted for diabetes, BMI, systolic blood pressure, C-reactive protein, and triglycerides, the apoB to apoA-1 ratio still remained significant with a value of 2.03, but the ratio of total cholesterol to HDL cholesterol (1.23) did not. The two ratios, however, were almost identical in discriminating cases from controls using receiver-operating curves adjusted for diabetes, BMI, smoking, systolic blood pressure, and C-reactive protein: 0.673 for the apoB to apoA-1 ratio and .670 for the ratio of total cholesterol to HDL cholesterol. In this population, however, few subjects had diabetes (3.2%), where apoB and the number of LDL particles might be a more discriminative measure, and adjustment for diabetes and BMI might have decreased the discriminatory ability even further.

Two 15-year prospective cohort studies of the Framingham Offspring population of of 3322 middle-aged persons (age 30–74 years; median age, 51 years) without coronary heart disease help quantify the relative predictive power of the LDL cholesterol level, the non-HDL cholesterol level, the apoB level, and the number of LDL particles measured by nuclear magnetic spectroscopy to predict CHD, MI, angina pectoris, coronary insufficiency, or death from CHD.[41,42] The first study shows increasing RRs per 1 SD in men and women of 1.12 (not significant) and 1.18 (not significant), respectively, for the LDL cholesterol level, of 1.22 and 1.28, respectively, for the non-HDL cholesterol level, of 1.37 and 1/38, respectively, for the apoB level, and of 1.39 and 1.39, respectively, for both the total cholesterol to HDL cholesterol ratio and the apoB to apoA-1 ratio.

In the same population, looking beyond CHD and including stroke, transient ischemic attack, intermittent claudication, and congestive heart failure as end points, the combined RR per SD was 1.06 (not significant) for LDL cholesterol level, 1.17 for non-HDL cholesterol level, and 1.24 for the number of LDL particles. The studies are not totally comparable given the different end points, and the 95% confidence intervals overlap for all the measurements, but both studies show LDL cholesterol level to be a nonsignificant predictor. They also suggest that both the apoB level and the number of LDL particles could be better predictors of CHD risk than non-HDL cholesterol and LDL cholesterol levels.

In the Women's Health Study, 15,632 women age 45 years and older were assigned randomly in a 2 × 2 factorial design to aspirin or vitamin E versus placebo and were followed for 10 years for the end points of MI, stroke, coronary revascularization, and cardiovascular death.[43] The HR adjusted for age, smoking status, blood pressure, diabetes, and BMI for the highest versus lowest quintile was 2.50 for the apoB level and was 2.51 for non-HDL cholesterol level; both were higher than the 1.62 for LDL cholesterol level.

After 3 years a nested case control study also was performed in the same Women's Health study, with 130 cases of nonfatal MI, stroke, or sudden death and 130 controls.[44] The mean age was 60 years, and the mean BMI was 27. Crude RR estimates by logistic regression analysis comparing quartile 4 versus quartile 1 were 2.06 for the LDL cholesterol level, 2.43 for the apoB level, 2.94 for the non-HDL cholesterol level, 4.17 for the number of LDL particles, and 3.11 for the total cholesterol to HDL cholesterol ratio (all P values ≤ .008). Even after adjustment for the total cholesterol to HDL cholesterol ratio or risk factors including smoking, hypertension, diabetes, BMI, and family history of MI, the RR for the number of LDL particles persisted significantly at values of 2.85 and 2.67, respectively. In two-lipid/lipoprotein models, including the number of LDL particles and the total cholesterol to HDL cholesterol ratio or the number of LDL particles and the apoB level, the RRs for the number of LDL particles remained significant at 1.44 and 1.57, respectively, but the RRs for the total cholesterol to HDL cholesterol ratio and for the apoB level were no longer significant. The AUROC for cardiovascular events was 0.64 for both the number of LDL particles and the total cholesterol to HDL cholesterol ratio.

The Veterans Affairs High-Density Lipoprotein Intervention Trial was a randomized, placebo-controlled study of gemfibrozil, 1200 mg/d, versus placebo in 2531 men under 74 years of age (mean age, 64 years) who had CHD with HDL cholesterol levels of 40 mg/dL or lower, LDL cholesterol levels of 140 mg/dL or lower, and triglycerides levels of 300 mg/dL or lower.[45] The mean BMI was 29; 25% of the subjects had diabetes, and 50% were insulin resistant. During the course of 5.1 years, gemfibrozil reduced nonfatal MI and CHD death by 22% (P = .006). Gemfibrozil did not change LDL cholesterol level but lowered the triglycerides level by 31% and raised HDL cholesterol level by 6%, which predicted the reduction in CHD events.[46]

In a nested case-control study,[47] ORs per 1 SD change for multiple on-trial lipid and lipoprotein measures, adjusted for treatment group, age, smoking, hypertension, BMI, and diabetes, were calculated for a population of 364 men who had died from MI or CHD death and for 697 age-matched controls. The OR was still significant for the number of LDL particles (1.28; 95% CI, 1.12–1.47), for the number of HDL particles (0.71; 95% CI, 0.61–0.81), and for the ratio of total cholesterol to HDL cholesterol (1.14; 95% CI, 1.01–1.30) but not for the LDL cholesterol level (1.08), the non-HDL cholesterol level (1.09), the apoB level (1.14), or the apoB to apoA-1 ratio (1.14). This trial has been one of the most important in indicating the lack of significance of the number of LDL particles in this group of older overweight men who had CHD.

Non–High-Density Lipoprotein Cholesterol, Low-Density Lipoprotein Cholesterol, and Apolipoprotein B Level as Predictors of the Risk for Cardiovascular Disease in Diabetic Patients

Two recent epidemiologic studies have examined the possible increased predictive power of non-HDL cholesterol and apoB over LDL cholesterol level in diabetic patient populations (**Table 6**). A recent study analysis of 2108 diabetic patients age 45 to 74 years (mean age, 58 years) who participated in the Strong Heart Study,[48] a 9-year prospective study of cardiovascular disease and its associated risk factors in 13 American Indian communities, demonstrated that the non-HDL cholesterol level and the ratio of total cholesterol to HDL cholesterol were significantly better predictors than the LDL cholesterol level of the risk of CVD. After adjustment for standard risk factors plus hemoglobin A1C, urinary microalbumin and creatinine levels, insulin, and fibrinogen, the HR for overall risk of CVD of tertile 3 versus tertile 1 LDL cholesterol levels for men and women was 1.71 and 1.61, respectively. For non-HDL cholesterol

Table 6
Predictive comparisons in cardiovascular trials: lipid and lipoprotein variables in persons who have diabetes

Trial/Study Population	Events	Trial Type	Years Follow-up	Comparison Groups	Lipid or Lipoprotein Measure	HR, RR, OR, or Change in IMT (μm)
Strong Heart Study[48] n = 2108 CVD-free diabetic American Indians, age 45–74 y Mean age, 58 y	Fatal and non-fatal MI, CVA, CHD, CHF and sudden cardiac death	Prospective cohort	9	HR T3:T1, m/f, RF adj plus adj for HbA1c, insulin, urinary microalbumin, fibrinogen	LDL-C Non–HDL-C TC:HDL-C	1.71/1.61 2.23/1.80 2.46/1.48
Health Professionals' Follow-Up Study[49] n = 746 diabetic men Mean age, 63 y	Fatal CHD, MI, CVA, CABG, PCI	Prospective cohort	6	RR Q4:Q1 AUROC Rf adj	LDL-C Non–HDL-C ApoB TC:HDL-C LDL-C Non–HDL-C ApoB TC:HDL-C	1.63 2.25 2.31 4.56 0.685 0.695 0.691 0.722

Abbreviations: AUROC, area under the receiver operating curve; CABG, coronary artery bypass grafting; CHD, coronary heart disease; CHF, congestive heart failure; CVA, stroke; HbA1c, hemoglobin A1c; HDL-C, high-density lipoprotein cholesterol; HR, hazard ratio; IMT, intima media thickness; LDL-C, low-density lipoprotein cholesterol; m/f, male/female; MI, myocardial infarction; OR, odds ratio; PCI, percutaneous coronary intervention; RF adj, adjusted risk factors (smoking, body mass index, and diabetes); RR, relative risk; TC, total cholesterol.

levels, the HRs for men and women were 2.23 and 1.80, respectively, and for the total cholesterol to HDL cholesterol ratio the HRs were 2.46 and 1.48, respectively.

The Health Professionals' Follow-Up Study prospectively followed 746 diabetic men age 46 to 81 years (mean age, 63 years) over 6 years for cardiovascular outcomes including fatal CHD, nonfatal MI, fatal and nonfatal stroke, and coronary revascularization.[49] Adjusted for age, the RR for incident cardiovascular events in the quartile 4 compared with quartile 1 for LDL cholesterol level was 1.63, significantly lower than the RR for the non-HDL cholesterol level (2.25), the apoB level (2.31), and the total cholesterol to HDL cholesterol ratio (4.56). When log likelihood ratio tests were used to compare two nested models with LDL and other risk factors for CVD, the addition of the non-HDL cholesterol level to the model significantly improved prediction of risk ($P = .01$), whereas adding the apoB level did not ($P = .37$). Risk factor–adjusted AUROC for predicting CVD outcome using deciles of LDL cholesterol, non-HDL cholesterol, apoB, and the ratio of total cholesterol to HDL cholesterol were 0.685, 0.695, 0.691, and 0.722, respectively, suggesting little difference except perhaps for the ratio of total cholesterol to HDL cholesterol.

SUMMARY OF ALL STUDIES

After looking at all the results in all the tables from many different studies, study methodologies, populations, and different biostatistical analytic techniques with differing adjustments for different risk factors, the following conclusions can be drawn:

1. The LDL cholesterol level almost always is bested in prediction of CHD and ischemic CVD by more discriminating lipid/apolipoprotein risk factors—non-HDL cholesterol level, apoB level, and the number of LDL particles.
   - RRs, HRs, and ORs are higher for the latter three variables than for the LDL cholesterol level.
   - The latter three variables may be statistically significant predictors, whereas the LDL cholesterol level often is not.
   - In two-model analyses including the LDL cholesterol level and one of the other lipid/apolipoprotein variables, the other variable remains significant, but the LDL cholesterol level becomes statistically insignificant.
   - In area-under-the-curve analyses, the other variables always provide larger values and thus better discriminating power than LDL cholesterol.
2. The ratios of total cholesterol to HDL cholesterol and of apoB to apoA-1, which include a measure of HDL cholesterol level, often are better in risk prediction than the non-HDL cholesterol level, apoB level, or the number of LDL particles.
3. The two previous statements are true in the few diabetic population studies but no more so than in the general population.
4. Adjustments for risk factors (obesity, diabetes, hypertension) associated with the more advanced atherogenic lipids and apolipoproteins (apoB level, number of LDL particles) generally reduce the predictive value, as expected.

RECOMMENDATIONS

As physicians investigate lipid and lipoprotein levels in a patient who has coronary ischemia and who has achieved the LDL cholesterol goal of less than 70 mg/dL, one often finds that although the patient is at goal by LDL cholesterol measurement, only 25% of patients at the same population percentile have achieved the goal for the number of LDL particles at the same population percentile (authors' unpublished data). In a recent study comparing the LDL cholesterol level measured by the

Friedewald formula and the number of LDL particles measured by NMR in patients who had type 2 diabetes, there was increased heterogeneity of LDL particle size and number even in patients who had low (70–99 mg/dL) or very low (< 70 mg/dL) LDL cholesterol levels.[50] The study revealed that only 16% of patients who had very low LDL cholesterol levels (< 70 mg/dL, fifth population percentile) had an LDL particle concentration of less than 700 nmol/L, (fifth population percentile), and 40% still had an LDL particle concentration greater than 1000 nmol/L (twentieth population percentile).[50]

A very comprehensive joint consensus statement has been published recently by the American Diabetes Association (ADA) and the American College of Cardiology (ACC) Foundation concerning preventive approaches for persons who have global cardiometabolic risk, the cluster of obesity, insulin resistance, hyperglycemia, hypertension, and the dyslipoproteinemia of elevated triglycerides and small, dense LDL particles with depressed HDL cholesterol levels.[51] That report endorses the use of non-HDL cholesterol as a more routine target of therapy that should be made available on all laboratory reports and suggests targets for standardized apoB levels in the patients at the very highest and high risk of CHD. Although the predictive studies mentioned in this article can suggest lipid and apolipoprotein goals, a randomized trial is needed to test whether a target goal of less than the fifth population percentile for apoB or number of LDL particles versus a target goal of less than the fifth population percentile for LDL cholesterol level will produce an incremental decrease in the incidence of CHD events.

Such a trial would be done best in those who have the most pronounced cardiometabolic risk (ie, in persons who have type 2 diabetes). Recently a significant difference in cardiovascular imaging between populations of diabetic patients who have reached LDL cholesterol targets of less than 70 mg/dL and those whose LDL cholesterol levels were less than 100 mg/dL was published. The Stop Atherosclerosis in Native Diabetics Study[52] was a 3-year randomized, end point–blinded trial using aggressive treatment (LDL cholesterol $\leq$ 70 mg/dL and systolic blood pressure $\leq$ 115 mm Hg) versus standard treatment (LDL cholesterol $\leq$ 100 mg/dL and systolic blood pressure $\leq$ 130 mm Hg) in 499 American Indian diabetic patients 40 years old or older. Although there was no difference in cardiac events in this small trial, carotid IMT regressed in those treated aggressively but progressed in those receiving standard treatment ($P < .001$). IMT changes were related to LDL cholesterol level, not to systolic blood pressure; changes in the latter affected left ventricular mass. This finding suggests that an LDL cholesterol goal of 70 mg/dL or less in middle-aged type 2 diabetic patients may be a more preventive goal than a target of 100 mg/dL or less, but it does not help answer the question of whether a goal of less than the fifth population percentile for the number of LDL particles (< 700 nmol/L) or apoB (< 65 mg/dL) would be better than a goal of less than the fifth population percentile for LDL cholesterol ($\leq$ 70 mg/dL).

These studies do support the implementation of aggressive LDL-lowering strategies in middle-aged diabetic patients at highest risk (those who have CHD or ischemic CVD) or who do not have CHD or CVD but who have additional major cardiovascular risk factors with targets for an LDL cholesterol level of less than 70 mg/dL, a non-HDL cholesterol level of less than 100 mg/dL, a standardized apoB level of less than 65 mg/dL (the NHANES fifth population percentile) or less than 80 mg/dL (the ADA/ACC consensus statement), or an NMR-measured LDL particle number lower than 700 nmol/L (MESA fifth percentile) (**Table 2**). The ADA/ACC consensus statement was hesitant to advise adopting the NMR-measured number of LDL particles as a target because of the need for data from more than the one study[53] to confirm its accuracy in assessing individual lipoprotein concentrations as separated and measured using standard ultracentrifugation techniques. Nevertheless the current studies demonstrating a higher predictive value for the LDL particle number have used the same technique consistently, which has shown coefficients of variation based on reproducibility studies of less than 4% for the total number of LDL particles, less than 0.5% for LDL particle size, and less than 8% for the numbers of large and small LDL particles.[7]

For persons who have less immediate short-term risk, that is, persons who do not have diabetes but who have two or more major cardiovascular risk factors (smoking, hypertension, or family history of premature CHD) or those who have diabetes with no other cardiometabolic risk factors, one would suggest less strict goals using twentieth percentile population figures such as LDL cholesterol levels less than 100 mg/dL, non-HDL cholesterol levels less than 130 mg/dL, apoB levels less than 85 mg/dL (< 90 mg/dL by the ADA/ACC consensus panel), and an NMR-measured number of LDL particles lower than 1000 nmol/L (see **Table 2**).

Such goals based on advanced lipoprotein tests do not yet have sufficient supporting evidence to serve as population guidelines. Although such goals may reduce clinical events, the magnitude of such reduction is unclear, and the cost of such an approach remains to be seen. In addition, to reach such LDL particle number and apoB goals, it often may be necessary to use combined therapy with agents other than pure LDL-lowering agents, which lower these values but often also raise HDL cholesterol values, thus confounding the issue of which is more valuable: raising the HDL cholesterol level or lowering the number of LDL particles and the apoB level. Nonetheless, when faced with patients who have new or progressive CHD and a cardiometabolic or mixed dyslipidemia, it may be reasonable to apply such goals with the support of at least one major consensus document.[51]

The theoretical utility of this approach was demonstrated in the Framingham Offspring Study,[42] in which the number of LDL particles, but not the LDL cholesterol level, determined cardiovascular event–free survival. If the number of LDL particles is below the median, survival curves are better than if the number of LDL particles is above the median, regardless of whether the LDL cholesterol level is above or below the median. Conversely, if the LDL cholesterol level is below the median, but the number of LDL particles remains above it, cardiovascular event–free survival remains poorer, as when the LDL cholesterol level was not at target level.

Populations other than those with obvious insulin resistance or diabetes may have the same discrepancies between LDL cholesterol level and LDL particle number. NMR data from the Framingham Offspring Study have demonstrated that concentrations of LDL subclasses vary according to HDL cholesterol and triglycerides levels.[54] The data suggest that as HDL cholesterol levels decrease below 50 mg/dL, there is a shift towards greater numbers of smaller LDL particles, thus increasing the total number of LDL particles. At HDL cholesterol levels less than 40 mg/dL, the LDL cholesterol value may underestimate the concentration of LDL particles considerably (**Fig. 1**A). The LDL cholesterol level also may underestimate the concentration of LDL particles at triglycerides levels higher than 150 mg/dL (**Fig. 1**B). In fact, the number of LDL particles continues to rise as HDL levels decrease and triglycerides levels increase. Thus in persons who have very low HDL levels (certainly < 40 mg/dL) and/or elevated triglycerides levels (> 150 mg/dL), LDL cholesterol values may underestimate true lipoprotein-associated risk of CHD; such patients therefore may benefit from using the more sensitive measures of the number of apoB particles or the number of LDL particles measured by NMR. Being aware of the changes in the size of the LDL particles may be important in helping patients understand what is happening but may not help in risk prediction beyond its effect on total number of LDL particles.[7]

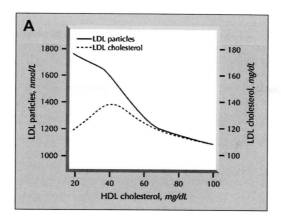

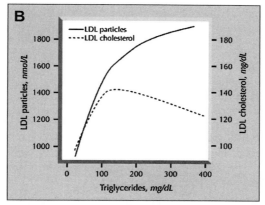

Fig. 1. Relationship of LDL cholesterol and NMR LDL particle number in the Framingham Offspring Study by (*A*) HDL cholesterol and (*B*) triglycerides levels. (*From* Cromwell WC, Otvos JD. Low-density lipoprotein particle number and risk for cardiovascular disease. Curr Atheroscler Rep 2004;6:385; with permission.)

SUMMARY

Today, many physicians, including cardiologists, endocrinologists, and clinical lipidologists, are ordering advanced lipoprotein tests, and marketing efforts have been intense. Enthusiasm for excessive testing must be tempered, however, because physicians and laboratories are in competition for shrinking dollars in health care financing. Hence, more clinical studies of these methods are needed to properly assess their incremental value in the management of patients who have lipid disorders.

Before going beyond the standard lipid profile with its non-HDL cholesterol level and ordering such advanced tests, the physician must understand with absolute clarity the purpose of the tests and how to interpret the results. Occasionally insurance companies force patients to change laboratories, so that different advanced lipoprotein tests are done on the same patient, adding possible confusion for both physician and patient.

Numerous studies have shown that the LDL cholesterol level as determined by the Friedewald formula is not the most sensitive measure of lipid- and lipoprotein-associated risk for ischemic CVD, especially in patients who have cardiometabolic risk factors including high triglycerides levels, low HDL cholesterol levels, and high numbers of LDL particles. The non-HDL cholesterol level is a better alternative goal, but the apoB level and the number of NMR-measured LDL particles are the most powerful single lipid and lipoprotein measures and should be ordered with discretion by physicians seeking to use them to improve lipid-altering therapies. This article has provided a detailed overview of the studies supporting this approach and has suggested possible lipid and lipoprotein goals that must be tested to evaluate their incremental preventive value.

REFERENCES

1. Illingworth DR. Management of hypercholesterolemia. Med Clin North Am 2000; 84(1):23–42.
2. LaRosa JC, Grundy SM, Waters DD, et al. Intensive lipid lowering with atorvastatin in patients with stable coronary disease. N Engl J Med 2005;352(14):1425–35.
3. Expert Panel on Detection EaToHBCiA. Executive Summary of the Third Report of the National Cholesterol Education Program (NCEP) Expert Panel on Detection, Evaluation, And Treatment of High Blood Cholesterol in Adults (Adult Treatment Panel III). JAMA 2001;285(19):2486–97.
4. Grundy SM, Cleeman JI, Merz CN, et al. Implications of recent clinical trials for the National Cholesterol Education Program Adult Treatment Panel III guidelines. J Am Coll Cardiol 2004;44(3):720–32.
5. Smith SC Jr, Allen J, Blair SN, et al. AHA/ACC guidelines for secondary prevention for patients with coronary and other atherosclerotic vascular disease: 2006 update: endorsed by the National Heart, Lung, And Blood Institute. Circulation 2006;113(19):2363–72.
6. Bachorik PS, Lovejoy KL, Carroll MD, et al. Apolipoprotein B and AI distributions in the United States, 1988–1991: results of the National Health and Nutrition Examination Survey III (NHANES III). Clin Chem 1997;43(12):2364–78.
7. Mora S, Szklo M, Otvos JD, et al. LDL particle subclasses, LDL particle size, and carotid atherosclerosis in the Multi-Ethnic Study of Atherosclerosis (MESA). Atherosclerosis 2007;192(1):211–7.
8. Friedewald WT, Levy RI, Fredrickson DS. Estimation of the concentration of low-density lipoprotein cholesterol in plasma, without use of the preparative ultracentrifuge. Clin Chem 1972;18(6):499–502.
9. Campos H, Khoo C, Sacks FM. Diurnal and acute patterns of postprandial apolipoprotein B-48 in VLDL, IDL, and LDL from normolipidemic humans. Atherosclerosis 2005;181(2):345–51.
10. Sniderman AD, Furberg CD, Keech A, et al. Apolipoproteins versus lipids as indices of coronary risk and as targets for statin treatment. Lancet 2003;361(9359):777–80.
11. Marcovina SM, Albers JJ, Kennedy H, et al. International Federation of Clinical Chemistry standardization project for measurements of apolipoproteins A-I and B. IV. Comparability of apolipoprotein B values by use of international reference material. Clin Chem 1994;40(4):586–92.
12. Grundy SM. Low-density lipoprotein, non-high-density lipoprotein, and apolipoprotein B as targets of lipid-lowering therapy. Circulation 2002;106(20):2526–9.
13. De Lalla OF, Gofman JW. Ultracentrifugal analysis of serum lipoproteins. Methods Biochem Anal 1954;1:459–78.

14. Chung BH, Wilkinson T, Geer JC, et al. Preparative and quantitative isolation of plasma lipoproteins: rapid, single discontinuous density gradient ultracentrifugation in a vertical rotor. J Lipid Res 1980;21(3):284–91.

15. Marcovina SM, Albers JJ, Scanu AM, et al. Use of a reference material proposed by the International Federation of Clinical Chemistry and Laboratory Medicine to evaluate analytical methods for the determination of plasma lipoprotein(a). Clin Chem 2000;46(12):1956–67.

16. Kulkarni KR, French KW. Determination of apolipoprotein B_{100} by the vertical auto profile method. Clinical Chemistry 2007;53(S6):A41.

17. Williams PT, Superko HR, Haskell WL, et al. Smallest LDL particles are most strongly related to coronary disease progression in men. Arterioscler Thromb Vasc Biol 2003;23(2):314–21.

18. St-Pierre AC, Ruel IL, Cantin B, et al. Comparison of various electrophoretic characteristics of LDL particles and their relationship to the risk of ischemic heart disease. Circulation 2001;104(19):2295–9.

19. Otvos JD, Jeyarajah EJ, Bennett DW, et al. Development of a proton nuclear magnetic resonance spectroscopic method for determining plasma lipoprotein concentrations and subspecies distributions from a single, rapid measurement. Clin Chem 1992;38(9):1632–8.

20. Summary of the second report of the National Cholesterol Education Program (NCEP) Expert Panel on Detection, Evaluation, and Treatment of High Blood Cholesterol in Adults (Adult Treatment Panel II). JAMA 1993;269(23):3015–23.

21. Liu J, Sempos CT, Donahue RP, et al. Non-high-density lipoprotein and very-low-density lipoprotein cholesterol and their risk predictive values in coronary heart disease. Am J Cardiol 2006;98(10):1363–8.

22. Farwell WR, Sesso HD, Buring JE, et al. Non-high-density lipoprotein cholesterol versus low-density lipoprotein cholesterol as a risk factor for a first nonfatal myocardial infarction. Am J Cardiol 2005;96(8):1129–34.

23. Rallidis LS, Pitsavos C, Panagiotakos DB, et al. Non-high density lipoprotein cholesterol is the best discriminator of myocardial infarction in young individuals. Atherosclerosis 2005;179(2):305–9.

24. Bittner V, Hardison R, Kelsey SF, et al. Non-high-density lipoprotein cholesterol levels predict five-year outcome in the Bypass Angioplasty Revascularization Investigation (BARI). Circulation 2002;106(20):2537–42.

25. von MD, Langer RD, Barrett-Connor E. Sex and time differences in the associations of non-high-density lipoprotein cholesterol versus other lipid and lipoprotein factors in the prediction of cardiovascular death (the Rancho Bernardo Study). Am J Cardiol 2003;91(11):1311–5.

26. Shai I, Rimm EB, Hankinson SE, et al. Multivariate assessment of lipid parameters as predictors of coronary heart disease among postmenopausal women: potential implications for clinical guidelines. Circulation 2004;110(18):2824–30.

27. Walldius G, Jungner I, Holme I, et al. High apolipoprotein B, low apolipoprotein A-I, and improvement in the prediction of fatal myocardial infarction (AMORIS study): a prospective study. Lancet 2001;358(9298):2026–33.

28. Benn M, Nordestgaard BG, Jensen GB, et al. Improving prediction of ischemic cardiovascular disease in the general population using apolipoprotein B: the Copenhagen City Heart Study. Arterioscler Thromb Vasc Biol 2007;27(3):661–70.

29. Pischon T, Girman CJ, Sacks FM, et al. Non-high-density lipoprotein cholesterol and apolipoprotein B in the prediction of coronary heart disease in men. Circulation 2005;112(22):3375–83.

30. Simes RJ, Marschner IC, Hunt D, et al. Relationship between lipid levels and clinical outcomes in the Long-Term Intervention with Pravastatin in Ischemic Disease (LIPID) trial: to what extent is the reduction in coronary events with pravastatin explained by on-study lipid levels? Circulation 2002;105(10):1162–9.

31. Gotto AM Jr, Whitney E, Stein EA, et al. Relation between baseline and on-treatment lipid parameters and first acute major coronary events in the Air Force/Texas Coronary Atherosclerosis Prevention Study (AFCAPS/TexCAPS). Circulation 2000;101(5):477–84.

32. Kastelein JJ, van der Steeg WA, Holme I, et al. Lipids, apolipoproteins, and their ratios in relation to cardiovascular events with statin treatment. Circulation 2008; 117(23):3002–9.

33. Hsia SH, Pan D, Berookim P, et al. A population-based, cross-sectional comparison of lipid-related indexes for symptoms of atherosclerotic disease. Am J Cardiol 2006;98(8):1047–52.

34. Sharrett AR, Ballantyne CM, Coady SA, et al. Coronary heart disease prediction from lipoprotein cholesterol levels, triglycerides, lipoprotein(a), apolipoproteins A-I and B, and HDL density subfractions: the Atherosclerosis Risk in Communities (ARIC) study. Circulation 2001;104(10):1108–13.

35. Kuller L, Arnold A, Tracy R, et al. Nuclear magnetic resonance spectroscopy of lipoproteins and risk of coronary heart disease in the cardiovascular health study. Arterioscler Thromb Vasc Biol 2002;22(7):1175–80.

36. Rosenson RS, Otvos JD, Freedman DS. Relations of lipoprotein subclass levels and low-density lipoprotein size to progression of coronary artery disease in the Pravastatin Limitation of Atherosclerosis in the Coronary Arteries (PLAC-I) trial. Am J Cardiol 2002;90(2):89–94.

37. St-Pierre AC, Cantin B, Dagenais GR, et al. Apolipoprotein-B, low-density lipoprotein cholesterol, and the long-term risk of coronary heart disease in men. Am J Cardiol 2006;97(7):997–1001.

38. St-Pierre AC, Cantin B, Dagenais GR, et al. Low-density lipoprotein subfractions and the long-term risk of ischemic heart disease in men: 13-year follow-up data from the Quebec cardiovascular study. Arterioscler Thromb Vasc Biol 2005;25(3): 553–9.

39. El HK, van der Steeg WA, Stroes ES, et al. Value of low-density lipoprotein particle number and size as predictors of coronary artery disease in apparently healthy men and women: the EPIC-Norfolk prospective population study. J Am Coll Cardiol 2007;49(5):547–53.

40. van der Steeg WA, Boekholdt SM, Stein EA, et al. Role of the apolipoprotein B-apolipoprotein A-I ratio in cardiovascular risk assessment: a case-control analysis in EPIC-Norfolk. Ann Intern Med 2007;146(9):640–8.

41. Ingelsson E, Schaefer EJ, Contois JH, et al. Clinical utility of different lipid measures for prediction of coronary heart disease in men and women. JAMA 2007;298(7):776–85.

42. Cromwell WC, Otvos JD, Keyes MJ, et al. LDL particle number and risk of future cardiovascular disease in the Framingham offspring study—implications for LDL management. Journal of Clinical Lipidology 2007;1:583–92.

43. Ridker PM, Rifai N, Cook NR, et al. Non-HDL cholesterol, apolipoproteins A-I and B100, standard lipid measures, lipid ratios, and CRP as risk factors for cardiovascular disease in women. JAMA 2005;294(3):326–33.

44. Blake GJ, Otvos JD, Rifai N, et al. Low-density lipoprotein particle concentration and size as determined by nuclear magnetic resonance spectroscopy as predictors of cardiovascular disease in women. Circulation 2002;106(15):1930–7.

45. Rubins HB, Robins SJ, Collins D, et al. Gemfibrozil for the secondary prevention of coronary heart disease in men with low levels of high-density lipoprotein cholesterol. Veterans Affairs High-Density Lipoprotein Cholesterol Intervention Trial Study Group. N Engl J Med 1999;341(6):410–8.
46. Robins SJ, Collins D, Wittes JT, et al. Relation of gemfibrozil treatment and lipid levels with major coronary events: VA-HIT: a randomized controlled trial. JAMA 2001;285(12):1585–91.
47. Otvos JD, Collins D, Freedman DS, et al. Low-density lipoprotein and high-density lipoprotein particle subclasses predict coronary events and are favorably changed by gemfibrozil therapy in the Veterans Affairs High-Density Lipoprotein Intervention Trial. Circulation 2006;113(12):1556–63.
48. Lu W, Resnick HE, Jablonski KA, et al. Non-HDL cholesterol as a predictor of cardiovascular disease in type 2 diabetes: the Strong Heart study. Diabetes Care 2003;26(1):16–23.
49. Jiang R, Schulze MB, Li T, et al. Non-HDL cholesterol and apolipoprotein B predict cardiovascular disease events among men with type 2 diabetes. Diabetes Care 2004;27(8):1991–7.
50. Cromwell WC, Otvos JD. Heterogeneity of low-density lipoprotein particle number in patients with type 2 diabetes mellitus and low-density lipoprotein cholesterol <100 mg/dL. Am J Cardiol 2006;98(12):1599–602.
51. Brunzell JD, Davidson M, Furberg CD, et al. Lipoprotein management in patients with cardiometabolic risk: consensus statement from the American Diabetes Association and the American College of Cardiology Foundation. Diabetes Care 2008;31(4):811–22.
52. Howard BV, Roman MJ, Devereux RB, et al. Effect of lower targets for blood pressure and LDL cholesterol on atherosclerosis in diabetes: the SANDS randomized trial. JAMA 2008;299(14):1678–89.
53. la-Korpela M, Lankinen N, Salminen A, et al. The inherent accuracy of 1H NMR spectroscopy to quantify plasma lipoproteins is subclass dependent. Atherosclerosis 2007;190(2):352–8.
54. Cromwell WC, Otvos JD. Low-density lipoprotein particle number and risk for cardiovascular disease. Curr Atheroscler Rep 2004;6(5):381–7.
55. Contois JH, McNamara JR, Lammi-Keefe CJ, et al. Reference intervals for plasma apolipoprotein B determined with a standardized commercial immunoturbidimetric assay: results from the framingham offspring study. Clin Chem 1996;42(4): 515–23.

Risk Scores for Prediction of Coronary Heart Disease: An Update

Peter W.F. Wilson, MD[a,b,c,*]

KEYWORDS

- Coronary heart disease • Risk factors • Prediction
- Cholesterol • Epidemiology

ORIGINS OF CORONARY HEART DISEASE ESTIMATION

The prediction of coronary heart disease (CHD) owes its origins to the development of epidemiologic and biostatistical methods that allowed the assessment of factors that might determine risk of a specific outcome over time. An appropriate study design involved recruiting individuals free of the particular vascular event of interest, obtaining baseline data on factors that might affect risk for the outcome, and following the participants prospectively for the development of the clinical outcome under investigation.[1] For example, prospective CHD studies that originated in the late 1940s considered the role of factors such as age, sex, high blood pressure, high blood cholesterol, diabetes mellitus, and smoking as risk factors for heart disease. Logistic regression methods become available on mainframe computers in the 1950s and 1960s.[2,3] This process involved assembling data for a population sample that had been followed prospectively for the occurrence of a dichotomous event such as clinical CHD.

BASELINE MEASUREMENTS AS PREDICTORS OF CORONARY HEART DISEASE RISK

To develop reliable CHD risk estimations, it is important to have a longitudinal study, standardized measurements at baseline, and adjudicated outcomes that are consistent over the follow-up interval. A prospective design is necessary because critical

[a] Division of Cardiology, Emory University School of Medicine, EPICORE, Suite 1 North, 1256 Briarcliff Road, Atlanta, GA 30306, USA
[b] Department of Epidemiology, Atlanta VAMC Epidemiology and Genetics Section, Atlanta, GA 30322, USA
[c] Department of Global Health, Rollins School of Public Health, Emory University, Atlanta, GA 30322, USA
* Division of Cardiology, Emory University School of Medicine, EPICORE, Suite 1 North, 1256 Briarcliff Road, Atlanta, GA 30306.
E-mail address: peter.wf.wilson@emory.edu

Endocrinol Metab Clin N Am 38 (2009) 33–44
doi:10.1016/j.ecl.2008.11.001
0889-8529/08/$ – see front matter © 2009 Elsevier Inc. All rights reserved.

endo.theclinics.com

risk factors may change after the occurrence of CHD, and such a design allows the inclusion of fatal events as outcomes. An example of the benefits of a prospective design is evident from literature related to tobacco use and risk of CHD. After experiencing a myocardial infarction, a person may stop smoking or underreport the amount of smoking that occurred before the occurrence of the myocardial infarction, which could lead to analyses that would show a smaller effect of smoking on myocardial infarction risk than is actually present.

It is important to standardize measurements when assessing the role of factors that might increase risk for vascular disease outcomes. For example, blood pressure levels are typically measured in the arm using an appropriate size arm cuff, inflating and deflating the arm cuff according to a protocol, maintaining the level of the arm near the level of heart, taking measurements in subjects who have been sitting in a room at ambient temperature for a specified number of minutes, using a sphygmomanometer that has been standardized, and having determinations made by properly trained personnel. There are several possibilities for inaccuracies and imprecision to be introduced into blood pressure measurements when such guidelines are not followed.

Standardization of lipid measurements, typically obtained in the fasting state, is an important component in the development of risk estimation for CHD. The Lipid Research Clinics Program that was initiated in the 1970s led to the formal development of such a program at the Centers for Disease Control and Prevention and the adoption of a standard protocol to measure cholesterol, HDL cholesterol, and triglycerides with accuracy and precision.[4–6] Methods were used to assure high quality determinations and this program updated the laboratory methodologies and techniques over time to accommodate newer methods of measurement.[7–9] Variability in laboratory results has several potential sources and include pre-analytic phases, analytic phases, and biological variability, as reviewed by Cooper and colleagues.[10,11] Preanalytic sources of error include fasting status, appropriate use of tourniquets during phlebotomy, room temperature, and sample transport conditions. Laboratory variability is kept lower with high quality instrumentation, reliable assays, performing replicate assays, and employing algorithms to repeat assays if the difference between replicates exceeds specified thresholds. Other methods to ensure that laboratory determinations are accurate and precise include use of external standards, batching samples, minimizing the number of lots for calibration. Biological variability should also be considered and sources of imprecision include fasting status, time of day, season of the year, and intervening illnesses.

Another key risk factor is diabetes status. Many of the older studies did not have fasting visits for each clinical visit, and an expert-derived diagnosis of diabetes mellitus was employed based on the available glucose information, medication use, and chart reviews. The American Diabetes Association has changed the criteria for diabetes over the last few decades. For example, in 1979 diabetes was considered present if fasting glucose was 140 mg/dL or higher, or if a casual glucose level was greater than 200 mg/dL.[12] These criteria were revised in 1997 so that a fasting glucose greater than or equal to 126 mg/dL was considered to be diagnostic of diabetes mellitus.[13]

CORONARY HEART DISEASE OUTCOMES

A variety of outcomes have been used to predict coronary heart disease events. Most study designs have centered on the initial occurrence of a CHD event in subjects who are known not to have clinical CHD at baseline. Total CHD (angina pectoris, myocardial infarction, and coronary heart disease death), or hard CHD (myocardial infarction and coronary heart disease death) are the outcomes that have been studied most frequently, but others have reported on risk of hard CHD and included subjects with a baseline history of angina pectoris,[14] and the European CHD risk estimates have focused on the occurrence of CHD death.[15]

PAST HISTORY OF CORONARY HEART DISEASE RISK ESTIMATION

In the early 1970s estimation of CHD risk was undertaken using logistic regression methods and cross-sectional pooling with the variables age, sex, blood pressure, cholesterol level, smoking, and diabetes.[16] With these approaches the results were reported as logistic regression analyses and the relative risk effects for each of the predictor variables were provided. Time-dependent regression methods and the addition of HDL cholesterol levels as an important predictor led to improved prediction models for CHD,[17] employing score sheets and regression equation information with intercepts to estimate absolute risk for coronary heart disease over a interval that typically spanned 8–12 years of follow-up.

Score sheets to estimate CHD risk were highlighted in a Framingham CHD risk publication in 1991 that predicted total CHD[18] and a variety of first cardiovascular events.[19] The outcome of interest was prediction of an initial vascular disease event using the independent variables age, sex, high blood pressure, high blood cholesterol, diabetes mellitus, smoking, and left ventricular hypertrophy on the electrocardiogram. Risk equations with coefficients were provided to allow estimation of CHD risk using score sheets, pocket calculators, and computer programs.[18]

In the mid-1990s the fifth report of the Joint National Committee on the Detection, Evaluation, and Treatment of High Blood Pressure (JNC V) contained guidelines that used categories of arterial pressure and a similar approach was undertaken by the National Cholesterol Education Program (NCEP) Adult Treatment Panel II for total cholesterol and HDL cholesterol categories.[20,21] These guidelines were followed by an updated Framingham publication on total CHD risk that used categories for all of the common variables and employed categories for the variables that were used by the blood pressure and cholesterol expert committees.[1]

The 1998 Framingham CHD risk estimation article showed little difference in the overall predictive capability of Total CHD when total cholesterol was replaced by LDL cholesterol, which suggested that an initial lipid screening with total cholesterol, HDL cholesterol, age, sex, systolic blood pressure, diabetes mellitus, and smoking had good overall predictive capabilities without lipid subgroup measurements. The 1998 CHD risk manuscript did not include information on ECG-LVH as a risk predictor because the JNC and the NCEP had not recommended that electrocardiograms be performed on asymptomatic middle-aged subjects.[22] The prevalence of ECG-LVH as a risk predictor was only a few percent in middle-aged white populations. On the other hand, ECG-LVH has been much more common in African Americans. It is thought that including ECGs might be particularly helpful to estimate CHD risk in African Americans and other racial and ethnic groups where ECG-LVH is more common and where the population burden of hypertension is greater.[20]

A workshop was convened by the National Heart, Lung, and Blood Institute in 2001 to assess the ability to estimate risk of first CHD events in middle-aged Americans. In summaries of the workshop proceedings, D'Agostino and colleagues[23] and Grundy and colleagues[24] compared the predictive results for CHD in several studies using Framingham equations or using equations that employed the same variables as the Framingham equation but used study-specific predictions. The summary findings included the following: (1) relative risks for the individual variables were similar to the Framingham experience; (2) the Framingham equations predicted CHD quite well when applied to other populations, and the c-statistic for the Framingham prediction was usually very similar to the c-statistic from the study-specific predictor equation; and (3) in African Americans and Japanese American men from the Honolulu Heart Study, the Framingham equation prediction had much lower discrimination capability.[23]

CORONARY HEART DISEASE RISK ALGORITHM DEVELOPMENT

It is helpful to understand how CHD risk algorithms are currently developed and performance criteria are used to evaluate prediction algorithms. The key starting point is the experience of a well-characterized prospective study cohort that is generally representative of a larger population group. That initial stipulation can help to assure the generalizability of the results. Only data from subjects with complete outcome and covariate information for a given endpoint are used in the analyses.

Risk estimates for CHD are usually derived from proportional hazards regression models according to methods developed by Cox.[25] The variables that are significant in the individual analyses are then considered for inclusion in multivariable prediction models using a fixed design or a stepwise model that selects the variables for inclusion using an iterative approach. Pairwise interactions can be considered for inclusion in the model, but it may be difficult to interpret those results and interactions may be less generalizable when tested in other population groups.

Traditional candidate variables considered for this analysis have often included systolic or diastolic blood pressure, blood pressure treatment, cholesterol level, diabetes mellitus, current smoking, and body mass index. Including information related to treatment, such as blood pressure medication, may be relevant, but caution should be exercised in this situation because the risk algorithm is typically being developed from an observational study with a prospective design, not from a clinical trial where treatments are randomly assigned (**Table 1**).

A validation group is used to test the usefulness of the risk prediction algorithm. One approach uses an internal validation sample within the study. By this method a fraction

Table 1
Examples of coronary heart disease event prediction with risk factor algorithms

Author (Reference) Year of Publication Item	Wilson[1] 1998	ATP III[46] 2001	Assmann[14] 2002	euroSCORE[15] 2003
Source	Framingham	Framingham	PROCAM	Europe
Age interval	5 years	5 years	5 years	5 years
Sex	Men, women	Men, women	Men	Men, women
BP levels	JNC-VI	BP systolic	BP systolic	BP systolic
BP therapy	No	Yes	No	No
Cholesterol	Yes	Yes	No	Yes
HDL cholesterol	Yes	Yes	Yes	No
LDL cholesterol	optional	No	Yes	No
Cigarettes	Yes	Yes	Yes	Yes
Diabetes mellitus	Yes	No	Yes	Yes
Baseline heart disease	ECG-LVH	No	Myocardial infarction history	No
Coronary heart disease event	Total CHD	Hard CHD	Next Hard CHD	CHD death

of the data are used for model development and the other fraction of the data are used for validation. An alternative to this approach is to take a very large fraction of the subjects in the study and successively develop models from near-complete data sets. External validation of a risk prediction model is especially useful, testing the use of the model in other population samples, and providing the first indication of whether it is possible to generalize the risk prediction model to other venues.

PERFORMANCE CRITERIA FOR CORONARY HEART DISEASE RISK ALGORITHMS

A variety of statistical evaluations are now available to evaluate the usefulness of CHD risk prediction and they are discussed successively in the section below.

Relative Risk

For each risk factor, proportional hazards modeling yields regression coefficients for a study cohort. The relative risk of a variable is computed by exponentiating the regression coefficient in the multivariable regression models. This measure estimates the difference in risk for someone with a given risk factor such as cigarette smoking compared with the risk for someone who does not smoke. An analogous approach can be undertaken to estimate effects for continuous variables by showing effects for a specific number of units for the variable or by identifying differences in risk associated with a difference in the number of units associated with a standard deviation for the factor.

Discrimination

Discrimination is the ability of a statistical model to separate those who experience clinical CHD events from those who do not. The c-statistic is the typical performance measure used, which is analogous to the area under a receiver-operator characteristic curve, and is a composite of the overall sensitivity and specificity of the prediction equation (**Fig. 1**).[26] The c-statistic represents an estimate of the probability that a model assigns a higher risk to those who develop CHD within a specified follow-up than to those who do not. The error associated with c-statistic estimates can be estimated.[26,27] Values for the c-statistic range from 0.00 to 1.00, and 0.50 reflects discrimination by chance. Higher values generally indicate a good level of agreement between observed and predicted risks. The average c-statistic for the prediction of CHD

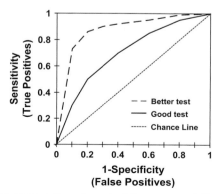

Fig. 1. Schematic for receiver operating characteristic curves and disease prediction based on sensitivity and specificity of multivariable prediction models.

is typically in the 0.70 range.[1,23] Using a large number of independent predictor variables can lead to better discrimination but may also overfit the prediction model.

Calibration

Calibration measures how closely predicted estimates agree with actual outcomes. To present calibration analyses, the data are separated into deciles of risk, and observed rates are tested for differences from the expected across the deciles using a version of the Hosmer-Lemeshow χ^2 statistic.[23] Smaller χ^2 values indicate good calibration and values greater than 20 generally indicate significant lack of calibration.

Recalibration

An existing CHD prediction model can be recalibrated if it provides relatively good ranking of risk for the population being studied, but the model systematically over- or underestimates CHD risk in the new population. For example, recalibrating the Framingham risk prediction equation would involve inserting the mean risk factor values and average incidence rate for the new population into the Framingham equation. Kaplan-Meier estimates can be used to determine average incidence rates.[28] This approach was undertaken for Framingham risk equations that were applied to the CHD experience of Japanese American men in the Honolulu Heart Study and for Chinese men and women.[23,28] In each of these instances the Framingham risk equation provided relatively good discrimination but did not provide reliable estimates of absolute risk. A schematic of such an approach is shown in **Fig. 2**, where the left panel shows

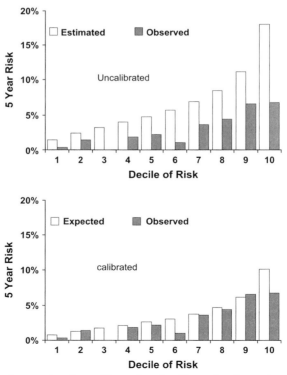

Fig. 2. Hypothetical example of uncalibrated and calibrated estimated and observed CHD risk according to deciles of CHD risk.

CHD risk is systematically overestimated when the Framingham equation is applied to another population. After calibration the estimation fits the observed experience much more closely and the Hosmer-Lemeshow χ^2 is much lower.

Reclassification

Specialized testing in subgroups has been used to reclassify risk for vascular disease. An example of such an approach is the use of exercise testing to upgrade, downgrade, or not change estimates of vascular disease risk in patients being evaluated for angina pectoris.[29] Coronary heart disease algorithms may do a reasonably good job in prediction of CHD risk, and the inclusion of a new variable may have minimal effects on c-statistic estimates.[30–33] Methods developed to assess this approach have used a multivariable estimation procedure and tested the utility of a new test to increase, decrease, or not change risk estimates.[29] Pencina and colleagues[34] has recently published an updated method to assess reclassification that takes into account the potential reclassification of both cases and noncases.

Reclassification has practical applications, as shown in **Fig. 3**, where an initial probability of CHD is estimated from a multivariable prediction equation, and additional information allows a posterior estimation of risk. If the new information did not provide any added value, the risk estimate would be the same as for the initial calculation and would lie close to the identity line. The schematic shows the hypothetical effects for a small number of patients. For some individuals the test was positive, increasing the posterior risk estimates. On the other hand, negative tests moved the risk estimates downward for some individuals. The magnitude of the effects can be shown graphically by the length of the vertical lines and how they differ from the identity line. Finally, a posterior risk estimate that would reclassify the individual to a lower or higher risk category is important to evaluate. For example, **Fig. 3** shows seven subjects with an initial probability of developing disease in the 10% to 20% range. Risk was increased in three subjects and decreased in four subjects with new variable information. Some of the risk differences did not differ appreciably from the initial estimates. Risk was reclassified into a higher category in only one subject and reclassified to a lower category in two subjects. Some authors have used performance measures such as the Bayesian Information Criteria as another method to interpret potential effects of reclassification.[31]

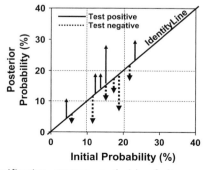

Fig. 3. Example of reclassification strategy and risk of disease according to initial and posterior probabilities. Gridlines represent potential levels that are associated with reclassification of risk.

PRESENT CORONARY HEART DISEASE RISK ESTIMATION

The current starting point for using a CHD risk prediction equation in subjects being screened for CHD is a medical history and clinical examination with standardized collection of key predictor (independent) risk factors: age, sex, fasting lipids (total, LDL, and HDL cholesterol, total/HDL ratio), systolic blood pressure, history of diabetes mellitus treatment, fasting or postprandial glucose levels, use of tobacco and other substances.[1,14] With this information it is possible to estimate risk of CHD over a 10-year interval using score sheets or computer programs.

Specialized models have been developed for subjects with type 2 diabetes that consider additional potential predictor variables. The experience of diabetic patients who participated in the United Kingdom Prospective Diabetes Study has been used to develop this prediction algorithm. The authors have reported that the key predictor variables for initial CHD events were age, sex, ethnic group, smoking status, time since diagnosis of diabetes, hemoglobin A1c, systolic blood pressure, and lipid levels.[35]

European groups have developed strategies to estimate risk of CHD using European data. Investigators from the Prospective Cardiovascular Münster (PROCAM) in Germany have followed a cohort for the development of CHD and their results are generally similar to what has been estimated from Framingham data.[14] Their analyses were restricted to men. The factors significantly associated with the development of a next CHD event included age, LDL cholesterol, smoking, HDL cholesterol, systolic blood pressure, family history of premature myocardial infarction, diabetes mellitus, and triglycerides. The Italian scientists undertook prediction analyses in middle-aged men who were followed 10 years for CHD events. They found that age, total cholesterol, systolic blood pressure, cigarette smoking, HDL cholesterol, diabetes mellitus, hypertension drug treatment, and family history of CHD were associated with initial CHD events.[36] The Italian team also tested the utility of Framingham and PROCAM estimating equations in Italy (CUORE). They generally found that both Framingham and PROCAM overestimated CHD risk in Italian men and after calibration of the Framingham equations it was possible to reliably predict CHD events in their study cohort.[36] Risk scores have also been developed in the United Kingdom (QRISK) and Scotland (ASSIGN) with consideration of the effects of social deprivation. The QRISK algorithm predicts total cardiovascular disease (QRISK) using age, sex, smoking status, systolic blood pressure, ratio of total serum cholesterol to high density lipoprotein, body mass index, family history of coronary heart disease in first degree relative aged less than 60, area measure of deprivation, and existing treatment with antihypertensive agent.

The euroSCORE algorithm is currently the most popular CHD prediction algorithm in Europe. It predicts CHD death outcomes and includes a data from a large number of studies across Europe to generate the predictions. The factors used in the prediction include age, sex, smoking, systolic blood pressure, and the ratio of total/HDL cholesterol. Unfortunately, not enough of the participating centers had data on CHD morbidity and a prediction algorithm for total CHD based on experience across Europe is still in development.

FUTURE OF CORONARY HEART DISEASE PREDICTION

The prediction of CHD has helped to guide clinical decisions for subjects free of clinical cardiovascular disease at baseline. It is especially helpful to identify subjects who middle-aged individuals who should be treated aggressively with management of cholesterol and blood pressure. As blood pressure and lipid treatment strategies become more widespread, more efficacious, and achievable at lower cost, it makes sense to try to prevent total cardiovascular events. For the preceding reasons it is likely that first cardiovascular disease (CVD) events (including total CHD, peripheral arterial disease, cerebrovascular disease, and cardiac failure), may become the clinical outcome of greatest interest and significance in the future.[19,37] Some investigations, especially large cardiovascular registries, have also been involved with the prediction of next cardiovascular events and bedside risk estimation of 6-month mortality in patients surviving admission for an acute coronary syndromes.[38,39]

It is possible to estimate risk of CHD, CVD, and other vascular disease events over a lifetime. The event rates are generally much greater than what is observed for 10-year intervals.[40] For instance, the lifetime risk for the development of CHD in a 40-year-oldwithout a history of CHD is approximately 50% over the rest of his life-time. If a man lives to age 80 and has not experienced CHD up to that point, his risk of developing CHD over the rest of his lifetime is approximately 25%. It is more difficult to provide multivariable risk estimations to subjects concerning their lifetime risks.[41] It is likely that lifetime estimates will be of greater interest in future estimations of risk for cardiovascular sequelae, and we can expect these formulations to be integrated into treatment strategies and consensus recommendations.

Coronary disease risk can be estimated using several methods, and recent reports have shown that simple prediction tools can potentially be self-administered. For example, analyses undertaken by Mainous and colleagues[42] for participants in the Atherosclerosis Risk in Communities Study showed that the variables age, diabetes, hypertension, hypercholesterolemia, smoking, physical activity, and family history were predictive of initial CHD events in men, and similar results were available for women. Similarly, Gaziano and colleagues[43] used data from the National Health and Nutrition Examination Survey and showed that a simple set of variables, including age, systolic blood pressure, smoking status, body mass index, reported diabetes status, and current treatment for hypertension were predictive of CHD risk. It has been suggested that such approaches may be useful in developing parts of the world where lower cost estimates of CHD risk would be particularly useful.

Imaging information related to atherosclerotic burden can be particularly helpful to predict risk of coronary heart disease events, but the cost of such procedures is relatively great compared with the low cost of health risk screening.[44] Atherosclerotic images may be particularly successful when coupled with reclassification that first identify subjects at intermediate risk by low-cost screening methods, then followed up with an imaging test of an arterial bed (coronary arteries, aorta, or carotid) to then reclassify risk, depending on the results of the imaging test. Genetic information can potentially be used to develop an estimate of CHD risk, and some analyses have been undertaken.[45] It is likely that this method will achieve greater efficacy when the genetic information is coupled with clinically useful information such as blood pressure and lipid levels.

REFERENCES

1. Wilson PW, D'Agostino RB, Levy D, et al. Prediction of coronary heart disease using risk factor categories. Circulation 1998;97(18):1837–47.
2. Walker SH, Duncan DB. Estimation of the probability of an event as a function of several independent variables. Biometrika 1967;54:167–79.
3. Truett J, Cornfield J, Kannel WB. A multivariate analysis of risk of coronary heart disease in Framingham. J Chronic Dis 1967;20:511–24.

4. Lipid Research Clinics Population Studies. Data book. 1st edition. In: The Prevalence Study 1980(NIH Publ 80-1527), vol. 1. Bethesda: NIH; 1990.

5. Lipid Research Clinics Program. Manual of Laboratory Operation. 1st edition. Bethesda: NIH; 1974.

6. Rifkind BM, Segal P. Lipid research clinics program reference values for hyperlipidemia and hypolipidemia. JAMA 1983;250:1869–72.

7. Warnick GR, Myers GL, Cooper GR, et al. Impact of the third cholesterol report from the adult treatment panel of the National Cholesterol Education Program on the clinical laboratory. Clin Chem 2002;48(1):11–7.

8. McNamara JR, Leary ET, Ceriotti F, et al. Point: status of lipid and lipoprotein standardization. Clin Chem 1997;43(8 Pt 1):1306–10.

9. Myers GL, Cooper GR, Sampson EJ. Traditional lipoprotein profile: clinical utility, performance requirement, and standardization. Atherosclerosis 1994;108(Suppl): S157–69.

10. Cooper GR, Myers GL, Smith J, et al. Blood lipid measurements: variations and practical utility. JAMA 1992;267:1652–60.

11. Cooper GR, Smith SJ, Myers GL, et al. Estimating and minimizing effects of biologic sources of variation by relative range when measuring the mean of serum lipids and lipoproteins. Clin Chem 1994;40:227–32.

12. National Diabetes Data Group. Classification and diagnosis of diabetes mellitus and other categories of glucose intolerance. Diabetes 1979;28:1039–57.

13. Report of the Expert Committee on the Diagnosis and Classification of Diabetes Mellitus. Diabetes Care 1997;20(7):1183–97.

14. Assmann G, Cullen P, Schulte H. Simple scoring scheme for calculating the risk of acute coronary events based on the 10-year follow-up of the prospective cardiovascular Münster (PROCAM) study. Circulation 2002;105(3):310–5.

15. Conroy RM, Pyorala K, Fitzgerald AP, et al. Estimation of ten-year risk of fatal cardiovascular disease in Europe: the SCORE project. Eur Heart J 2003;24(11): 987–1003.

16. Kannel WB, Castelli WP, Gordon T, et al. Serum cholesterol, lipoproteins, and the risk of coronary heart disease: the Framingham Study. Ann Intern Med 1971;74: 1–12.

17. Wilson PWF, Castelli WP, Kannel WB. Coronary risk prediction in adults: The Framingham heart study. Am J Cardiol 1987;59(G):91–4.

18. Anderson KM, Wilson PWF, Odell PM, et al. An updated coronary risk profile. A statement for health professionals. Circulation 1991;83:357–63.

19. Anderson KM, Odell PM, Wilson PWF, et al. Cardiovascular disease risk profiles. Am Heart J 1991;121:293–8.

20. Joint National Committee. The fifth report of the Joint National Committee on detection, evaluation, and treatment of high blood pressure (JNC V). Arch Intern Med 1993;153:154–83.

21. The Expert Panel. National cholesterol education program. Second report. The expert panel on detection, evaluation, and treatment of high blood cholesterol in adults (adult treatment panel II). Circulation 1994;89(3):1333–45.

22. National High Blood Pressure Education Program. The 1988 report of the Joint National Committee on detection, evaluation, and treatment of high blood pressure. Arch Intern Med 1988;148:1023–38.

23. D'Agostino RB Sr, Grundy S, Sullivan LM, et al. Validation of the Framingham coronary heart disease prediction scores: results of a multiple ethnic groups investigation. JAMA 2001;286(2):180–7.

24. Grundy SM, D'Agostino RB Sr, Mosca L, et al. Cardiovascular risk assessment based on US cohort studies: findings from a National Heart, Lung, and Blood Institute workshop. Circulation 2001;104(4):491–6.
25. Cox DR. Regression models and life tables. J R Stat Soc(B) 1972;34:187–220.
26. Pencina MJ, D'Agostino RB. Overall C as a measure of discrimination in survival analysis: model specific population value and confidence interval estimation. Stat Med 2004;23(13):2109–23.
27. D'Agostino RB Sr, Nam BH. Evaluation of the performance of survival analysis models: discrimination and calibration measures. Handbook of Statistics (vol 23): Advances in Survival Analysis. Amsterdam: Elsevier; 2004. p. 1–26.
28. Liu J, Hong Y, D'Agostino RB Sr, et al. Predictive value for the Chinese population of the Framingham CHD risk assessment tool compared with the Chinese Multi-Provincial Cohort Study. JAMA 2004;291(21):2591–9.
29. Diamond GA, Hirsch M, Forrester JS, et al. Application of information theory to clinical diagnostic testing. The electrocardiographic stress test. Circulation 1981;63(4):915–21.
30. Wilson PW, Nam BH, Pencina M, et al. C-reactive protein and risk of cardiovascular disease in men and women from the Framingham heart study. Arch Intern Med 2005;165(21):2473–8.
31. Cook NR, Buring JE, Ridker PM. The effect of including C-reactive protein in cardiovascular risk prediction models for women. Ann Intern Med 2006;145(1):21–9.
32. Pepe MS, Thompson ML. Combining diagnostic test results to increase accuracy. Biostatistics 2000;1(2):123–40.
33. Pepe MS, Janes H, Longton G, et al. Limitations of the odds ratio in gauging the performance of a diagnostic, prognostic, or screening marker. Am J Epidemiol 2004;159(9):882–90.
34. Pencina MJ, D'Agostino RB Sr, D'Agostino RB Jr, et al. Evaluating the added predictive ability of a new marker: from area under the ROC curve to reclassification and beyond. Stat Med 2008;27(2):157–72.
35. Stevens RJ, Kothari V, Adler AI, et al. The UKPDS risk engine: a model for the risk of coronary heart disease in type II diabetes (UKPDS 56). Clin Sci (Lond) 2001; 101(6):671–9.
36. Ferrario M, Chiodini P, Chambless LE, et al. Prediction of coronary events in a low incidence population. Assessing accuracy of the CUORE cohort study prediction equation. Int J Epidemiol 2005;34(2):413–21.
37. D'Agostino RB Sr, Vasan RS, Pencina MJ, et al. General cardiovascular risk profile for use in primary care: the Framingham heart study. Circulation 2008;117(6): 743–53.
38. Califf RM, Armstrong PW, Carver JR, et al. 27th Bethesda Conference: matching the intensity of risk factor management with the hazard for coronary disease events. Task force 5. Stratification of patients into high, medium and low risk subgroups for purposes of risk factor management. J Am Coll Cardiol 1996;27(5):1007–19.
39. Eagle KA, Lim MJ, Dabbous OH, et al. A validated prediction model for all forms of acute coronary syndrome: estimating the risk of 6-month post-discharge death in an international registry. JAMA 2004;291(22):2727–33.
40. Lloyd-Jones DM, Larson MG, Beiser A, et al. Lifetime risk of developing coronary heart disease. Lancet 1999;353(9147):89–92.
41. Lloyd-Jones DM, Leip EP, Larson MG, et al. Prediction of lifetime risk for cardiovascular disease by risk factor burden at 50 years of age. Circulation 2006;113: 791–8.

42. Mainous AG III, Koopman RJ, Diaz VA, et al. A coronary heart disease risk score based on patient-reported information. Am J Cardiol 2007;99(9):1236–41.

43. Gaziano TA, Young CR, Fitzmaurice G, et al. Laboratory-based versus non-laboratory-based method for assessment of cardiovascular disease risk: the NHANES I Follow-up Study cohort. Lancet 2008;371(9616):923–31.

44. Detrano R, Guerci AD, Carr JJ, et al. Coronary calcium as a predictor of coronary events in four racial or ethnic groups. N Engl J Med 2008;358(13):1336–45.

45. Humphries SE, Yiannakouris N, Talmud PJ. Cardiovascular disease risk prediction using genetic information (gene scores): is it really informative? Curr Opin Lipidol 2008;19(2):128–32.

46. Executive summary of the Third Report of the National Cholesterol Education Program (NCEP) expert panel on detection, evaluation, and treatment of high blood cholesterol in adults (adult treatment panel III). JAMA 2001;285(19):2486–97.

Lifestyle Approaches and Dietary Strategies to Lower LDL-Cholesterol and Triglycerides and Raise HDL-Cholesterol

Heather I. Katcher, PhD, RD[a,d], Alison M. Hill, PhD[a],
Julie L.G. Lanford, MPH, RD[b], Janey S. Yoo, MS, RD[c],
Penny M. Kris-Etherton, PhD, RD[a,*]

KEYWORDS

- Nutrition • Diet • Lifestyle • Weight loss
- Cardiovascular disease • Lipids • Lipoproteins

Risk factor reduction has been the long-standing cornerstone in the prevention and treatment of coronary heart disease (CHD). Implementing healthy lifestyle behaviors including diet is a foundation for reducing CHD risk.[1] Epidemiologic studies and controlled clinical trials consistently have demonstrated cardioprotective benefits of dietary patterns high in vegetables, fruits, legumes, whole grains, fiber, fish, lean meats and poultry, and low-fat dairy products.[1,2] Other healthy lifestyle behaviors such as nonsmoking, maintaining a waist-to-hip ratio below the 75th percentile, and regular exercise, in concert with a healthy dietary pattern that includes moderate alcohol consumption, are associated with a 92% decrease in heart attack risk.[3] Given the magnitude of the benefits that a healthy dietary pattern and lifestyle behaviors can have, these are the first steps in the prevention and treatment of CHD.[4]

Low-density lipoprotein-cholesterol (LDL-C) is the primary target for cholesterol-lowering therapy because of strong evidence in humans and animal models that high LDL-C levels initiate and promote atherogenesis, and that LDL-C lowering reduces CHD risk.[4] It is estimated that each 1.8 mg/dL decrease in LDL-C reduces

The authors have no conflicts of interest to report.

[a] Department of Nutritional Sciences, Pennsylvania State University, 119 Chandlee Lab, University Park, PA 16802, USA

[b] Cancer Services, Inc., 3175 Maplewood Avenue, Winston-Salem, NC 27103, USA

[c] Children's Hospital, 518 Octavia Street, New Orleans, LA 70115, USA

[d] Washington Center for Clinical Research, Washington, DC 20016, USA

* Corresponding author.

E-mail address: pmk3@psu.edu (P.M. Kris-Etherton).

Endocrinol Metab Clin N Am 38 (2009) 45–78
doi:10.1016/j.ecl.2008.11.010
0889-8529/08/$ – see front matter © 2009 Elsevier Inc. All rights reserved.

endo.theclinics.com

the risk of a cardiovascular event (heart attack, stroke, hospitalization for unstable angina, or revascularization) by 1%.[5] Based on subsequent modifications of ATP III Guidelines, the recommended LDL-C goal for high-risk patients is less than 100 mg/dL; when risk is very high, an LDL-C goal of less than 70 mg/dL is a therapeutic option.[6] Consistent with this recommendation is that even for very high risk patients who have a baseline LDL-C less than 100 mg/dL, an LDL-C goal of less than 70 mg/dL is a therapeutic option. In addition, an LDL-C goal of less than 100 mg/dL is a therapeutic option for moderately high-risk patients over the recommended LDL-C of less than 130 g/dL.[6] As a result of these recommendations, the goal for LDL-C is to have levels as low as possible.

Diet and lifestyle patterns affect many CHD risk factors by a variety of mechanisms beyond LDL-C lowering.[4] Several other major, independent lipid risk factors have been identified, including elevated triglycerides (TG) and low high-density lipoprotein-cholesterol (HDL-C). These lipid risk factors are two of the five criteria for clinically defining metabolic syndrome, and can present with normal LDL-C levels.[7] Because metabolic syndrome is related to obesity and physical inactivity, diet and lifestyle practices also are the first line of treatment.[4] This article discusses specific dietary factors as well as dietary patterns that affect the major CHD lipid risk factors, ie, LDL-C, HDL-C, and TG. Based on a very large evidence base, it is clear that diet and lifestyle practices can markedly affect these major CHD lipid risk factors, and consequently decrease CHD risk substantively.

DIETARY FACTORS THAT INCREASE LOW-DENSITY LIPOPROTEIN-CHOLESTEROL
Saturated Fatty Acids

Saturated fatty acids (SFA) raise LDL-C in a dose-dependent manner.[8] The major sources of SFA in the United States are fatty red meats and full-fat dairy products.[8] Tropical oils, including palm oil, palm kernel oil, and coconut oil, also are high in SFA. SFA intake has been positively correlated with CHD risk in several observational studies.[9] In the Seven Countries Study, collective intake of the four major long-chain saturated fatty acids (eg, lauric, myristic, palmitic, and stearic acid) had a strong positive correlation with 25-year death rates from CHD ($r > 0.80$).[10]

Meta-analyses of clinical trial data indicate that for every 1% increase in energy from SFA, LDL-C increases by 1.8 mg/dL.[11] Reducing SFA intake to less than 7% of energy and cholesterol intake to less than 200 mg per day reduces LDL-C by 9% to 12% compared with baseline or a Western diet.[12] In conjunction with a 3- to 6-kg weight loss, LDL-C can be reduced by 16%.[12]

The Institute of Medicine (IOM) recommendations are to consume as little SFA as possible along with a diet that is adequate in all essential nutrients.[8] The American Heart Association (AHA) recommends that less than 7% of energy come from SFA.[1] Substituting unsaturated fats, carbohydrates, or protein for SFA all are effective means for decreasing total- and LDL-C. Replacing SFA with unsaturated fats also lowers the total cholesterol (TC):HDL-C ratio and prevents or attenuates an increase in TG that can occur when SFA are replaced by carbohydrates.[12] However, choosing foods high in fiber and complex carbohydrates can attenuate or prevent the TG-raising effect of increasing carbohydrate intake.[13] Although individual SFA have different effects on LDL-C (eg, stearic acid has a neutral effect versus the other long-chain SFA), at the present time it is not appropriate to focus on specific SFA when selecting food containing a mixture of individual SFA. The presence of a variety of SFA in foods makes it challenging to emphasize or limit individual SFA.[14] **Table 1** lists simple strategies for reducing SFA in the diet.[2]

Table 1
Comparisons of the saturated fat content of different forms of commonly consumed foods, illustrating that lower saturated fat choices can be made within the same food group

Food Category	Portion	Saturated Fat Content, g	Calories
Cheese			
Regular cheddar cheese	1 oz	6.0	114
Low-fat cheddar cheese	1 oz	1.2	49
Ground beef			
Regular ground beef (25% fat)	3 oz (cooked)	6.1	236
Extra lean ground beef (5% fat)	3 oz (cooked)	2.6	148
Milk			
Whole milk (3.25%)	1 cup	4.6	146
Low-fat milk (1%)	1 cup	1.5	102
Breads			
Croissant	1 medium	6.6	231
Bagel, oat bran (4")	1 medium	0.2	227
Frozen desserts			
Regular ice cream	0.5 cup	4.9	145
Frozen yogurt, low fat	0.5 cup	2.0	110
Table spreads			
Butter	1 tsp	2.4	34
Soft margarine with zero trans fats	1 tsp	0.7	25
Chicken			
Fried chicken (leg with skin)	3 oz (cooked)	3.3	212
Roasted chicken (breast with no skin)	3 oz (cooked)	0.9	140
Fish			
Fried cat fish	3 oz	2.8	195
Baked cat fish	3 oz	1.5	129

Data from United States Department of Health and Human Services and United States Department of Agriculture. Dietary guidelines for Americans. Washington, DC: U.S. Government Printing Office; 2005.

Trans Fatty Acids

Trans fatty acids (TFA) adversely affect serum lipid and lipoprotein levels. Compared with *cis*-unsaturated fatty acids, TFA raise TC and LDL-C, lower HDL-C, and increase the ratios of TC:HDL-C and LDL-C:HDL-C.[15] Compared with saturated fatty acids (SFA), *trans* fatty acids increase LDL-C similarly, but lower HDL-C. As a result, the increase in the LDL-C:HDL-C ratio following TFA consumption is twofold higher than for saturated fat (**Fig. 1**).[16] Randomized clinical trials have demonstrated a positive linear relationship between TFA intake and the LDL-C:HDL-C ratio (see **Fig. 1**). Based on these data, each 2% increase in TFA intake raises the LDL-C:HDL-C ratio by 0.1 unit (see **Fig. 1**).[16]

In prospective studies, the incidence of CHD in individuals with the highest TFA intake is greater than predicted by lipid levels alone,[15,17] suggesting that there are adverse effects of TFA beyond their effects on lipids. Likewise, individuals with the highest levels of TFA in plasma phospholipids, adipose tissue, and red blood cell

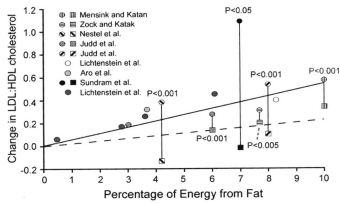

Fig. 1. Results of randomized studies of the effects of a diet high in *trans* fatty acids (TFA) (*circles*) or saturated fatty acids (SFA) (*squares*) on the ratio of LDL:HDL cholesterol.[199–207] A diet with isocaloric amounts of *cis* fatty acids was used as the comparison group. The solid line indicates the best-fit regression for TFA. The dashed line indicates the best-fit regression for SFA. (*Adapted from* Ascherio A, Katan MB, Zock PL, et al. Trans fatty acids and coronary heart disease. N Engl J Med 1999;340(25):1994–8; with permission. Copyright © 1999, Massachusetts Medical Society.)

membranes had up to a 3-fold greater increase myocardial infarction risk and approximately a 1.5-fold greater risk of cardiac arrest and fatal ischemic heart disease (IHD) compared with individuals with the lowest TFA levels.[18–21] Based on data from four prospective studies of 140,000 participants, it is estimated that a 2% increase in energy intake from TFA increases the incidence of CHD by 23% (Pooled relative risk [RR] 1.23; 95% confidence interval [CI] 1.11–1.37, $P<.001$).[15] Because TFA make up 2% to 3% of daily energy intake, a reduction in TFA in the diet to less than 1% of energy intake, as recommended by the AHA,[1] can significantly reduce CHD risk.[22,23]

TFA are formed by partial hydrogenation of vegetable oils, resulting in semisolid fats. The most common sources of TFA are margarines, shortenings, commercially fried foods, baked goods, and savory snack foods (**Table 2**).[2] Thus, limiting

Table 2
Contribution of various foods to trans fatty acid (TFA) intake in the American diet

Food Group	Contribution (% of Total TFA Consumed)
Cakes, cookies, crackers, pies, bread	40
Animal products	21
Margarine	17
Fried potatoes	8
Potato chips, corn chips, popcorn	5
Household shortening	4
Other[a]	5

The major dietary sources of TFA are listed in decreasing order. Processed foods and oils provide approximately 80% of TFA in the diet, compared with 20% that occur naturally in food from animal sources. The TFA content of certain processed foods has changed and is likely to continue to change as the industry reformulates its products.[2]

[a] Includes breakfast cereal and candy. USDA analysis reported 0 g of TFA in salad dressing.

consumption of fried foods, commercial baked goods, and other foods made with partially hydrogenated oils are an effective means of reducing TFA intake. Naturally occurring TFA produced by biohydrogenation of fatty acids in the rumen are found in full and reduced fat milk and dairy products. In clinical trials, moderate amounts (1.5% of energy) of ruminant TFA had a neutral effect on lipids,[24] whereas higher doses ($\geq$ 2% of energy) had an adverse effect.[24–26] In contrast, the majority of observational trials that have been conducted indicate a neutral or even protective effect of ruminant TFA.[27–31] Further studies are needed to clarify the effects of ruminant TFA on CVD risk factors. In the meantime, clinicians and health professionals should focus on recommending that industrial sources of TFA be avoided to facilitate lowering total- and LDL-C. In addition, the focus on reducing TFA should not detract from efforts to decrease SFA.

Dietary Cholesterol

Epidemiologic studies have reported a positive[32,33] or neutral[28,34–36] relationship between dietary cholesterol intake and CHD risk. Clinical studies have shown that dietary cholesterol raises total- and LDL-C, but to a lesser extent than saturated and *trans* fatty acids.[11,37] Consuming an additional 100 mg per day of cholesterol raises TC by about 2.4 mg/dL and LDL-C by 2.1 mg/dL.[38] Food sources of dietary cholesterol are animal products (eg, eggs, dairy products, and meats), with eggs contributing the most cholesterol to the diet (approximately 213 mg cholesterol per egg). A decrease in dietary cholesterol is recommended to reduce LDL-C, especially in persons with elevated LDL-C levels. The AHA recommends consuming less than 300 mg of cholesterol per day[1] and the National Cholesterol Education Program Adult Treatment Panel (NCEP ATP) III recommends less than 200 mg per day to maximize cholesterol lowering with diet.[4]

Numerous controlled clinical trials have shown that whole egg and egg yolk consumption increases total- and LDL-C.[11,37,39,40] In contrast, most observational studies have not demonstrated a positive relationship between egg consumption and incidence of CHD.[41–45] However, a recent, 20-year follow-up of the Physicians Health Study reported that although consumption of up to six eggs per week was not associated with incident heart failure, consumption of seven or more eggs per week was associated with an increased risk of heart failure.[46] Compared with subjects who reported egg consumption of less than one per week, hazard ratios for heart failure risk were 1.28 (95% CI 1.02–1.61) and 1.64 (95% CI 1.08–2.49) for egg consumption of 1 per day and 2 or more per day, respectively. Two other studies have reported a twofold increased risk of CHD or CAD in individuals with diabetes who eat more than six to seven eggs per week compared with those who eat less than one egg per week.[44,47] No adverse effects were associated with egg consumption in these studies in individuals without diabetes.

Because plant foods (eg, fruits, vegetables, beans, grains, nuts, and seeds) do not contain cholesterol, dietary cholesterol can be reduced by replacing meats and other animal products with plant foods.[1] This is recommended for high-risk patients and individuals with diabetes as one dietary strategy for significantly lowering total- and LDL-C.

DIET AND LIFESTYLE FACTORS THAT LOWER LOW-DENSITY LIPOPROTEIN-CHOLESTEROL
Soluble Fiber

Dietary fiber is the nondigestible carbohydrate components of plants. Observational studies have demonstrated an inverse association between dietary fiber and CHD risk,[48] and clinical trials have shown an LDL-C lowering effect of dietary fiber.[49] The primary mechanism for the reduction in LDL-C is via decreased absorption of cholesterol and bile acids.[50-52] Soluble fiber is present in foods such as beans, oats, barley, and some fruits and vegetables.[49] Based on observational and clinical trial evidence, the Food and Drug Administration (FDA) has approved a health claim that foods containing 1.7 g per serving of psyllium husk soluble fiber or 0.75 g of oat or barley soluble fiber as β-glucans may reduce the risk of heart disease as part of a diet low in saturated fat and cholesterol. The NCEP ATP III recommends 10 to 25 g per day of soluble fiber as a therapeutic option to enhance LDL-C lowering. Adding as little as 5 to 10 g of soluble fiber to a Therapeutic Lifestyle Change (TLC) diet (< 7% SFA, < 200 mg cholesterol per day) is expected to reduce LDL-C by approximately 5%.[4]

The most common soluble fibers are β-glucan, pectin, guar gum, and psyllium. De Groot and colleagues[53] were first to report a decrease in serum cholesterol (−11%) following 3-week daily consumption of 300 g of bread containing 140 g of rolled oats. Davy and colleagues[54] subsequently reported that soluble fiber also favorably affects LDL particle size. In a randomized controlled trial, 36 overweight men consumed 14 g of fiber daily for 12 weeks, including two large servings of high-fiber oat cereal (5.5 g β-glucan). At the end of the diet period, subjects had a 17% reduction in small LDL-C, a 5% reduction in LDL-C particle number, and a 2.5% reduction in LDL-C concentration. Similar results were reported by Shrestha and colleagues.[55] Recently, Moreyra and colleagues[56] reported that psyllium supplementation also reduces LDL-C in men when taken in combination with a statin. After 8 weeks of treatment, LDL-C levels in the group receiving 10 mg of simvastatin plus a fiber placebo fell by 55 mg/dL compared with 63 mg/dL in the group receiving 10 mg of simvastatin plus 15 g of psyllium (Metamucil) daily (P = .03). The popularity of β-glucan has led to its supplementation in other foods such as orange juice, where it also is effective in reducing LDL-C.[57,58]

In a meta-analysis conducted to evaluate the efficacy of various soluble fibers to lower total- and LDL-C, Brown and colleagues[59] reported similar effects of oats, psyllium, pectin, and guar gum. In this study, each gram of oats lowered total- and LDL-C by 1.42 mg/dL and 1.23 mg/dL, each gram of psyllium lowered total- and LDL-C by 1.10 mg/dL and 1.11 mg/dL, each gram of pectin lowered total- and LDL-C by 2.69 mg/dL and 1.96 mg/dL, and each gram of guar gum decreased total- and LDL-C by 1.13 mg/dL and 1.20 mg/dL, respectively. The similar efficacy of different soluble fibers can help achieve current recommendations for dietary fiber.

Stanols/Sterols

Phytosterols, ie, sterols and stanols, are structurally similar to cholesterol (**Fig. 2**). Stanols are saturated sterols and are much less abundant in nature than sterols.[60] Phytosterols are present in small amounts in nuts, seeds, and vegetable oils. More than 40 different phytosterols have been identified,[60] of which β-sitosterol, campesterol, and stigmasterol are the most abundant.[61] Phytosterols lower LDL-C independent of dietary cholesterol intake,[62] and different phytosterols (ie, β-sitosterol versus campesterol) are equally effective in lowering LDL-C.[63]

Numerous studies have shown that phytosterols lower LDL-C in a dose-dependent fashion in amounts up to 2.5 g per day,[64] with an LDL-C lowering effect in both normocholesterolemic and hypercholesterolemic adults.[12] A meta-analysis of 41 trials reported that intake of 2 g per day of phytosterols reduces LDL-C by 10%, and higher intakes confer little additional benefit.[60] The NCEP ATP III recommends 2 g per day of phytosterols to acheive about a 10% reduction in LDL-C.[4,65] The typical daily intake

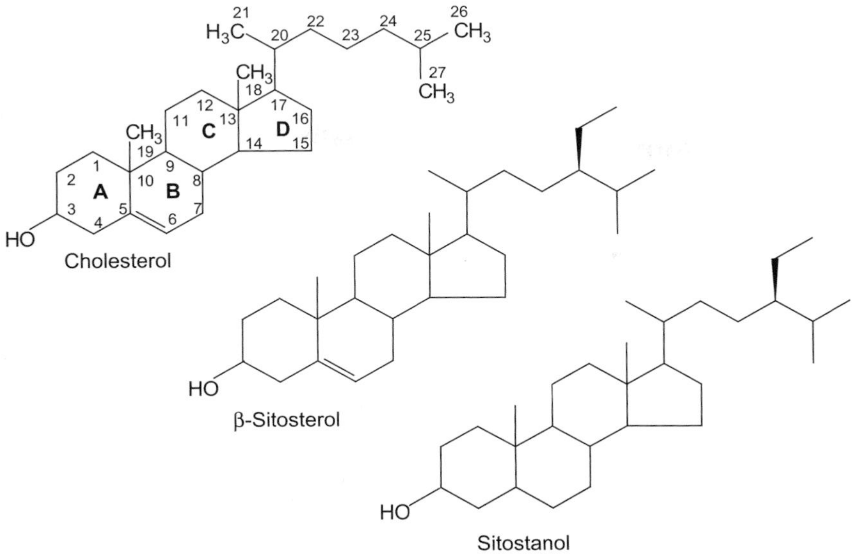

Fig. 2. Structures of sterols. Cholesterol is the sterol of mammalian cells. β-sitosterol is the most common sterol in plants; it differs from cholesterol by having an ethyl group attached at C-24. Hydrogenation of the 5,6 double bond of β-sitosterol converts it into sitostanol. Campesterol and campestanol carry a methyl instead of ethyl group at C-24. (*Reprinted from* Katan MB, Grundy SM, Jones P, et al. Efficacy and safety of plant stanols and sterols in the management of blood cholesterol level. Mayo Clin Proc 2003;78(8):965–78.)

of phytosterols in western cultures ranges from 150 mg per day to 400 mg per day,[60] making supplementation necessary to achieve the recommended intake.

Observational studies have investigated whether there is a relationship between plasma phytosterol levels and CVD risk.[66–69] Most studies have not reported adverse associations. However, in the Prospective Cardiovascular Münster (PROCAM) study, there was a 1.8-fold increased risk of coronary events in subjects with sitosterol levels in the upper quartile compared with the lower three quartiles ($P<.05$).[66] In contrast, in the European Prospective Investigation into Cancer and Nutrition (EPIC)-Norfolk Population study, there was a 21% reduced risk of future CAD in subjects in the highest tertile of sitosterol concentration (ns, non-significant) after adjusting for traditional risk factors.[67] The Longitudinal Aging Study Amsterdam (LASA) study reported that high plasma concentrations of sitosterol were associated with a significant 22% reduced risk of CHD ($P<.05$).[68] In the Dallas Heart Study, there was no relationship between plant sterol levels and family history of CHD or coronary calcium.[69] Long-term randomized clinical trials will be a useful adjunct to the epidemiologic evidence base to learn about the effect of phytosterol supplementation on CVD events.

There are many products on the market that contain phytosterols for total- and LDL-C lowering. These products include orange juice, yogurt, margarine spreads, salad dressings, breads, cereals, milk, and granola bars. Phytosterols also are available in soft-gel pills. A meta-analysis of supplementation studies in familial hypercholesterolemic subjects reported that fat spreads enriched with 2.3 ± 0.5 g phytosterols per day significantly reduced TC by 7% to 11% ($P<.001$) and LDL-C by 10% to 15% ($P<.001$) in 6.5 ± 1.9 weeks compared with control treatment.[70] Other studies using foods fortified with 1.6 to 2.6 g per day of phytosterols have resulted in an LDL-C reduction of 9.4%,[71] 12.4%,[72] 5% to 10%,[73] 9.8%,[74] and 7.8%.[75] The lowest calorie strategy for achieving maximum LDL-C lowering with phytosterols is to use soft-gel capsules that are consumed with a meal that contains fat. Alternatively, other foods including the lite margarines can be incorporated into a low calorie meal to achieve maximum LDL-C lowering.

Phytosterols inhibit cholesterol absorption by displacing cholesterol from mixed micelles.[60] This mechanism of action is different from statin drugs, which inhibit cholesterol synthesis. Consequently, phytosterols can be used in conjunction with statins for greater LDL-C lowering.[76–79] Moreover, this strategy may be more effective for LDL-C lowering than doubling the statin dose.[60] Phytosterols also elicit additional lipid lowering when combined with a heart-healthy diet using other LDL-lowering strategies.[60] Phytosterols are well tolerated, and no adverse effects have been reported.[12] A decrease in blood levels of β-carotene and other carotenoids has been reported following plant sterol consumption,[60] but does not appear to be associated with any adverse outcomes.[80] A diet high in carotenoids (high-carotenoid fruits or vegetables include carrots, pumpkin, apricots, spinach, and broccoli) can prevent this decrease in plasma levels, and is recommended when consuming phytosterols.[12,81]

Soy

Epidemiologic studies have shown that dietary soy is inversely related to TC [82,83] and LDL-C[83] in some Asian populations. More recently, the Shanghai Women's Health Study found that increased consumption of soy foods was associated with a significantly reduced risk of nonfatal myocardial infarction and CHD.[84]

Soy protein is the major component of soybeans and typically accounts for 36% of the total bean. Nutritionally, soy protein is considered to be a complete protein because it provides all essential amino acids. A component of soy protein of interest is isoflavones, which are bioactive molecules that act as phytoestrogens. Isoflavones are present in whole soy foods in inactive forms as glucosides. Metabolism of the glucoside forms of isoflavones produces the biologically active aglycones: genistein, daidzein, and glycitein.[85] The conversion of isoflavones by intestinal flora is an area of scientific interest, as individuals with intestinal capacity to convert daidzein to equol may benefit from its greater biological activity and superior antioxidant activity.[86] The estimated prevalence of equol producers ranges between 30% and 50% of the population.[86,87]

The potential for soy protein to decrease serum cholesterol levels has been studied extensively. An earlier meta-analysis (published in 1995) of 38 controlled trials reported that consumption of soy protein (average 47 g per day) significantly reduced TC (9.3%), LDL-C (12.9%), and TG (10.5%).[88] These changes in TC and LDL-C were a function of initial serum cholesterol concentrations; the greatest reductions were observed in individuals with higher levels at baseline. In 1999, the FDA approved a soy protein health claim that authorized the following label on qualified soy foods: "Diets low in saturated fat and cholesterol that include 25 g of soy protein a day may reduce the risk of heart disease." For a food to qualify for the health claim, the FDA requires that a serving contain at least 6.25 g of soy protein, which is 25% of the recommended daily amount (25 g).[89]

More recent evidence indicates that soy protein is not as effective at reducing LDL-C as initially reported. In a 2005 meta-analysis, Zhan and Ho[90] reported that soy protein with isoflavones (median 80 mg per day isoflavones) reduced TC (3.8%), LDL-C (5.3%), and TG (7.3%), and increased HDL-C (3.0%), with higher intakes of soy isoflavones (> 80 mg per day) eliciting greater effects. In a more recent meta-analysis prepared by the Agency for Health care Research and Quality (AHRQ), Balk and colleagues[91] reported that consumption of soy protein (median intake 36 g) was associated with a modest TC (−5 mg/dL, 2.5%), LDL-C (−5 mg/dL, 3%) and TG (−8 mg/dL, 6%) lowering effect. Similar effects of soy protein on LDL-C were reported by Sacks and colleagues[92] who reviewed 22 randomized trials conducted between 1998 and 2005 as part of an AHA Science Advisory. In this analysis, intake of soy protein (25 to 135 g per day) and isoflavones (40 to 318mg per day) varied considerably among studies; 50 g per day (average intake) of soy protein was associated with a 3% reduction in LDL-C. These effects of soy protein on LDL-C are substantially lower than those reported by Anderson and colleagues[88] in 1995, but are consistent with more recent meta-analyses.

As first reported by Anderson and colleagues[88] and illustrated in **Fig. 3**, baseline LDL-C concentration is an important determinant of the effectiveness of soy protein. Also evident is a dose-response relationship between changes in LDL-C and soy protein intake, but not isoflavone intake. Other factors that may influence the magnitude of changes in LDL-C include the bioavailability of isoflavones, the type and preparation of the soy foods, and the population studied (eg, hypercholesterolemic individuals).[91]

The effect of isoflavones on LDL-C is less clear. Data supporting an independent cholesterol-lowering effect of soy isoflavones are inconsistent, and several meta-analyses have been conducted in an attempt to explain these differences. Wegemans and Trautwein[93] reported that daily consumption of soy protein (average 36 g)

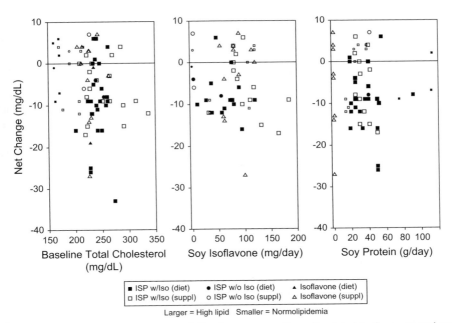

Fig. 3. Change in LDL-C concentration following consumption of isolated isoflavones and soy protein with (ISP w/Iso) or without (ISP w/o Iso) isoflavones, compared with control, by baseline level, isoflavone content, and soy protein content. Suppl, supplement. (*Reprinted from* Balk E, Chung M, Chew P, et al. Effects of soy on health outcomes. Evidence Report/Technology Assessment No. 126. AHRQ Publication No. 05-E024-2. Agency for Health care Research and Quality. August 2005; with permission.)

+ isoflavones (average 52 mg) reduced LDL-C by 6.6 mg/dL (−4%) and increased HDL-C by 1.2 mg/dL (+3%). However the absence of a dose-response relationship between changes in isoflavone concentration and changes in LDL-C and HDL-C suggested that these bioactive compounds had no independent effects on lipids/lipoproteins. In comparison, another meta-analysis showed that high (96 mg per day) intakes of isoflavones were associated with greater reductions (−5.8 mg/dL) in LDL-C than lower (6 mg per day) intakes, with standard amounts of soy protein (50 g per day).[94] This was supported by another recent meta-analysis of 11 studies that showed differential effects of the same amount of soy protein, if it were enriched or depleted of isoflavones.[95] Isoflavone-enriched soy-protein lowered TC by 1.8% and LDL-C by 3.6% compared with isoflavone-depleted soy protein. When compared with animal protein, there is some evidence that soy protein combined with isoflavones work synergistically or additively to lower LDL-C (−4.98% for soy protein + isoflavones versus −2.77% for soy protein without isoflavones). However, both the AHRQ Report[91] and the AHA Science Advisory on Soy Protein[96] concluded that isoflavones have no effect on LDL-C or other lipids.

Although yet to be fully elucidated, there are animal and cell culture data supporting several mechanisms by which soy protein and isoflavones may influence lipids, including modulation of transcription factors and regulation of expression of genes involved in lipid metabolism (reviewed by Torres and colleagues[97] and Xiao and colleagues).[98] For example, soy protein may down-regulate the activity of sterol regulatory element binding protein (SREBP)-1, which leads to a "downstream" reduction in serum and liver TG and LDL-C. However, as discussed previously, these molecular and biochemical changes do not necessarily translate to clinically relevant benefits, particularly at doses likely to be consumed.[95]

In conclusion, recent meta-analyses demonstrate that 30 to 50 g per day of soy protein can reduce LDL-C by 3% to 5%. For individuals trying to achieve this LDL-C lowering effect, the most concentrated sources of soy protein are isolated soy protein powders (typically 80% to 90% protein), soy nuts (40% protein), and full-fat soy flour (35% protein). Other manufactured food products such as protein bars and breakfast patties also are modest sources of soy protein, although the protein in these products is not always exclusively from soy. The following is one example of how to achieve an intake of 50 g per day of soy protein using traditional and nontraditional soy products: one breakfast patty (eg, Morningstar Farms organic soy breakfast patty, 9.8 g protein), an 8-ounce glass of soy milk (7.3 g), 3 ounces of Tofu (6 g), 1 ounce of soy nuts (11 g), and two heaping tablespoons (20 g) of soy protein powder (17 g). It is important to note that some soy protein foods are high in sodium. For example, a 70-g soy burger provides about 400 mg of sodium, and an 85-g vegan soy burger provides approximately 550 mg of sodium.

Weight Loss

Weight loss has favorable affects on TC, LDL-C, HDL-C, and triglycerides.[99] Weight loss of 5% to 10% of body weight results in approximately a 15% reduction in LDL-C, a 20% decrease in triglycerides, and an 8% to 10% increase in HDL-C.[100] Although HDL-C generally decreases during weight loss, HDL-C increases following weight maintenance in proportion to the amount of weight that is lost.[101] The magnitude of decrease in total- and LDL-C, as well as triglycerides, is directly related to the amount of weight loss ($r = 0.89$, 0.90, and 0.83, respectively, all $P < .001$).[102] In contrast, there is a weaker, indirect relationship between HDL-C and weight loss ($r = -0.31$, n.s.) (**Fig. 4**).

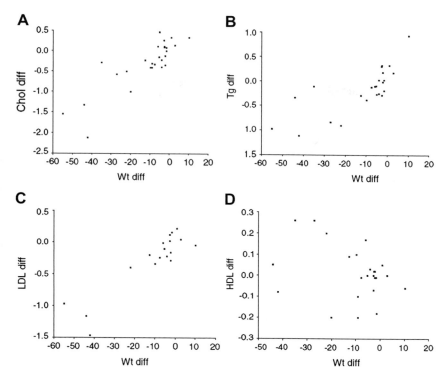

Fig. 4. Mean differences (diff) of weight versus (*A*) cholesterol (Chol), (*B*) triglyceride (Tg), (*C*) low-density lipoprotein (LDL) and (*D*) high-density lipoprotein (HDL). (*Reprinted from Pooblan A, Aucott L, Smith WC, et al. Effects of weight loss in overweight/obese individuals and long-term lipid outcomes—a systematic review. Obes Rev 2004;5(1):43–50; with permission.*)

Weight loss provides health benefits beyond lipid lowering by improving glycemic control, systolic and diastolic blood pressure, inflammation, and fibrinolysis. In addition, sustained weight loss also may increase life expectancy. In a prospective analysis of 43,457 overweight, never-smoking US white women age 40 to 64, intentional weight loss of any amount was associated with a 20% reduction in all-cause mortality, a 40% to 50% reduction in mortality from obesity-related cancers, and a 30% to 40% decrease in diabetes-associated mortality.[103]

Several clinical trials have reported a greater decrease in total and LDL-C cholesterol in men compared with women following a similar amount of weight loss.[104] However, these sex differences are generally accounted for by differences in baseline body weight and lipid levels. Importantly, diet adherence is a strong predictor of weight loss.[105] Therefore, it is important to individualize weight loss advice to match patient food preferences and lifestyle to achieve weight loss that can be sustained in the long term.[105]

DIETARY PATTERNS THAT LOWER LOW-DENSITY LIPOPROTEIN-CHOLESTEROL
Therapeutic Lifestyle Change Diet

The NCEP ATP III guidelines recommend the Therapeutic Lifestyle Change (TLC) diet with therapeutic options for maximal LDL-C lowering (**Table 3**).[4] The estimated

Table 3
Components of a Therapeutic Lifestyle Changes diet

Component	Recommendation
LDL-raising nutrients	—
Saturated fat[a]	Less than 7% of total calories
Dietary cholesterol	Less than 200 mg/d
Therapeutic options for LDL lowering	—
Plant stanols/sterols	2 g/d
Increased viscous (soluble) fiber	10–25 g/d
Total calories (energy)	Adjust total caloric intake to maintain desirable body weight/prevent weight gain
Physical activity	Include enough moderate exercise to expend at least 200 kcal/d

Abbreviation: LDL, low-density lipoprotein.
    [a] *Trans* fatty acids are another LDL-raising fat that should be kept at a low intake.
    Reprinted from Third Report of the National Cholesterol Education Program (NCEP) Expert Panel on Detection, Evaluation, and Treatment of High Blood Cholesterol in Adults (Adult Treatment Panel III) final report. Circulation 2002;106(25):3143–421; with permission.

reduction in LDL-C for the TLC diet is shown in **Table 4**. Lichtenstein and colleagues[106] evaluated the effects of the TLC diet (15% protein, 58% carbohydrate, 30% fat) versus a typical Western diet (15% protein, 47% carbohydrate, 38% fat) on lipids and lipoproteins in a controlled setting. Thirty-six participants with LDL-C higher than 130 mg/dL and not taking lipid-lowering medications were studied. The Western diet was higher in saturated fat (16% versus 7%) and monounsaturated fat (16% versus 10%) and lower in polyunsaturated fat (6% versus 10%). The TLC diet decreased LDL-C and HDL-C by 11% and 7%, respectively, over 32 days versus the Western diet. There were no significant changes in TG or the TC:HDL-C ratio. In another study, by Welty and colleagues,[107] combining the TLC diet with aerobic exercise (30 to 60 minutes three to six times per week) for 6 months resulted in a 9.3% reduction in LDL-C ($P = .02$), an 18.8% reduction in triglycerides ($P<.05$), and

Table 4
Approximate and cumulative LDL-C reduction achievable by dietary modification

Dietary Component	Dietary Change	Approximate LDL-C Reduction
Major		
Saturated fat	<7% of calories	8%–10%
Dietary cholesterol	<200 mg/d	3%–5%
Weight reduction	Lose 10 lbs	5%–8%
Other LDL-lowering options		
Viscous fiber	5–10 g/d	3%–5%
Plant sterol/stanol esters	2 g/d	6%–15%
Cumulative estimate		20%–30%

Abbreviation: LDL-C, low-density lipoprotein cholesterol.
    Reprinted from Third Report of the National Cholesterol Education Program (NCEP) Expert Panel on Detection, Evaluation, and Treatment of High Blood Cholesterol in Adults (Adult Treatment Panel III) final report. Circulation 2002;106(25):3143–421; with permission.

a 2.6% increase in HDL-C (ns). In this study, physical activity beneficially affected HDL-C and TG in subjects on a TLC diet.

Portfolio Diet

The Portfolio Diet is a plant-based TLC diet that is low in saturated fat (< 7% of calories) and cholesterol (< 200 mg per day) with four LDL-C lowering components: viscous fiber (9.8 g/1000 calories), soy and other vegetable proteins (21.4 g/1000 calories), plant sterols (1.0 g/1000 calories), and almonds (14 g/1000 calories).[108] A 35% reduction in LDL-C was predicted in response to the portfolio diet, which is similar to the reduction attainable with statin drugs.[108]

In three randomized clinical trials of the Portfolio Diet, all meals were provided to hypercholesterolemic adults (LDL-C >158 mg/dL); the portfolio diet reduced LDL-C by 29% to 35% in 4 weeks versus an 8% to 12% reduction in the control group on a traditional diet low in saturated fat and cholesterol (ATP III).[109–111] The LDL-C lowering effect with the Portfolio Diet was comparable to the 31% reduction in LDL-C in participants who followed the low saturated fat and cholesterol diet with statin treatment (ie, 20 mg per day lovastatin).[110] Participants on the portfolio diet also had a 28% reduction in C-reactive protein, which also was comparable to the effect seen with statin treatment (−33%),[110] suggesting a similar reduction in CVD risk.

In a recent study, the efficacy of the Portfolio Diet was tested in a free-living setting with subjects on self-selected diets for 1 year.[112] LDL-C decreased 14.0% ± 1.6% at 3 months, which was maintained at 1 year (−12.8% ± 2.0%). Although the overall reduction in LDL-C at 3 months was significantly less than in previous studies where meals were provided, 32% of participants achieved LDL-C reductions greater than 20% after 1 year. Adherence to the diet was significantly correlated with the change in LDL-C ($r = -0.42$, $P<.001$). There also was a significant increase in HDL-C (3%) and a decrease in TG (−14%) and the TC:HDL-C (−13%) and LDL-C:HDL-C (−15%) ratios after 1 year compared with baseline.[112] This study demonstrates that the Portfolio Diet is one effective means for achieving a long-term reduction in LDL-C using diet in a free-living setting, especially for individuals who are able to adhere to this dietary pattern.

Very Low Fat Diet

Very low fat diets (VLFD) contain 15% or less fat and are effective in lowering total- and LDL-C.[113] A VLFD diet frequently is accompanied by weight loss because of a reduced energy-density of the diet resulting in a negative calorie balance. Decreasing the fat content of the diet from 35% to 40% of energy to 15% to 20% of energy reduces total- and LDL-C by 10% to 20%, which reflects a decrease in saturated fat intake.[113] There is an increase in TG and decrease in HDL-C following short-term consumption of a VLFD, regardless of whether the diet is high in simple or complex carbohydrates.[113] These changes may be attenuated by a high fiber intake or weight loss.

The Ornish Lifestyle Heart Trial reported that a VLFD, when combined with other lifestyle changes, also reduces cardiac event rates and induces regression of atherosclerosis.[114] In this study, 48 patients with moderate to severe CHD were randomized to receive intensive lifestyle changes or usual care. The intensive lifestyle changes included a vegetarian diet with 7% of calories from total fat, moderate aerobic exercise, stress management training, smoking cessation, and group psychosocial support. In the intensive lifestyle group, LDL-C decreased 40% at 1 year and remained 20% below baseline at 5 years. In the control group, LDL-C decreased by 1.2% at 1 year and by 19.3% at 5 years. The similar results between groups after 5 years likely reflects the fact that 9 (60%) of 15 of the control patients took lipid-lowering medications between year 1 and year 5 of the study. Overall, 82% of the experimental group experienced lesion regression; the average percent diameter stenosis decreased 3% in the intervention group, whereas the control group showed an 11% increase. At 5 years there also was a 60% decrease in relative risk in cardiac events in the intervention group. Likewise, Esselstyn and colleagues[115,116] reported disease arrest (measured by angiographic analysis) in all patients (n = 11) with severe CAD who followed a plant-based diet containing less than 10% fat after 5 years. In addition, the investigators reported regression in 8 (73%) adherent patients and no extension of clinical disease or coronary events after 12 years.

The Multisite Cardiac Lifestyle Intervention Program is a comprehensive lifestyle intervention program administered by insurance companies.[117] Participants in an initial report were 869 nonsmoking CHD patients who attended an onsite program two times per week for 3 months for a total of 104 hours. Participants received diet instruction on a very low fat (10% of energy), plant-based, whole foods diet high in complex carbohydrates and low in simple sugars. They also were provided with demonstrations (eg, cooking), supervised exercise, stress management, and group support. Over a 3-month period, LDL-C decreased approximately 15%, and reduced dietary fat intake was the only predictor of improvement in LDL-C ($P<.001$). Improvements in weight, TC, TG, exercise capacity, and hemoglobin A1c also were reported. In 108 patients reporting mild angina and 174 reporting limiting angina at baseline, 74% of these patients were angina free by 12 weeks, and an additional 9% moved from limiting to mild angina.[118]

Clinical trial evidence indicates that a VLFD is effective in reducing total- and LDL-C in the short and long term. Although shown to be effective for reducing total and LDL-C, food and nutrient intake should be monitored in certain population subgroups following a VLFD including growing children, pregnant and lactating women, and the elderly because of the relatively high nutrient and calorie needs for some individuals.[113] More information about a very low fat diet and the Lifestyle Heart Program can be found at www.ornish.com.

DIET AND LIFESTYLE COMPONENTS THAT LOWER TRIGLYCERIDES AND RAISE HIGH-DENSITY LIPOPROTEIN-CHOLESTEROL
Omega 3 Fatty Acids

Omega-3 (n-3) fatty acids are polyunsaturated fatty acids of marine (primarily eicosapentaenoic acid [EPA] and docosahexaenoic acid [DHA]) and plant (principally alpha-linolenic acid [ALA]) origin. Direct sources of EPA and DHA are fatty fish, fish oil, fortified foods, and more recently, DHA-rich algal oil supplements. EPA, and to some extent DHA, also can be derived from ALA. ALA is an essential fatty acid because it cannot be synthesized by humans and therefore must be consumed in the diet. Major dietary sources of ALA are vegetable oils, nuts, and seeds, with particularly high levels found in flaxseed. Other sources of ALA include canola and soybean oils, and walnuts.

ALA is the precursor to the n-3 fatty acid family and through a series of elongation and desaturation steps can be converted to EPA and DHA. However, this biochemical pathway is relatively inefficient, with low conversion of dietary ALA to EPA, and especially DHA.[119–121] Metabolic conversion studies in humans estimate that 5% of ALA is converted to EPA and 0.5% to DHA.[122] Nonetheless, there is some epidemiologic evidence of ALA having a benefit on CHD risk.[123,124] The evidence to date suggests that ALA beneficially affects CVD risk via nonlipid and lipoprotein risk factors.[125]

The Institute of Medicine of the National Academies recommends 0.6% to 1.2% of total energy from ALA (up to 10% of which can be from EPA + DHA). The lower boundary of this range meets the adequate intake for ALA. The upper boundary corresponds to the highest intakes from foods consumed by individuals in the United States and Canada. The inclusion of 1 to 2 teaspoons per day of flaxseed oil or 1 tablespoon per day of ground flaxseed meets the current recommendations for ALA. Additionally, 500 mg per day EPA + DHA is recommended for CVD risk reduction, which is equivalent to 8 ounces or 2 servings (4 ounces) of fatty fish per week.

Numerous epidemiologic studies have demonstrated that intake of fish and marine-derived n-3 fatty acids, specifically EPA and DHA, is associated with a reduced risk of fatal and nonfatal CV events.[126–131] Further evidence for a cardioprotective effect of n-3 fatty acids is provided by two secondary prevention intervention studies: the Diet and Reinfarction Trial (DART) and the Gruppo Italiano per lo Studio della Sopravvivenza nell'Infarto Miocardico (GISSI)-Prevenzione Study.[132,133] The DART trial demonstrated a 29% reduction in 2-year all-cause mortality in recovered myocardial infarction (MI) patients advised to increase their intake of fatty fish to two servings per week.[132] After 2 years, intake of EPA had increased fourfold and averaged 2.4 g per week, compared with 0.6 g per week in the control group. The GISSI Prevenzione Study was designed to investigate the independent and combined effects of fish oil and vitamin E (300 mg per day) on morbidity and mortality after a heart attack[133] Patients supplemented with 1 g per day of fish oil (0.85 to 0.88 mg EPA + DHA) had a 20% reduction in risk of overall mortality, a 30% reduction in risk of mortality from CVD, and 47% decrease in risk of sudden death.[134] In the GISSI Prevenzione Study there was no benefit of vitamin E supplementation. More recently, the Japan EPA Lipid Intervention Study (JELIS) reported that combined statin + EPA treatment (1.8 g per day) in patients with existing CAD significantly reduced major coronary events (19%) and the incidence of unstable angina (28%) compared with statin-only controls.[135] These cardioprotective benefits largely have been attributed to the antiarrhythmic effects of EPA and DHA, but also relate to improvements in other CV risk factors.

When considering effects on lipids and lipoproteins, marine-derived n-3 fatty acids are known for their hypotriglyceridemic effects. A comprehensive review by Harris[136] summarized the results of placebo-controlled trials administering less than 7 g per day of n-3 fatty acids (EPA + DHA) from fish oil in individuals with normal (TG < 177 mg/dL) and elevated (TG ≥ 177 mg/dL) TG. Omega-3 fatty acid supplementation (from fish oil) consistently lowered TG in both populations; approximately 4 g per day of EPA + DHA decreased serum TG by 25% to 30%. Furthermore, other studies conducted during this time showed that fish oil lowers TG in a dose-dependent manner (**Fig. 5**),[137] with the greatest reductions in TG occurring in individuals with higher TG levels at baseline.[138] The results from these early studies are supported by data from numerous clinical trials. In a systematic analysis of 21 studies, Balk and colleagues[139] reported an average reduction in TG of 15% with n-3 fatty acid supplementation from fish oil (0.045 to 5.9 g per day EPA + DHA). A dose-dependent relationship also was apparent; every 1 g per day increase in fish oil (EPA + DHA not reported) resulted in an 8 mg/dL reduction in TG.

In comparison to their effects on TG, the extent to which marine-derived n-3 fatty acids induce clinically significant changes in LDL-C and HDL-C is still under question. Generally, fish oil supplementation is associated with small increases in LDL-C and HDL-C.[136] This LDL-C and HDL-C response typically is seen in response to high doses of marine-derived n-3 fatty acids that are used to treat hypertriglyceridemia. Harris[136] reported that daily supplementation with approximately 4 g per day n-3 fatty acids (EPA + DHA) was associated with a 5% to 10% increase in LDL-C and a 1% to 3% increase in HDL-C. The observed increase in LDL-C was greater in

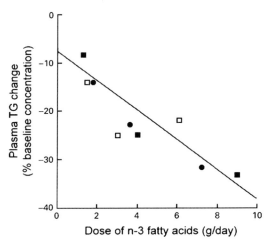

Fig. 5. Dose-dependent hypotriglyceridemic effect of omega-3 fatty acids. □, Blonk et al. (1990); ●, Sanders et al. (1983); ■, Schmidt et al. (1990). TG, triglycerides. Regression equation: $y = -7\cdot67 - 3\cdot05x$; R^2 0·87. (*Reprinted from* Roche HM. Unsaturated fatty acids. Proc Nutr Soc 1999;58(2):397–401; with permission.)

hypertriglyceridemic patients (TG ≥ 177 mg/dL), and in those with the greatest TG-lowering response. Similarly, Balk and colleagues[139] concluded that n-3 fatty acids from fish oil (0.045 to 5.9 g per day EPA + DHA) increased HDL-C and LDL-C by 1.6 mg/dL and 6 mg/dL, respectively. In a meta-analysis of 27 studies, Robinson and Stone[140] summarized and updated the findings of an AHRQ commissioned review of the CV effects of n-3 fatty acids. They reported a 10 mg/dL net increase in LDL-C, with smaller changes in HDL-C (3 to 5 mg/dL), following supplementation with n-3 fatty acids from fish oil (0.045 to 5.4 g per day EPA + DHA). It has been suggested that the increase in LDL-C with fish oil supplementation is because of an increase in LDL-C particle size,[141,142] although not all studies have reported such an effect.[143] Although marine-derived n-3 fatty acids have modest effects on total HDL-C, there is some evidence that they also alter HDL subfractions toward a more favorable, cardioprotective profile (increased HDL-2, decreased HDL-3).[141,144]

Monounsaturated Fatty Acids

There is evidence from both epidemiologic and clinical studies that dietary monounsaturated fatty acids (MUFA) have a protective effect on CVD risk. Compared with saturated fats, MUFA have a small total- and LDL-C lowering effect, and relative to carbohydrate, they increase HDL-C and decrease TG.[145] In a study by Kris-Etherton and colleagues[146] comparing high-MUFA diets (34% to 36% fat, 17% to 21% MUFA) with a low-fat, Step 2 diet (25% fat, 12% MUFA) and an average American diet (AAD) (34% fat, 11% MUFA), TG were 13% lower in subjects consuming the high-MUFA diets compared with the AAD. In contrast, TG were 11% higher following the low-fat, Step 2 diet compared with the AAD. The high-MUFA diet did not lower HDL-C compared with the AAD, whereas the low-fat diet lowered HDL-C by 4%. Both the high-MUFA diets and low-fat Step 2 diet lowered LDL-C by 10% to 15%. Likewise, a recent study by Berglund and colleagues[147] compared an AAD (36% fat) with two diets in which 7% of energy from SFA was replaced with either carbohydrate (CHO) or MUFA. Relative to the AAD, LDL-C decreased similarly after the CHO

(−7.0%) and MUFA (−6.3%) diets. However, the decrease in HDL-C was less during the MUFA diet (−4.3%) versus the CHO diet (−7.2%) (P<.01) In addition, TG were not affected by the MUFA diet compared with the AAD; however, compared with the AAD and the MUFA diet, they were higher on the CHO diet (7.4% and 12%, respectively, P<.01 for both).

These reports that MUFA are more effective than carbohydrates at maintaining HDL-C and lowering TG are consistent with other studies comparing a low-fat versus a moderate-fat diet. A 2008 meta-analysis by Cao and colleagues[148] of 30 controlled feeding studies reported that moderate-fat (MF) and low-fat (LF) blood cholesterol–lowering diets decreased LDL-C similarly. However, although both blood cholesterol–lowering diets decreased HDL-C, the MF diet decreased HDL-C less than the LF diet (difference 2.28 mg/dL, 95% CI 1.66, 2.90, P<.001). The MF diet decreased TG versus the LF diet (−9.36 mg/dL, 95% CI −12.26, −6.08, P<.001 for MF versus LF).

The OmniHeart study compared a diet high in MUFA (37% fat, 21% MUFA) with a carbohydrate-rich (58% carbohydrate, 27% fat, 13% MUFA) and protein-rich (25% protein, 27% fat, 13% MUFA) diet in a randomized, crossover design. HDL-C significantly decreased on the high-carbohydrate and high-protein blood cholesterol–lowering diets (−1.4, and −2.6 mg/dL), but not on the high-MUFA diet (−0.3 mg/dL). In addition, TG significantly decreased following the high-MUFA and high-protein diets (−9.3 and −16.4 mg/dL), but not on the high-carbohydrate diet (+0.1 mg/dL). LDL-C decreased similarly on all three blood cholesterol-lowering diets (−13.1, −14.2 mg/dL, and −11.6, respectively).

Although human studies have reported a favorable effect of MUFA on the lipid profile, a primate study has demonstrated an adverse effect of MUFA on atherosclerosis progression.[149] In this report by Rudel and colleagues,[149] monkeys fed MUFA developed equivalent amounts of coronary artery atherosclerosis (measured by intimal area) as those fed saturated fat, whereas coronary artery atherosclerosis was less in monkeys fed polyunsaturated fat. Further human studies with long-term CVD end points are needed to conclusively determine the effect of MUFA on CVD risk. Long-term studies of a Mediterranean diet, which is high in MUFA and described later in this article, suggests there is, in fact, a favorable effect of a dietary pattern that emphasizes a high-MUFA vegetable oil (ie, olive oil).

Physical Activity

Several notable studies provided early evidence for an association between increased physical activity and reduced total mortality.[150,151] Since then, epidemiologic studies have sought to clarify the relationship between physical activity and CHD, and have confirmed a reduced risk of overall and/or CVD mortality in physically active compared with sedentary individuals.[152,153] The Framingham Study provides additional support for the prevention of CVD and an increase in life expectancy in physically active individuals.[154] In this longitudinal study, data collected over 12 years of follow-up showed that men and women in the highest tertile for physical activity had 3.7 and 3.5 years more total life expectancy, respectively, than those with a low physical activity level. Furthermore, men who had a high level of physical activity lived 3.2 more years without CV disease and women 3.3 more years than those in the lowest tertile. More objective measures of physical activity, ie, physical or cardiorespiratory fitness (CRF), also are associated with a reduced incidence of all-cause and CVD mortality.[155–157] An increase in energy expenditure of 1000 kcal per week (equivalent to 30 minutes of moderate-intensity walking on most days of the week) is associated with a 20% to 30% reduction in risk of all-cause mortality.[158] It is probable that this risk reduction is influenced by improvements in CVD risk factors, including plasma lipids and lipoproteins.

The effects of regular aerobic exercise training on lipids and lipoproteins have been reviewed in several meta-analyses.[159–162] Carroll and Dudfield[159] reported that regular aerobic exercise was effective in reducing TG (−18.7 mg/dL, −12%) and increasing HDL-C (1.6 mg/dL, +4.1%) in overweight and obese, sedentary adults with dyslipidemia. Although not clinically significant, exercise was associated with a small reduction in body weight (range −1.5 to 1.9 kg). Similar changes in HDL-C (+4.6%) were reported by Leon and Sanchez,[162] primarily because of an increase in HDL-2. However, they noted that the effect of regular exercise on other parameters such as TG, total- and LDL-C, and body weight was far less consistent and induced only modest improvements (−3.7%, −1.0% (ns), −5.0%, and −0.82 kg, respectively). A meta-analysis by Kelley and colleagues[161] concluded that regular aerobic exercise was effective in reducing TG (−11%) and TC (−2%), but had no significant effects on LDL-C or HDL-C in previously sedentary, overweight, and obese adults. Exercise training was associated with a small reduction in body weight (−1.6 kg).

Interestingly, there is evidence that regular moderate exercise changes LDL-C particle size without any change in total LDL-C concentration.[163] Other reviews have suggested that changes in lipids are dependent on training volume, which can be determined by the number calories expended during physical activity. Durstine and colleagues[160] reported that a regular training program with a minimum expenditure of 1200 kcal per week reduces TG by 4% to 22% and increases HDL-C by 4% to 37%, but has limited effects on LDL-C and TC. Kodama and colleagues[164] recently reported that a minimum energy expenditure of 900 kcal per week (or 120 min/wk) from physical activity was required to elicit changes in HDL-C. For energy expended above this threshold, there existed a dose-response relationship; every 10-minute prolongation of exercise per session (ie, above 120 min/wk) was associated with a 1.4-mg/dL increase in HDL-C.

Although variable, these reviews indicate that regular aerobic exercise can induce favorable changes in TG and HDL-C, but is less effective in lowering total- and LDL-C. Without concomitant energy restriction, exercise training produces only small changes in body weight (generally 1 to 2 kg), and therefore the associated improvements in TG and HDL-C are relatively independent of weight loss. Regular physical activity is recognized by the AHA as an effective therapeutic strategy for the management of abnormal blood lipids, particularly for reducing TG and increasing HDL-C.[165] The exercise-induced improvements in TG and HDL-C are likely mediated by changes in the activity of lipoprotein lipase (LPL), which is increased following aerobic exercise.[166] Interestingly, there is emerging evidence that LPL also is strongly influenced by inactivity. Studies have shown that reducing normal spontaneous standing and ambulatory time (ie, increased sitting) suppresses LPL activity more than it is increased by a bout of vigorous exercise (reviewed by Hamilton and colleagues).[167] With this in mind, individuals aiming to improve their TG and HDL-C levels should increase their participation in regular structured physical activity and reduce their time spent in sedentary activities. The recently updated physical activity guidelines from the AHA and American College of Sports Medicine[168] recommend that adults spend a minimum of 30 minutes, 5 days per week engaged in moderate aerobic activity, or 20 minutes, 3 days per week in vigorous aerobic activity (a combination of the two is also acceptable) to promote and maintain health. Such aerobic activity is in addition to other light physical tasks such as household chores, gardening, and activities lasting less than 10 minutes. Individuals also are advised to perform muscle strength and endurance activities on 2 days per week.

Alcohol

Population and cohort studies have reported an inverse relationship between daily consumption of one to two alcoholic beverages and CVD risk.[169–171] One mechanism by which alcohol reduces CVD risk is by lowering fibrinogen levels and increasing protein tissue type plasminogen activator, thereby decreasing blood clot formation.[172] In addition, moderate alcohol consumption (one to two drinks per day) is associated with higher levels of HDL–C.[173] The AHA defines a drink as 12 ounces of beer, 4 ounces of wine, 1.5 ounces of 80-proof spirits, or 1 ounce of 100-proof spirits.[1] The Dietary Guidelines for Americans, 2005 similarly defines alcoholic beverages, however, a serving of wine is defined as 5 ounces.[2] A meta-analysis of 26 retrospective and prospective observational studies reported a lower risk of CVD for wine and beer drinkers who consume one to two alcoholic beverages daily.[174] The RR for wine drinkers was 0.68 (95% CI 0.59–0.77) and 0.78 (95% CI 0.70–0.86) for beer drinkers compared with nondrinkers.

A cross-sectional analysis of data from the Third National Health and Nutrition Examination Survey (NHANES III) evaluated the relationship between alcohol consumption and the prevalence of the metabolic syndrome and its components in the US population.[175] This analysis was performed on 8125 men and women age 20 or older, of which 22% met the NCEP criteria for metabolic syndrome. After adjusting for age, sex, race/ethnicity, education, income, tobacco use, physical activity, and diet, a lower prevalence of metabolic syndrome was observed with mild to moderate alcohol consumption, as was more favorable lipid levels, waist circumference, and fasting insulin (**Table 5**).

Randomized clinical trials consistently have demonstrated an HDL-raising effect of alcohol. In a randomized crossover study performed by Baer and colleagues,[176] 51 postmenopausal women were given a controlled diet with zero, one (15 g), or two (30 g) alcoholic drinks per day for 8 weeks. The alcohol, Everclear, was provided with orange juice and participants were instructed to consume their beverage with their evening snack. When compared with the control diet, the alcohol-consuming

Table 5
Multivariate adjusted odds ratio for the prevalence of metabolic syndrome and selected components in 8125 subjects from NHANES III stratified by increasing quantities of alcohol consumption

<1 Alcoholic Drink/d	< Alcoholic Drink/d	1–19 Alcoholic Drinks/Month	≥20 Alcoholic Drinks/Month
Metabolic syndrome[a]	1.0	0.65 (0.54–0.79)	0.34 (0.26–0.47)
Low serum HDL-C[b]	1.0	0.69 (0.60–0.78)	0.22 (0.16–0.29)
Elevated triglycerides[c]	1.0	0.73 (0.62–0.87)	0.56 (0.43–0.74)
Increased waist circumference[d]	1.0	0.74 (0.62–0.89)	0.41 (0.32–0.52)
Elevated fasting insulin[e]	1.0	0.64 (0.46–0.88)	0.39 (0.24–0.62)

Abbreviations: HDL-C, high-density lipoprotein-cholesterol; NHANES III, Third National Health and Nutrition Examination Survey.
[a] Meet at least three of five National Cholesterol Education Program Adult Treatment Panel III criteria for metabolic syndrome.
[b] Men < 40 mg/dL, Women < 50 mg/dL.
[c] Triglycerides ≥ 150 mg/dL.
[d] Men >102 cm, Women >88 cm.
[e] Fasting serum insulin ≥ 90th percentile (116 pmol/L).
Data from Freiberg MS, Cabral HJ, Heeren TC, et al. Alcohol consumption and the prevalence of the metabolic syndrome in the US: a cross-sectional analysis of data from the Third National Health and Nutrition Examination Survey. Diabetes Care 2004;27(12):2954–9.

groups exhibited a small decrease in triglycerides (−6% to −10%) and LDL-C (−3% to −5%). In addition, HDL-C increased with increasing alcohol consumption: mean HDL-C levels were 54.1 mg/dL with no alcohol intake, 55.3 mg/dL (2.1% increase, ns) with one drink per day, and 57.2 mg/dL (5.7% increase, P = .02) with two drinks per day (P<.05). Likewise, in a study by Naissides and colleagues,[177] consumption of red wine for 4 weeks decreased LDL-C by 8% and increased HDL-C by 17%, whereas there were no significant changes in the control group. Hansen and colleagues[178] randomized 69 men and women to one of four groups: (1) red wine (males 300 mL per day, females 200 mL per day), (2) water + red grape extract tablets (wine-equivalent dose), (3) water + red grape extract tablets (half dose), or (4) water + placebo tablets for a period of 4 weeks. An increase in HDL-C (+6%) was observed only in the red wine group. Finally, Sierksma and colleagues[179] conducted a randomized crossover study with 18 healthy postmenopausal women. The study participants consumed 24 g of white wine or white grape juice daily for 3 weeks, resulting in a 5% increase in HDL-C in the white wine group (P<.05).

In summary, multiple studies have demonstrated a beneficial influence of alcohol on HDL-C and CVD risk. As a result, the AHA supports moderate alcohol consumption (one to two drinks per day for men and one drink per day for women) in persons who routinely consume alcohol responsibly. However, the AHA acknowledges that drinking larger quantities of alcohol increases the risk of alcoholism, high blood pressure, obesity, stroke, breast cancer, suicide, and accidents, and cautions people not to start drinking if they do not already drink alcohol.

DIETARY PATTERNS THAT LOWER TRIGLYCERIDES AND RAISE HIGH-DENSITY LIPOPROTEIN-CHOLESTEROL
Very Low Carbohydrate Diet

Some scientists have begun advocating a very low carbohydrate diet (VLCD) for treatment of dyslipidemia because it is effective in lowering TG and raising HDL-C (**Fig. 6**).[180] In contrast, a low-fat, high-carbohydrate diet tends to raise TG and lower HDL-C. There generally is a small decrease or no change in total- or LDL-C following a VLCD; however, there is a shift in the distribution of LDL particle size resulting in a decreased number of atherogenic small, dense LDL particles, and an increase in the number of large, buoyant LDL particles,[181–183] which are considered to be less atherogenic.

A VLCD generally provides 50 g or less per day of carbohydrate or has less than 10% of total energy from carbohydrate.[184] The consumption of protein and fat is thus increased in a VLCD to compensate for the limited amount of carbohydrate. This results in an average intake of 60% to 65% of calories from fat and 20% to 25% of calories from protein.[184] Food choices compatible with this level of carbohydrate intake include vegetables, beef, poultry, fish, oils, nuts, seeds, and cheese. Despite a high intake of dietary fat on a VLCD, there are few reported adverse effects on lipid levels.[181,185,186] The adverse effects that have been reported for VLCDs in the short term (1 year) include constipation, headaches, muscle cramps, diarrhea, weakness, and skin rash.[180] In addition, a VLCD limits fruits, whole grains, and skim milk dairy products, all of which provide important nutrients, and are specific food groups recommended in the Dietary Guidelines for Americans, 2005.[2]

Following a VLCD typically leads to a reduced calorie intake because of appetite suppression and hunger reduction that is the result of the satiating effects of protein and/or ketosis from the high intake of fat.[180] In clinical trials, a VLCD consistently results in a greater amount of weight loss than a low-fat diet over 6 months,[187–191]

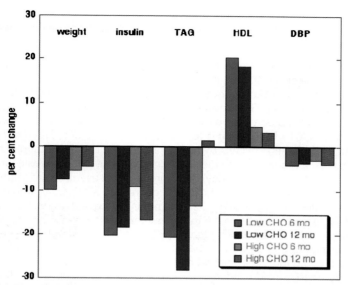

Fig. 6. Comparison of features of metabolic syndrome on low-carbohydrate versus high-carbohydrate diets. TAG, triglycerides; DBP, diastolic blood pressure. (*Reprinted from* Volek JS, Feinman RD. Carbohydrate restriction improves the features of metabolic syndrome. Metabolic syndrome may be defined by the response to carbohydrate restriction. Nutr Metab (Lond) 2005;2:31; with permission.)

but at 12 months weight loss is similar.[187,189,192] A decrease in TG and increase in HDL-C also is reported with a VLCD in the absence of weight loss.[193]

In summary, a VLCD diet appears to be as effective in reducing body weight over the long term (ie, 1 year) as a low-fat diet. With respect to effects on the lipid profile, a VLCD diet appears to confer benefits on TG lowering. However, achieving nutrient adequacy via food-based dietary recommendations is not possible for a VLCD because of limitations in foods allowed (eg, milk, fruits, and whole grains). Thus, long-term safety studies of this dietary pattern are needed before recommendations can be made.

Mediterranean Diet

There are many countries in the Mediterranean region that have distinct dietary patterns. Nonetheless, there are a number of similar characteristics of diets in this region. The Mediterranean diet is associated with a low incidence of CHD, which is attributed in part to a high consumption of MUFA (primarily from olive oil) and low consumption of saturated fat. The International Conference on the Diet of the Mediterranean summarized the key dietary components in 1993. They are:

1. An abundance of plant foods (eg, fruits, vegetables, potatoes, breads, grains, beans, nuts, and seeds)
2. Minimally processed and, whenever possible, seasonally fresh foods
3. Fresh fruits as the typical daily dessert
4. Olive oil as the principal source of dietary fat
5. Dairy, poultry, and fish in low to moderate amounts
6. Less than five eggs per week

7. Red meat in low frequency and amounts
8. Wine in low to moderate amounts (one to two glasses per day for men and one glass per day for women)

The Mediterranean diet, being largely plant based, also includes a high intake of fiber and phytosterols (~400 mg per day).[64,194]

The Mediterranean diet is effective in reducing triglycerides and increasing HDL-C in randomized clinical trials. The Prevención con Dieta Mediterránea (PREDIMED) study is a large (n = 9000) randomized, clinical trial that is being conducted in Spain and will be completed in 2010.[195] The aim is to evaluate the effects of the Mediterranean diet on the primary prevention of CVD by comparing three diets: a low-fat diet that meets AHA Guidelines, a Mediterranean diet with virgin olive oil (1 L per week), and a Mediterranean diet with nuts (30 g per day). A subgroup of 772 asymptomatic subjects ages 55 to 80 were followed for 3 months. LDL-C decreased significantly in both Mediterranean diet groups (−3.8 to −5.8 mg/dL) but not in the low-fat group. Both Mediterranean diets increased HDL-C relative to the low-fat diet (1.6 to 2.5 mg/dL, $P<.001$). In addition, triglycerides decreased significantly in the Mediterranean diet with nuts group (−7.6 mg/dL) compared with baseline, but not in the Mediterranean diet with virgin olive oil (−3.0 mg/dL) or low-fat diet (+2.4 mg/dL) groups.

In a randomized, single-blind trial by Esposito and colleagues,[196] 180 men and women with metabolic syndrome were randomized to a control or Mediterranean style diet for 2 years. The intervention group received detailed advice about how to increase daily consumption of whole grains, fruits, vegetables, nuts, and olive oil; the control group followed a prudent diet (50% to 60% carbohydrate; 15% to 20% proteins, < 30% fat). Compared with the control group, the Mediterranean diet group had a significant decrease in triglycerides (−19 mg/dL; 95% CI −6 to −32; $P = .001$) and a significant increase in HDL-C (3 mg/dL; 95% CI 0.8 to 5.2; $P = .03$).

The benefits of the Mediterranean diet go beyond its effects on HDL-C and triglycerides, as it has also been shown to reduce inflammatory markers and body weight, and improve endothelial function.[196–198] In addition, the Lyon Diet Heart Study reported a dramatic decrease in recurrent heart disease in patients following a Mediterranean diet. The Lyon Diet Heart Study was a randomized, controlled trial in which patients who survived a first myocardial infarction were randomized to a Mediterranean-style diet (30% fat, high in alpha-linolenic acid, 13% MUFA, 8% SFA) or

Table 6
Examples of daily dietary patterns consistent with AHA-recommended dietary goals at 2000 calories[1]

Eating Pattern	DASH	TLC
Grains	6–8 sv/d	7 sv/d
Vegetables	4–5 sv/d	5 sv/d
Fruits	4–5 sv/d	4 sv/d
Fat-free or low-fat dairy products	2–3 sv/d	2–3 sv/d
Lean meats, poultry and fish	<6oz./d	≤5 oz./d
Nuts, seeds, legumes	4–5 sv/wk	Counted in vegetable servings
Fats and oils	2–3 sv/d	Amount depends on calorie level
Sweets and added sugars	5 or less sv/wk	No recommendation

Abbreviations: AHA, American Heart Association; DASH, dietary approaches to stop hypertension; TLC, Therapeutic Lifestyle Changes; sv, serving.

a prudent Western diet for an average of 46 months.[125] Subjects following the Mediterranean-style diet had a 50% to 70% lower risk of recurrent heart disease, despite no change in lipids and lipoproteins during the study period. Collectively, there is considerable evidence that a Mediterranean-style diet favorably affects HDL-C, TG, and CVD risk. The ongoing PREDIMED study will provide new data on the long-term CV effects of a Mediterranean diet.

SUMMARY

Food-based dietary guidelines have been issued that meet the recommended levels of nutrients described herein (**Table 6**). Adhering to these guidelines is expected to lower TC, LDL-C, and TG, and increase HDL-C, and, thereby reduce CVD risk. This dietary pattern is low in SFA, TFA, and dietary cholesterol, and emphasizes unsaturated fats. It also promotes consumption of fruits, vegetables, whole grains, low-fat/skim dairy products, lean meats, poultry, and fish (ie, two servings per week with emphasis on fatty fish), and liquid vegetable oils, nuts, and seeds. For maximum LDL-C reduction, emphasis on viscous fiber is recommended, as well as inclusion of plant sterols/stanols. In addition, weight loss and a program of regular physical activity will beneficially affect these major lipid and lipoprotein CVD risk factors. Adhering to a healthy diet is an important tool for combating heart disease through lipid and lipoprotein modulation. Major public health efforts are needed to help people adhere to this dietary pattern with recommended lifestyle behaviors to markedly reduce CVD risk.

REFERENCES

1. Lichtenstein AH, Appel LJ, Brands M, et al. Diet and lifestyle recommendations revision 2006: a scientific statement from the American Heart Association Nutrition Committee. Circulation 2006;114(1):82–96.
2. United States Department of Health and Human Services and United States Department of Agriculture. Dietary guidelines for Americans. Washington, DC: U.S. Government Printing Office; 2005.
3. Akesson A, Weismayer C, Newby PK, et al. Combined effect of low-risk dietary and lifestyle behaviors in primary prevention of myocardial infarction in women. Arch Intern Med 2007;167(19):2122–7.
4. Third Report of the National Cholesterol Education Program (NCEP) Expert Panel on Detection, Evaluation, and Treatment of High Blood Cholesterol in Adults (Adult Treatment Panel III) final report. Circulation 2002;106(25):3143–421.
5. Cannon CP, Steinberg BA, Murphy SA, et al. Meta-analysis of cardiovascular outcomes trials comparing intensive versus moderate statin therapy. J Am Coll Cardiol 2006;48(3):438–45.
6. Grundy SM, Cleeman JI, Merz CN, et al. Implications of recent clinical trials for the National Cholesterol Education Program Adult Treatment Panel III guidelines. Circulation 2004;110(2):227–39.
7. Doelle GC. The clinical picture of metabolic syndrome. An update on this complex of conditions and risk factors. Postgrad Med Jul 2004;116(1):30–2, 35–8.
8. Dietary reference intakes for energy, carbohydrate, fiber, fat, fatty acids, cholesterol, protein, and amino acids. Washington, DC: National Academy of Sciences; 2002.
9. Woodside JV, Kromhout D. Fatty acids and CHD. Proc Nutr Soc 2005;64(4): 554–64.

10. Kromhout D, Menotti A, Bloemberg B, et al. Dietary saturated and trans fatty acids and cholesterol and 25-year mortality from coronary heart disease: the Seven Countries Study. Prev Med 1995;24(3):308–15.

11. Howell WH, McNamara DJ, Tosca MA, et al. Plasma lipid and lipoprotein responses to dietary fat and cholesterol: a meta-analysis. Am J Clin Nutr 1997;65(6):1747–64.

12. Van Horn L, McCoin M, Kris-Etherton PM, et al. The evidence for dietary prevention and treatment of cardiovascular disease. J Am Diet Assoc 2008; 108(2):287–331.

13. Anderson JW. Dietary fiber prevents carbohydrate-induced hypertriglyceride-mia. Curr Atheroscler Rep 2000;2(6):536–41.

14. Kris-Etherton PM, Innis S, American Dietetic Association, et al. Position of the American Dietetic Association and Dietitians of Canada: dietary fatty acids. J Am Diet Assoc 2007;107(9):1599–611.

15. Mozaffarian D, Katan MB, Ascherio A, et al. Trans fatty acids and cardiovascular disease. N Engl J Med 2006;354(15):1601–13.

16. Ascherio A, Katan MB, Zock PL, et al. Trans fatty acids and coronary heart disease. N Engl J Med 1999;340(25):1994–8.

17. Katan MB. Regulation of trans fats: the gap, the Polder, and McDonald's French fries. Atheroscler Suppl 2006;7(2):63–6.

18. Clifton PM, Keogh JB, Noakes M. Trans fatty acids in adipose tissue and the food supply are associated with myocardial infarction. J Nutr 2004;134(4):874–9.

19. Baylin A, Kabagambe EK, Ascherio A, et al. High 18:2 trans-fatty acids in adipose tissue are associated with increased risk of nonfatal acute myocardial infarction in Costa Rican adults. J Nutr 2003;133(4):1186–91.

20. Lemaitre RN, King IB, Raghunathan TE, et al. Cell membrane trans-fatty acids and the risk of primary cardiac arrest. Circulation 2002;105(6):697–701.

21. Lemaitre RN, King IB, Mozaffarian D, et al. Plasma phospholipid trans fatty acids, fatal ischemic heart disease, and sudden cardiac death in older adults: the cardiovascular health study. Circulation 2006;114(3):209–15.

22. Allison DB, Egan SK, Barraj LM, et al. Estimated intakes of trans fatty and other fatty acids in the US population. J Am Diet Assoc 1999;99(2):166–74 [quiz 175–66].

23. Willett WC. Trans fatty acids and cardiovascular disease—epidemiological data. Atheroscler Suppl 2006;7(2):5–8.

24. Motard-Belanger A, Charest A, Grenier G, et al. Study of the effect of trans fatty acids from ruminants on blood lipids and other risk factors for cardiovascular disease. Am J Clin Nutr 2008;87(3):593–9.

25. Chardigny JM, Destaillats F, Malpuech-Brugere C, et al. Do trans fatty acids from industrially produced sources and from natural sources have the same effect on cardiovascular disease risk factors in healthy subjects? Results of the trans Fatty Acids Collaboration (TRANSFACT) study. Am J Clin Nutr 2008;87(3):558–66.

26. Tholstrup T, Sandstrom B, Hermansen JE, et al. Effect of modified dairy fat on postprandial and fasting plasma lipids and lipoproteins in healthy young men. Lipids 1998;33(1):11–21.

27. Willett WC, Stampfer MJ, Manson JE, et al. Intake of trans fatty acids and risk of coronary heart disease among women. Lancet 1993;341(8845):581–5.

28. Pietinen P, Ascherio A, Korhonen P, et al. Intake of fatty acids and risk of coronary heart disease in a cohort of Finnish men. The Alpha-Tocopherol, Beta-Carotene Cancer Prevention Study. Am J Epidemiol 1997;145(10):876–87.

29. Ascherio A, Hennekens CH, Buring JE, et al. Trans-fatty acids intake and risk of myocardial infarction. Circulation 1994;89(1):94–101.
30. Oomen CM, Ocke MC, Feskens EJ, et al. Association between trans fatty acid intake and 10-year risk of coronary heart disease in the Zutphen Elderly Study: a prospective population-based study. Lancet 2001;357(9258):746–51.
31. Jakobsen MU, Overvad K, Dyerberg J, et al. Intake of ruminant trans fatty acids and risk of coronary heart disease. Int J Epidemiol 2008;37(1):173–82.
32. McGee DL, Reed DM, Yano K, et al. Ten-year incidence of coronary heart disease in the Honolulu Heart Program. Relationship to nutrient intake. Am J Epidemiol 1984;119(5):667–76.
33. Shekelle RB, Shryock AM, Paul O, et al. Diet, serum cholesterol, and death from coronary heart disease. The Western Electric study. N Engl J Med 1981;304(2): 65–70.
34. Ascherio A, Rimm EB, Giovannucci EL, et al. Dietary fat and risk of coronary heart disease in men: cohort follow up study in the United States. BMJ 1996; 313(7049):84–90.
35. Posner BM, Cobb JL, Belanger AJ, et al. Dietary lipid predictors of coronary heart disease in men. The Framingham Study. Arch Intern Med 1991;151(6):1181–7.
36. Esrey KL, Joseph L, Grover SA. Relationship between dietary intake and coronary heart disease mortality: lipid research clinics prevalence follow-up study. J Clin Epidemiol 1996;49(2):211–6.
37. Clarke R, Frost C, Collins R, et al. Dietary lipids and blood cholesterol: quantitative meta-analysis of metabolic ward studies. BMJ 1997;314(7074):112–7.
38. McNamara DJ. The impact of egg limitations on coronary heart disease risk: do the numbers add up? J Am Coll Nutr 2000;19(5 Suppl):540S–8S.
39. McGill HC Jr. The relationship of dietary cholesterol to serum cholesterol concentration and to atherosclerosis in man. Am J Clin Nutr 1979;32(12 Suppl):2664–702.
40. Hopkins PN. Effects of dietary cholesterol on serum cholesterol: a meta-analysis and review. Am J Clin Nutr 1992;55(6):1060–70.
41. Dawber TR, Nickerson RJ, Brand FN, et al. Eggs, serum cholesterol, and coronary heart disease. Am J Clin Nutr 1982;36(4):617–25.
42. Fraser GE. Diet and coronary heart disease: beyond dietary fats and low-density-lipoprotein cholesterol. Am J Clin Nutr 1994;59(5 Suppl):1117S–23S.
43. Gramenzi A, Gentile A, Fasoli M, et al. Association between certain foods and risk of acute myocardial infarction in women. BMJ 1990;300(6727):771–3.
44. Hu FB, Stampfer MJ, Rimm EB, et al. A prospective study of egg consumption and risk of cardiovascular disease in men and women. JAMA 1999;281(15):1387–94.
45. Nakamura Y, Iso H, Kita Y, et al. Egg consumption, serum total cholesterol concentrations and coronary heart disease incidence: Japan Public Health Center-based prospective study. Br J Nutr 2006;96(5):921–8.
46. Djousse L, Gaziano JM. Egg consumption and risk of heart failure in the Physicians' Health Study. Circulation 2008;117(4):512–6.
47. Qureshi AI, Suri FK, Ahmed S, et al. Regular egg consumption does not increase the risk of stroke and cardiovascular diseases. Med Sci Monit 2007;13(1): CR1–8.
48. Pereira MA, O'Reilly E, Augustsson K, et al. Dietary fiber and risk of coronary heart disease: a pooled analysis of cohort studies. Arch Intern Med 2004; 164(4):370–6.
49. Theuwissen E, Mensink RP. Water-soluble dietary fibers and cardiovascular disease. Physiol Behav 2008;94(2):285–92.

50. Lia A, Hallmans G, Sandberg AS, et al. Oat beta-glucan increases bile acid excretion and a fiber-rich barley fraction increases cholesterol excretion in ileostomy subjects. Am J Clin Nutr 1995;62(6):1245–51.
51. Marlett JA, Hosig KB, Vollendorf NW, et al. Mechanism of serum cholesterol reduction by oat bran. Hepatology 1994;20(6):1450–7.
52. Lia A, Andersson H, Mekki N, et al. Postprandial lipemia in relation to sterol and fat excretion in ileostomy subjects given oat-bran and wheat test meals. Am J Clin Nutr 1997;66(2):357–65.
53. de Groot A, Luyken R, Pikaar NA. Cholesterol-lowering effect of rolled oats. Lancet 1963;2(7302):303–4.
54. Davy BM, Davy KP, Ho RC, et al. High-fiber oat cereal compared with wheat cereal consumption favorably alters LDL-cholesterol subclass and particle numbers in middle-aged and older men. Am J Clin Nutr 2002;76(2):351–8.
55. Shrestha S, Freake HC, McGrane MM, et al. A combination of psyllium and plant sterols alters lipoprotein metabolism in hypercholesterolemic subjects by modifying the intravascular processing of lipoproteins and increasing LDL uptake. J Nutr 2007;137(5):1165–70.
56. Moreyra AE, Wilson AC, Koraym A. Effect of combining psyllium fiber with simvastatin in lowering cholesterol. Arch Intern Med 2005;165(10):1161–6.
57. Naumann E, van Rees AB, Onning G, et al. Beta-glucan incorporated into a fruit drink effectively lowers serum LDL-cholesterol concentrations. Am J Clin Nutr 2006;83(3):601–5.
58. Kerckhoffs DA, Hornstra G, Mensink RP. Cholesterol-lowering effect of beta-glucan from oat bran in mildly hypercholesterolemic subjects may decrease when beta-glucan is incorporated into bread and cookies. Am J Clin Nutr 2003;78(2):221–7.
59. Brown L, Rosner B, Willett WW, et al. Cholesterol-lowering effects of dietary fiber: a meta-analysis. Am J Clin Nutr 1999;69(1):30–42.
60. Katan MB, Grundy SM, Jones P, et al. Efficacy and safety of plant stanols and sterols in the management of blood cholesterol levels. Mayo Clin Proc 2003; 78(8):965–78.
61. Neil HA, Huxley RR. Efficacy and therapeutic potential of plant sterols. Atheroscler Suppl 2002;3(3):11–5.
62. Kassis AN, Vanstone CA, AbuMweis SS, et al. Efficacy of plant sterols is not influenced by dietary cholesterol intake in hypercholesterolemic individuals. Meta 2008;57(3):339–46.
63. Clifton PM, Mano M, Duchateau GS, et al. Dose-response effects of different plant sterol sources in fat spreads on serum lipids and C-reactive protein and on the kinetic behavior of serum plant sterols. Eur J Clin Nutr 2008;62(8):968–77.
64. Poli A, Marangoni F, Paoletti R, et al. Non-pharmacological control of plasma cholesterol levels. Nutr Metab Cardiovasc Dis 2008;18(2):S1–16.
65. Grundy SM. Stanol esters as a component of maximal dietary therapy in the National Cholesterol Education Program Adult Treatment Panel III report. Am J Cardiol 2005;96(1A):47D–50D.
66. Assmann G, Cullen P, Erbey J, et al. Plasma sitosterol elevations are associated with an increased incidence of coronary events in men: results of a nested case-control analysis of the Prospective Cardiovascular Munster (PROCAM) study. Nutr Metab Cardiovasc Dis 2006;16(1):13–21.
67. Pinedo S, Vissers MN, von Bergmann K, et al. Plasma levels of plant sterols and the risk of coronary artery disease: the prospective EPIC-Norfolk Population Study. J Lipid Res 2007;48(1):139–44.

68. Fassbender K, Lutjohann D, Dik MG, et al. Moderately elevated plant sterol levels are associated with reduced cardiovascular risk—the LASA study. Atherosclerosis 2008;196(1):283–8.
69. Wilund KR, Yu L, Xu F, et al. No association between plasma levels of plant sterols and atherosclerosis in mice and men. Arterioscler Thromb Vasc Biol 2004;24(12):2326–32.
70. Moruisi KG, Oosthuizen W, Opperman AM. Phytosterols/stanols lower cholesterol concentrations in familial hypercholesterolemic subjects: a systematic review with meta-analysis. J Am Coll Nutr 2006;25(1):41–8.
71. Devaraj S, Autret BC, Jialal I. Reduced-calorie orange juice beverage with plant sterols lowers C-reactive protein concentrations and improves the lipid profile in human volunteers. Am J Clin Nutr 2006;84(4):756–61.
72. Devaraj S, Jialal I, Vega-Lopez S. Plant sterol-fortified orange juice effectively lowers cholesterol levels in mildly hypercholesterolemic healthy individuals. Arterioscler Thromb Vasc Biol 2004;24(3):e25–8.
73. Noakes M, Clifton PM, Doornbos AM, et al. Plant sterol ester-enriched milk and yoghurt effectively reduce serum cholesterol in modestly hypercholesterolemic subjects. Eur J Nutr 2005;44(4):214–22.
74. Shrestha S, Volek JS, Udani J, et al. A combination therapy including psyllium and plant sterols lowers LDL cholesterol by modifying lipoprotein metabolism in hypercholesterolemic individuals. J Nutr 2006;136(10):2492–7.
75. Hansel B, Nicolle C, Lalanne F, et al. Effect of low-fat, fermented milk enriched with plant sterols on serum lipid profile and oxidative stress in moderate hypercholesterolemia. Am J Clin Nutr 2007;86(3):790–6.
76. Goldberg AC, Ostlund RE Jr, Bateman JH, et al. Effect of plant stanol tablets on low-density lipoprotein cholesterol lowering in patients on statin drugs. Am J Cardiol 2006;97(3):376–9.
77. Vuorio AF, Gylling H, Turtola H, et al. Stanol ester margarine alone and with simvastatin lowers serum cholesterol in families with familial hypercholesterolemia caused by the FH-North Karelia mutation. Arterioscler Thromb Vasc Biol 2000;20(2):500–6.
78. De Jong A, Plat J, Bast A, et al. Effects of plant sterol and stanol ester consumption on lipid metabolism, antioxidant status and markers of oxidative stress, endothelial function and low-grade inflammation in patients on current statin treatment. Eur J Clin Nutr 2008;62(2):263–73.
79. Castro Cabezas M, de Vries JH, Van Oostrom AJ, et al. Effects of a stanol-enriched diet on plasma cholesterol and triglycerides in patients treated with statins. J Am Diet Assoc 2006;106(10):1564–9.
80. Richelle M, Enslen M, Hager C, et al. Both free and esterified plant sterols reduce cholesterol absorption and the bioavailability of beta-carotene and alpha-tocopherol in normocholesterolemic humans. Am J Clin Nutr 2004;80(1):171–7.
81. Noakes M, Clifton P, Ntanios F, et al. An increase in dietary carotenoids when consuming plant sterols or stanols is effective in maintaining plasma carotenoid concentrations. Am J Clin Nutr 2002;75(1):79–86.
82. Nagata C, Takatsuka N, Kurisu Y, et al. Decreased serum total cholesterol concentration is associated with high intake of soy products in Japanese men and women. J Nutr 1998;128(2):209–13.
83. Ho SC, Woo JLF, Leung SSF, et al. Intake of soy products is associated with better plasma lipid profiles in the Hong Kong Chinese population. J Nutr 2000;130(10):2590–3.
84. Zhang X, Shu XO, Gao Y-T, et al. Soy food consumption is associated with lower risk of coronary heart disease in Chinese women. J Nutr 2003;133(9):2874–8.

85. Tham DM, Gardner CD, Haskell WL. Clinical review 97: potential health benefits of dietary phytoestrogens: a review of the clinical, epidemiological, and mechanistic evidence. J Clin Endocrinol Metab 1998;83(7):2223–35.
86. Atkinson C, Frankenfeld CL, Lampe JW. Gut bacterial metabolism of the soy isoflavone daidzein: exploring the relevance to human health. Exp Biol Med (Maywood) 2005;230(3):155–70.
87. Yuan JP, Wang JH, Liu X. Metabolism of dietary soy isoflavones to equol by human intestinal microflora—implications for health. Mol Nutr Food Res 2007; 51(7):765–81.
88. Anderson JW, Johnstone BM, Cook-Newell ME. Meta-analysis of the effects of soy protein intake on serum lipids. N Engl J Med 1995;333(5):276–82.
89. Food and Drug Administration. Food labeling: health claims; soy protein and coronary heart disease. Fed Regist 1999;64(206):57700–33.
90. Zhan S, Ho SC. Meta-analysis of the effects of soy protein containing isoflavones on the lipid profile. Am J Clin Nutr 2005;81(2):397–408.
91. Balk E, Chung M, Chew P, et al. Effects of soy on health outcomes. Evidence Report/Technology Assessment No. 126. AHRQ Publication No. 05-E024-2. Rockland (MD): Agency for Healthcare Research and Quality; 2005.
92. Sacks FM, Lichtenstein A, Van Horn L, et al. Soy protein, isoflavones, and cardiovascular health: an American Heart Association science advisory for professionals from the nutrition committee. Circulation 2006;113(7):1034–44.
93. Weggemans RM, Trautwein EA. Relation between soy-associated isoflavones and LDL and HDL cholesterol concentrations in humans: a meta-analysis. Eur J Clin Nutr 2003;57(8):940–6.
94. Zhuo X-G, Melby MK, Watanabe S. Soy isoflavone intake lowers serum LDL cholesterol: a meta-analysis of 8 randomized controlled trials in humans. J Nutr 2004;134(9):2395–400.
95. Taku K, Umegaki K, Sato Y, et al. Soy isoflavones lower serum total and LDL cholesterol in humans: a meta-analysis of 11 randomized controlled trials. Am J Clin Nutr 2007;85(4):1148–56.
96. Sacks FM, Lichtenstein A, Van Horn L, et al. Soy protein, isoflavones, and cardiovascular health: a summary of a statement for professionals from the American Heart Association Nutrition Committee. Arterioscler Thromb Vasc Biol 2006; 26(8):1689–92.
97. Torres N, Torre-Villalvazo I, Tovar AR. Regulation of lipid metabolism by soy protein and its implication in diseases mediated by lipid disorders. J Nutr Biochem 2006;17(6):365–73.
98. Xiao CW, Mei J, Wood CM. Effect of soy proteins and isoflavones on lipid metabolism and involved gene expression. Front Biosci 2008;13:2660–73.
99. Pasanisi F, Contaldo F, de Simone G, et al. Benefits of sustained moderate weight loss in obesity. Nutr Metab Cardiovasc Dis 2001;11(6):401–6.
100. Van Gaal LF, Mertens IL, Ballaux D. What is the relationship between risk factor reduction and degree of weight loss. Eur Heart J Suppl 2005;7(Suppl L):L21–6.
101. Dattilo AM, Kris-Etherton PM. Effects of weight reduction on blood lipids and lipoproteins: a meta-analysis. Am J Clin Nutr 1992;56(2):320–8.
102. Poobalan A, Aucott L, Smith WC, et al. Effects of weight loss in overweight/ obese individuals and long-term lipid outcomes—a systematic review. Obes Rev 2004;5(1):43–50.
103. Williamson DF, Pamuk E, Thun M, et al. Prospective study of intentional weight loss and mortality in never-smoking overweight US white women aged 40-64 years. Am J Epidemiol 1995;141(12):1128–41.

104. Noakes M, Clifton PM. Weight loss and plasma lipids. Curr Opin Lipidol 2000; 11(1):65–70.
105. Dansinger ML, Gleason JA, Griffith JL, et al. Comparison of the Atkins, Ornish, Weight Watchers, and Zone diets for weight loss and heart disease risk reduction: a randomized trial. JAMA 2005;293(1):43–53.
106. Lichtenstein AH, Ausman LM, Jalbert SM, et al. Efficacy of a therapeutic lifestyle change/step 2 diet in moderately hypercholesterolemic middle-aged and elderly female and male subjects. J Lipid Res 2002;43(2):264–73.
107. Welty FK, Stuart E, O'Meara M, et al. Effect of addition of exercise to therapeutic lifestyle changes diet in enabling women and men with coronary heart disease to reach Adult Treatment Panel III low-density lipoprotein cholesterol goal without lowering high-density lipoprotein cholesterol. Am J Cardiol 2002;89(10):1201–4.
108. Kendall CW, Jenkins DJ. A dietary portfolio: maximal reduction of low-density lipoprotein cholesterol with diet. Curr Atheroscler Rep 2004;6(6):492–8.
109. Jenkins DJ, Kendall CW, Marchie A, et al. The effect of combining plant sterols, soy protein, viscous fibers, and almonds in treating hypercholesterolemia. Meta 2003;52(11):1478–83.
110. Jenkins DJ, Kendall CW, Marchie A, et al. Effects of a dietary portfolio of cholesterol-lowering foods vs lovastatin on serum lipids and C-reactive protein. JAMA 2003;290(4):502–10.
111. Jenkins DJ, Kendall CW, Faulkner D, et al. A dietary portfolio approach to cholesterol reduction: combined effects of plant sterols, vegetable proteins, and viscous fibers in hypercholesterolemia. Meta 2002;51(12):1596–604.
112. Jenkins DJ, Kendall CW, Faulkner DA, et al. Assessment of the longer-term effects of a dietary portfolio of cholesterol-lowering foods in hypercholesterolemia. Am J Clin Nutr 2006;83(3):582–91.
113. Lichtenstein AH, Van Horn L. Very low fat diets. Circulation 1998;98(9):935–9.
114. Ornish D, Scherwitz LW, Billings JH, et al. Intensive lifestyle changes for reversal of coronary heart disease. JAMA 1998;280(23):2001–7.
115. Esselstyn CB Jr. Updating a 12-year experience with arrest and reversal therapy for coronary heart disease (an overdue requiem for palliative cardiology). Am J Cardiol 1999;84(3):339–41, A338.
116. Esselstyn CB Jr, Ellis SG, Medendorp SV, et al. A strategy to arrest and reverse coronary artery disease: a 5-year longitudinal study of a single physician's practice. J Fam Pract 1995;41(6):560–8.
117. Daubenmier JJ, Weidner G, Sumner MD, et al. The contribution of changes in diet, exercise, and stress management to changes in coronary risk in women and men in the multisite cardiac lifestyle intervention program. Ann Behav Med 2007;33(1):57–68.
118. Frattaroli J, Weidner G, Merritt-Worden TA, et al. Angina pectoris and atherosclerotic risk factors in the multisite cardiac lifestyle intervention program. Am J Cardiol 2008;101(7):911–8.
119. Pawlosky RJ, Hibbeln JR, Novotny JA, et al. Physiological compartmental analysis of {alpha}-linolenic acid metabolism in adult humans. J Lipid Res 2001; 42(8):1257–65.
120. Goyens PL, Spilker ME, Zock PL, et al. Compartmental modeling to quantify alpha-linolenic acid conversion after longer term intake of multiple tracer boluses. J Lipid Res 2005;46(7):1474–83.
121. Hussein N, Ah-Sing E, Wilkinson P, et al. Long-chain conversion of [13C]linoleic acid and {alpha}-linolenic acid in response to marked changes in their dietary intake in men. J Lipid Res 2005;46(2):269–80.

122. Plourde M, Cunnane SC. Extremely limited synthesis of long chain polyunsaturates in adults: implications for their dietary essentiality and use as supplements. Appl Physiol Nutr Metab 2007;32(4):619–34.

123. Hu FB, Stampfer MJ, Manson JE, et al. Dietary intake of alpha-linolenic acid and risk of fatal ischemic heart disease among women. Am J Clin Nutr 1999;69(5):890–7.

124. Albert CM, Oh K, Whang W, et al. Dietary alpha-linolenic acid intake and risk of sudden cardiac death and coronary heart disease. Circulation 2005;112(21):3232–8.

125. de Lorgeril M, Salen P, Martin JL, et al. Mediterranean diet, traditional risk factors, and the rate of cardiovascular complications after myocardial infarction: final report of the Lyon Diet Heart Study. Circulation 1999;99(6):779–85.

126. Albert CM, Hennekens CH, O'Donnell CJ, et al. Fish consumption and risk of sudden cardiac death. JAMA 1998;279(1):23–8.

127. Hu FB, Bronner L, Willett WC, et al. Fish and omega-3 fatty acid intake and risk of coronary heart disease in women. JAMA 2002;287(14):1815–21.

128. Lemaitre RN, King IB, Mozaffarian D, et al. n-3 Polyunsaturated fatty acids, fatal ischemic heart disease, and nonfatal myocardial infarction in older adults: the Cardiovascular Health Study. Am J Clin Nutr 2003;77(2):319–25.

129. Daviglus ML, Stamler J, Orencia AJ, et al. Fish consumption and the 30-year risk of fatal myocardial infarction. N Engl J Med 1997;336(15):1046–53.

130. Zhang J, Sasaki S, Amano K, et al. Fish consumption and mortality from all causes, ischemic heart disease, and stroke: an ecological study. Prev Med 1999;28(5):520–9.

131. Iso H, Kobayashi M, Ishihara J, et al. Intake of fish and n3 fatty acids and risk of coronary heart disease among Japanese: the Japan Public Health Center-Based (JPHC) Study Cohort I. Circulation 2006;113(2):195–202.

132. Burr ML, Fehily AM, Gilbert JF, et al. Effects of changes in fat, fish, and fibre intakes on death and myocardial reinfarction: diet and reinfarction trial (DART). Lancet 1989;2(8666):757–61.

133. GISSI-Prevenzione Investigators. Dietary supplementation with n-3 polyunsaturated fatty acids and vitamin E after myocardial infarction: results of the GISSI-Prevenzione trial. Gruppo Italiano per lo Studio della Sopravvivenza nell'Infarto miocardico. Lancet 1999;354(9177):447–55.

134. Marchioli R, Barzi F, Bomba E, et al. Early protection against sudden death by n-3 polyunsaturated fatty acids after myocardial infarction: time-course analysis of the results of the Gruppo Italiano per lo Studio della Sopravvivenza nell'Infarto Miocardico (GISSI)-Prevenzione. Circulation 2002;105(16):1897–903.

135. Yokoyama M, Origasa H, Matsuzaki M, et al. Effects of eicosapentaenoic acid on major coronary events in hypercholesterolaemic patients (JELIS): a randomised open-label, blinded endpoint analysis. Lancet 2007;369(9567):1090–8.

136. Harris WS. n-3 fatty acids and serum lipoproteins: human studies. Am J Clin Nutr 1997;65(5 Suppl):1645S–54S.

137. Roche HM. Unsaturated fatty acids. Proc Nutr Soc 1999;58(2):397–401.

138. Schmidt EB, Kristensen SD, De Caterina R, et al. The effects of n-3 fatty acids on plasma lipids and lipoproteins and other cardiovascular risk factors in patients with hyperlipidemia. Atherosclerosis 1993;103(2):107–21.

139. Balk EM, Lichtenstein AH, Chung M, et al. Effects of omega-3 fatty acids on serum markers of cardiovascular disease risk: a systematic review. Atherosclerosis 2006;189(1):19–30.

140. Robinson JG, Stone NJ. Antiatherosclerotic and antithrombotic effects of omega-3 fatty acids. Am J Cardiol 2006;98(4 Suppl 1):39–49.

141. Mori TA, Burke V, Puddey IB, et al. Purified eicosapentaenoic and docosahexaenoic acids have differential effects on serum lipids and lipoproteins, LDL particle size, glucose, and insulin in mildly hyperlipidemic men. Am J Clin Nutr 2000;71(5):1085–94.
142. Suzukawa M, Abbey M, Howe PR, et al. Effects of fish oil fatty acids on low density lipoprotein size, oxidizability, and uptake by macrophages. J Lipid Res 1995;36(3):473–84.
143. Rivellese AA, Maffettone A, Vessby B, et al. Effects of dietary saturated, mono-unsaturated and n-3 fatty acids on fasting lipoproteins, LDL size and post-pran-dial lipid metabolism in healthy subjects. Atherosclerosis 2003;167(1):149–58.
144. Lungershausen YK, Abbey M, Nestel PJ, et al. Reduction of blood pressure and plasma triglycerides by omega-3 fatty acids in treated hypertensives. J Hyper-tens 1994;12(9):1041–5.
145. Kris-Etherton PM. AHA science advisory: monounsaturated fatty acids and risk of cardiovascular disease. J Nutr 1999;129(12):2280–4.
146. Kris-Etherton PM, Pearson TA, Wan Y, et al. High-monounsaturated fatty acid diets lower both plasma cholesterol and triacylglycerol concentrations. Am J Clin Nutr 1999;70(6):1009–15.
147. Berglund L, Lefevre M, Ginsberg HN, et al. Comparison of monounsaturated fat with carbohydrates as a replacement for saturated fat in subjects with a high metabolic risk profile: studies in the fasting and postprandial states. Am J Clin Nutr 2007;86(6):1611–20.
148. Cao Y, Mauger DT, Christine L, et al. Effects of moderate-fat (MF) versus lower-fat (LF) diets on lipids and lipoproteins: A meta-analysis of clinical trials in subjects with and without Diabetes. Journal of Clinical Lipidology [in Press].
149. Rudel LL, Parks JS, Sawyer JK. Compared with dietary monounsaturated and saturated fat, polyunsaturated fat protects African green monkeys from coro-nary artery atherosclerosis. Arterioscler Thromb Vasc Biol 1995;15(12):2101–10.
150. Morris JN, Heady JA. Mortality in relation to the physical activity of work: a prelim-inary note on experience in middle age. Br J Ind Med 1953;10(4):245–54.
151. Paffenbarger RS, Hale WE. Work activity and coronary heart mortality. N Engl J Med 1975;292(11):545–50.
152. Berlin JA, Colditz GA. A meta-analysis of physical activity in the prevention of coronary heart disease. Am J Epidemiol 1990;132(4):612–28.
153. Powell KE, Thompson PD, Caspersen CJ, et al. Physical activity and the inci-dence of coronary heart disease. Annu Rev Public Health 1987;8:253–87.
154. Franco OH, de Laet C, Peeters A, et al. Effects of physical activity on life expec-tancy with cardiovascular disease. Arch Intern Med 2005;165(20):2355–60.
155. Blair SN, Kohl HWR, Barlow CE, et al. Changes in physical fitness and all-cause mortality. A prospective study of healthy and unhealthy men. JAMA 1995;273(14):1093–8.
156. Laukkanen JA, Lakka TA, Rauramaa R, et al. Cardiovascular fitness as a predictor of mortality in men. Arch Intern Med 2001;161(6):825–31.
157. Lee CD, Blair SN, Jackson AS. Cardiorespiratory fitness, body composition, and all-cause and cardiovascular disease mortality in men. Am J Clin Nutr 1999;69(3):373–80.
158. Lee IM, Skerrett PJ. Physical activity and all-cause mortality: what is the dose-response relation? Med Sci Sports Exerc 2001;33(6 Suppl):S459–71 [discus-sion: S493–54].
159. Carroll S, Dudfield M. What is the relationship between exercise and metabolic abnormalities? A review of the metabolic syndrome. Sports Med 2004;34(6):371–418.

160. Durstine JL, Grandjean PW, Davis PG, et al. Blood lipid and lipoprotein adaptations to exercise: a quantitative analysis. Sports Med 2001;31(15):1033–62.

161. Kelley GA, Kelley KS, Vu Tran Z. Aerobic exercise, lipids and lipoproteins in overweight and obese adults: a meta-analysis of randomized controlled trials. Int J Obes (Lond) 2005;29(8):881–93.

162. Leon AS, Sanchez OA. Response of blood lipids to exercise training alone or combined with dietary intervention. Med Sci Sports Exerc 2001;33(6 Suppl): S502–15 [discussion: S528–09].

163. Kraus WE, Houmard JA, Duscha BD, et al. Effects of the amount and intensity of exercise on plasma lipoproteins. N Engl J Med 2002;347(19):1483–92.

164. Kodama S, Tanaka S, Saito K, et al. Effect of aerobic exercise training on serum levels of high-density lipoprotein cholesterol: a meta-analysis. Arch Intern Med 2007;167(10):999–1008.

165. Fletcher B, Berra K, Ades P, et al. Managing abnormal blood lipids: a collaborative approach. Circulation 2005;112(20):3184–209.

166. Haskell WL. The influence of exercise on the concentrations of triglyceride and cholesterol in human plasma. Exerc Sport Sci Rev 1984;12:205–44.

167. Hamilton MT, Hamilton DG, Zderic TW. Role of low energy expenditure and sitting in obesity, metabolic syndrome, type 2 diabetes, and cardiovascular disease. Diabetes 2007;56(11):2655–67.

168. Haskell WL, Lee IM, Pate RR, et al. Physical activity and public health: updated recommendation for adults from the American College of Sports Medicine and the American Heart Association. Med Sci Sports Exerc 2007;39(8):1423–34.

169. Mukamal KJ, Conigrave KM, Mittleman MA, et al. Roles of drinking pattern and type of alcohol consumed in coronary heart disease in men. N Engl J Med 2003; 348(2):109–18.

170. Rimm EB, Giovannucci EL, Willett WC, et al. Prospective study of alcohol consumption and risk of coronary disease in men. Lancet 1991;338(8765): 464–8.

171. van Tol A, Hendriks HF. Moderate alcohol consumption: effects on lipids and cardiovascular disease risk. Curr Opin Lipidol 2001;12(1):19–23.

172. Rimm EB, Williams P, Fosher K, et al. Moderate alcohol intake and lower risk of coronary heart disease: meta-analysis of effects on lipids and haemostatic factors. BMJ 1999;319(7224):1523–8.

173. Rimm E. Alcohol and cardiovascular disease. Curr Atheroscler Rep 2000;2(6): 529–35.

174. Di Castelnuovo A, Rotondo S, Iacoviello L, et al. Meta-analysis of wine and beer consumption in relation to vascular risk. Circulation 2002;105(24):2836–44.

175. Freiberg MS, Cabral HJ, Heeren TC, et al. Alcohol consumption and the prevalence of the metabolic syndrome in the US: a cross-sectional analysis of data from the Third National Health and Nutrition Examination Survey. Diabetes Care 2004;27(12):2954–9.

176. Baer DJ, Judd JT, Clevidence BA, et al. Moderate alcohol consumption lowers risk factors for cardiovascular disease in postmenopausal women fed a controlled diet. Am J Clin Nutr 2002;75(3):593–9.

177. Naissides M, Mamo JC, James AP, et al. The effect of chronic consumption of red wine on cardiovascular disease risk factors in postmenopausal women. Atherosclerosis 2006;185(2):438–45.

178. Hansen AS, Marckmann P, Dragsted LO, et al. Effect of red wine and red grape extract on blood lipids, haemostatic factors, and other risk factors for cardiovascular disease. Eur J Clin Nutr 2005;59(3):449–55.

179. Sierksma A, Vermunt SH, Lankhuizen IM, et al. Effect of moderate alcohol consumption on parameters of reverse cholesterol transport in postmenopausal women. Alcohol Clin Exp Res 2004;28(4):662–6.
180. Westman EC, Feinman RD, Mavropoulos JC, et al. Low-carbohydrate nutrition and metabolism. Am J Clin Nutr 2007;86(2):276–84.
181. Krauss RM, Blanche PJ, Rawlings RS, et al. Separate effects of reduced carbohydrate intake and weight loss on atherogenic dyslipidemia. Am J Clin Nutr 2006;83(5):1025–31 [quiz 1205].
182. Seshadri P, Iqbal N, Stern L, et al. A randomized study comparing the effects of a low-carbohydrate diet and a conventional diet on lipoprotein subfractions and C-reactive protein levels in patients with severe obesity. Am J Med 2004;117(6):398–405.
183. Westman EC, Yancy WS Jr, Olsen MK, et al. Effect of a low-carbohydrate, ketogenic diet program compared to a low-fat diet on fasting lipoprotein subclasses. Int J Cardiol 2006;110(2):212–6.
184. Volek JS, Sharman MJ, Forsythe CE. Modification of lipoproteins by very low-carbohydrate diets. J Nutr 2005;135(6):1339–42.
185. Last AR, Wilson SA. Low-carbohydrate diets. Am Fam Physician 2006;73(11):1942–8.
186. Larosa JC, Fry AG, Muesing R, et al. Effects of high-protein, low-carbohydrate dieting on plasma lipoproteins and body weight. J Am Diet Assoc 1980;77(3):264–70.
187. Gardner CD, Kiazand A, Alhassan S, et al. Comparison of the Atkins, Zone, Ornish, and LEARN diets for change in weight and related risk factors among overweight premenopausal women: the A TO Z Weight Loss Study: a randomized trial. JAMA 2007;297(9):969–77.
188. Brehm BJ, Seeley RJ, Daniels SR, et al. A randomized trial comparing a very low carbohydrate diet and a calorie-restricted low fat diet on body weight and cardiovascular risk factors in healthy women. J Clin Endocrinol Metab 2003;88(4):1617–23.
189. Foster GD, Wyatt HR, Hill JO, et al. A randomized trial of a low-carbohydrate diet for obesity. N Engl J Med 2003;348(21):2082–90.
190. Samaha FF, Iqbal N, Seshadri P, et al. A low-carbohydrate as compared with a low-fat diet in severe obesity. N Engl J Med 2003;348(21):2074–81.
191. Yancy WS Jr, Olsen MK, Guyton JR, et al. A low-carbohydrate, ketogenic diet versus a low-fat diet to treat obesity and hyperlipidemia: a randomized, controlled trial. Ann Intern Med 2004;140(10):769–77.
192. Stern L, Iqbal N, Seshadri P, et al. The effects of low-carbohydrate versus conventional weight loss diets in severely obese adults: one-year follow-up of a randomized trial. Ann Intern Med 2004;140(10):778–85.
193. Volek JS, Feinman RD. Carbohydrate restriction improves the features of metabolic syndrome. Metabolic syndrome may be defined by the response to carbohydrate restriction. Nutr Metab (Lond) 2004;2:1.
194. Biesalski HK. Diabetes preventive components in the Mediterranean diet. Eur J Nutr 2004;43(Suppl 1):I/26–30.
195. Estruch R, Martinez-Gonzalez MA, Corella D, et al. Effects of a Mediterranean-style diet on cardiovascular risk factors: a randomized trial. Ann Intern Med 2006;145(1):1–11.
196. Esposito K, Marfella R, Ciotola M, et al. Effect of a Mediterranean-style diet on endothelial dysfunction and markers of vascular inflammation in the metabolic syndrome: a randomized trial. JAMA 2004;292(12):1440–6.

197. Fuentes F, Lopez-Miranda J, Perez-Martinez P, et al. Chronic effects of a high-fat diet enriched with virgin olive oil and a low-fat diet enriched with alpha-linolenic acid on postprandial endothelial function in healthy men. Br J Nutr 2008;100(1):159–65.

198. Esposito K, Pontillo A, Di Palo C, et al. Effect of weight loss and lifestyle changes on vascular inflammatory markers in obese women: a randomized trial. JAMA 2003;289(14):1799–804.

199. Aro A, Jauhiainen M, Partanen R, et al. Stearic acid, trans fatty acids, and dairy fat: effects on serum and lipoprotein lipids, apolipoproteins, lipoprotein(a), and lipid transfer proteins in healthy subjects. Am J Clin Nutr 1997;65(5):1419–26.

200. Judd JT, Baer D, Clevidence B. Blood lipid and lipoprotein modifying effects of trans monounsaturated fatty acids compared to carbohydrate, oleic acid, stearic acid, and C 12:0-16:0 saturated fatty acids in men fed controlled diets. FASEB J 1998;12:A229 [abstract].

201. Judd JT, Clevidence BA, Muesing RA, et al. Dietary trans fatty acids: effects on plasma lipids and lipoproteins of healthy men and women. Am J Clin Nutr 1994; 59(4):861–8.

202. Lichtenstein AH, Ausman LM, Carrasco W, et al. Hydrogenation impairs the hypolipidemic effect of corn oil in humans. Hydrogenation, trans fatty acids, and plasma lipids. Arterioscler Thromb 1993;13(2):154–61.

203. Lichtenstein AH, Ausman LM, Jalbert SM, et al. Effects of different forms of dietary hydrogenated fats on serum lipoprotein cholesterol levels. N Engl J Med 1999;340(25):1933–40.

204. Mensink RP, Katan MB. Effect of dietary trans fatty acids on high-density and low-density lipoprotein cholesterol levels in healthy subjects. N Engl J Med 1990;323(7):439–45.

205. Nestel P, Noakes M, Belling B, et al. Plasma lipoprotein lipid and Lp[a] changes with substitution of elaidic acid for oleic acid in the diet. J Lipid Res 1992;33(7): 1029–36.

206. Sundram K, Ismail A, Hayes KC, et al. Trans (elaidic) fatty acids adversely affect the lipoprotein profile relative to specific saturated fatty acids in humans. J Nutr 1997;127(3):514S–20S.

207. Zock PL, Katan MB. Hydrogenation alternatives: effects of trans fatty acids and stearic acid versus linoleic acid on serum lipids and lipoproteins in humans. J Lipid Res 1992;33(3):399–410.

Lowering Low-Density Lipoprotein Cholesterol: Statins, Ezetimibe, Bile Acid Sequestrants, and Combinations: Comparative Efficacy and Safety

Runhua Hou, MD[a], Anne Carol Goldberg, MD, FACP[b],*

KEYWORDS

- LDL-C • Statins • Ezetimibe • Bile acid sequestrants
- Efficacy • Safety

Cardiovascular disease (CVD) is the leading cause of death in the United States and accounts for 80% of deaths in diabetic patients.[1,2] It correlates strongly with the levels of plasma cholesterol- and triglyceride-containing particles. Besides transporting lipids between tissues, these lipid-containing particles promote plaque formation and induce atherosclerosis. Elevated levels of low-density lipoprotein cholesterol (LDL-C), decreased levels of high-density lipoprotein cholesterol (HDL-C), and increased triglyceride levels are independent risk factors for CVD, and improving these levels is an important intervention to reduce CVD.

ACG has received grant and/or research support from Abbott, Aegerion, Astra Zeneca, Glaxo-Smith-Kline, ISIS, Merck, Pfizer, Sanofi-Aventis, Sankyo, and Takeda. ACG has served as a consultant to Abbott, Unilever, Roche, and Sanofi-Aventis. ACG has served on the Merck-Schering-Plough Speaker's Bureau. ACG has received travel support from Sanofi-Aventis and speaking honoraria from Abbott.

[a] Endocrine Unit, University of Rochester, 601 Elmwood Avenue, Box 693, Rochester, NY 14642, USA
[b] Division of Endocrinology, Metabolism, and Lipid Research, Washington University School of Medicine, Campus Box 8127, 660 South Euclid, St. Louis, MO 63110, USA
* Corresponding author.
E-mail address: agoldber@im.wustl.edu (A.C. Goldberg).

Endocrinol Metab Clin N Am 38 (2009) 79–97
doi:10.1016/j.ecl.2008.11.007
0889-8529/08/$ – see front matter © 2009 Elsevier Inc. All rights reserved.

Lowering LDL-C levels has been shown to decrease the risk of cardiovascular events in patients with and without coronary artery disease.[3–7] The National Cholesterol Education Program Adult Treatment Panel III (NCEP ATP III)[8] set LDL-C as the primary target for treatment of hyperlipidemia. In 2004, the NCEP recommended an optional LDL-C goal of less than 70 mg/dL for patients considered at very high-risk as well as more aggressive therapy in patients at moderate to high risk.[9] Several classes of medications are useful for lowering LDL-C. They have differing mechanisms of action, efficacy, and side effect profiles. In general, the goal of drug treatment should be a reduction in the LDL-C level of at least 30% from baseline. Therapy with a single drug may be adequate for many patients, but multiple lipid-lowering medications may be needed to reach the target LDL-C level in some. This article discusses the statins, ezetimibe, and bile acid sequestrants (BAS) as well as combinations of drugs to lower LDL-C.

TARGETS OF THERAPY FOR HYPERLIPIDEMIA

Lowering LDL-C is the primary goal of treatment of hyperlipidemia. Current guidelines from the NCEP ATP III recommend that the target LDL-C should be based on the patient's risk for developing coronary heart disease (CHD).[8,9] Risk factors include age, gender, family history of premature CHD, hypertension, current cigarette smoking, and low HDL-C levels (**Table 1**). HDL-C levels $\geq$ 60 mg/dL count as a negative risk factor and remove one risk factor from the total number. Patients who have two or more risk factors are categorized further by assessing their 10-year risk using the Framingham score.

For patients who have a history of CHD or CHD equivalent such as diabetes, peripheral vascular disease, carotid artery stenosis, or abdominal aneurysm or who have a calculated 10-year risk greater than 20%, the LDL-C goal should be a level less than 100 mg/dL. In patients at very high risk, a goal of LDL-C less than 70 mg/dL is optional.[9] Very high risk is defined as established vascular disease and any additional

Table 1
National Cholesterol Education Program Adult Treatment Panel III major risk factors (exclusive of LDL-C) that modify LDL-C goals

Risk Factors	Description
Age and gender	Men: $\geq$ 45 years Women: $\geq$ 55 years
Family history of premature coronary heart disease	Men: <55 years in a first-degree male relative Women: <65 years in a first-degree female relative
Hypertension	Blood pressure $\geq$ 140/90 mm Hg or taking medication
Smoking	Any cigarette smoking
HDL-C[a]	<40 mg/dL

[a] If the HDL-C level is $\geq$ 60 mg/dL, subtract one risk factor, because high HDL-C levels decrease the risk of coronary heart disease.

Data from Expert Panel on Detection, Evaluation and Treatment of High Blood Cholesterol in Adults. Executive summary of the third report of the National Cholesterol Education Program (NCEP) Expert Panel on Detection, Evaluation, and Treatment of High Blood Cholesterol in Adults (Adult Treatment Panel III). JAMA 2001;285(19):2486–97.

conditions including multiple risk factors (such as diabetes), severe and poorly controlled risk factors (eg, cigarette smoking), metabolic syndrome (high triglyceride, low HDL-C levels), and acute coronary syndromes. The American Diabetes Association also recommends a target LDL-C level of less than 70 mg/dL in diabetic patients who have CVD.[10] The NCEP guidelines recommend that for patients who have more than two risk factors but a 10-year risk $\leq$ 20%, the target LDL-C level should be less than 130 mg/dL. For patients who have no or one risk factor, an LDL-C level less than 160 mg/dL should be the goal. **Table 2** lists the NCEP III guidelines in detail.

Therapeutic lifestyle changes should be initiated whenever a person's LDL-C level is above the target based on the risk assessment. In general, drug therapy should be started in conjunction with therapeutic lifestyle changes without delay when the LDL-C level is above target in high-risk or moderately high-risk groups, including patients who have CHD or CHD equivalents and those who have two or more risk factors and a 10-year risk score between 10% and 20%. For the other patients at low or moderately low risk, medical treatment should be initiated together with therapeutic lifestyle changes if the LDL-C level is more than 30 mg/dL above the target. For patients who have an LDL-C level less than 30 mg/dL above the target, therapeutic lifestyle changes alone may be adequate to lower the cholesterol into the target range, obviating the need for drug therapy. The 2004 NCEP update states that drug therapy to obtain a 30% reduction in LDL-C level from baseline can be considered even when the LDL-C level is less than 30 mg/dL above the target.[9] Once the LDL-C goal is reached, the non-HDL-C goal, which is 30 mg/dL above the LDL-C goal, and the HDL-C (> 40 mg/dL) and triglyceride (< 150 mg/dL) goals can be targeted (see **Table 2**).

STATINS

Before the introduction of the 3-hydroxy-3-methylglutaryl-coenzyme A (HMG-CoA) reductase inhibitors or "statins," lowering LDL-C often was difficult because of the

Table 2
National Cholesterol Education Program Adult Treatment Panel III guidelines for LDL-C reduction

Risk Factor	Target LDL-C (mg/dL)	Target Non–HDL-C (mg/dL)	LDL-C Threshold for Therapeutic Lifestyle Changes (mg/dL)	LDL-C Threshold for Drug Therapy (mg/dL)
Coronary heart disease or equivalent	<100 or <70 if very high-risk	<130	$\geq$ 100	$\geq$ 100 (<100 optional)
Two or more risk factors (10-year risk $\leq$ 20%)	<130	<160	$\geq$ 130	10-year risk 10%–20%: $\geq$ 130 (100–129 optional drug treatment)10-year risk <10%: $\geq$ 160
0–1 risk factor	<160	<190	$\geq$ 160	$\geq$ 190 (160–189 optional)

Data from Expert Panel on Detection, Evaluation and Treatment of High Blood Cholesterol in Adults. Executive summary of the third report of the National Cholesterol Education Program (NCEP) Expert Panel on Detection, Evaluation, and Treatment of High Blood Cholesterol in Adults (Adult Treatment Panel III). JAMA 2001;285(19):2486–97; Grundy SM, Cleeman JI, Merz CN, et al. Implications of recent clinical trials for the national cholesterol education program adult treatment panel III guidelines. Circulation 2004;110(2):227–39.

overall poor tolerability or insufficient efficacy of the available therapies. The development and marketing of the statins allowed greater reductions of LDL-C and with greater ease than with previous drugs. The large clinical trials using statins in a variety of patients for both primary and secondary prevention of cardiovascular events contributed to evidence-based clinical guidelines. The NCEP ATP III guidelines emphasize the importance of the statins in the therapeutic armamentarium for the management of lipid disorders.

Numerous event trials using statin therapy have shown a beneficial effect on rates of cardiovascular events for both primary and secondary prevention and in a wide variety of patients.[11] Early trials in patients who had pre-existing coronary heart disease include the Cholesterol and Recurrent Events Study (CARE) using pravastatin[6] and the Scandinavian Simvastatin Survival Study (4S).[4] Because the primary end point for the 4S was total mortality, the positive outcome of this study had a significant influence on the perception of the benefit of lowering the LDL-C level.[12]

This benefit also extends to patients who have a relatively low baseline LDL-C level. In the Heart Protection Study, simvastatin decreased the first occurrence of a major vascular event by 24% in high-risk patients even when the LDL-C level was below 3.0 mmol/L (116 mg/dL).[13] Evidence for lower LDL-C targets came from the Pravastatin or Atorvastatin Evaluation and Infection Therapy Study (PROVE-IT) showing a benefit of atorvastatin, 80 mg/d, compared with pravastatin, 40 mg/d, in patients who had acute coronary syndromes[14] and from the Treating to New Targets (TNT) study comparing atorvastatin, 80 mg versus 10 mg, in patients who had stable coronary disease.[15]

Clinical trials designed for primary prevention, such as the West of Scotland study,[5] the Air Force/Texas Coronary Atherosclerosis Protection study,[7] and the Collaborative Atorvastatin Diabetes Study (CARDS),[16] demonstrated the benefits of lowering LDL-C in decreasing the incidence of coronary artery events in patients who did not have a history of CHD but who had high LDL-C levels, low HDL-C levels, and type 2 diabetes, respectively.

Clinical trials with statins have shown an effect on the progression of atherosclerosis. In an uncontrolled study, rosuvastatin was associated with a 6.8% reduction in total atheroma volume as determined by intravascular ultrasound.[17] In the Reversal of Atherosclerosis with Aggressive Lipid Lowering trial, treatment with atorvastatin, 80 mg/d, (mean on-treatment LDL-C level, 79 mg/dL) was associated with no progression of coronary artery disease, whereas patients treated with pravastatin, 40 mg/d, (mean on-treatment LDL-C, 110 mg/dL) showed progression of disease.[18]

Mechanism of Action

The statins work by inhibiting HMG-CoA reductase, which catalyzes the conversion of the substrate, HMG-CoA, to mevalonate; this reaction is an early and rate-limiting step in the biosynthesis of cholesterol.[19] Structurally, the statins are similar to HMG-CoA and occupy a portion of the active binding site on the enzyme, blocking access of the substrate to the binding site.[20] This competitive inhibition leads to decreased production of cholesterol and thus to a decrease of intracellular cholesterol levels, causing up-regulation of LDL receptors and a reduction in LDL-C levels because of the increased clearance by the LDL receptor.[21] Statins also reduce the release of lipoproteins from the liver into the circulation.[22,23] At high doses, statins decrease triglyceride levels through the clearance of very low-density lipoprotein (VLDL) as well as by decreasing the production of lipoproteins.[24,25]

Indications for Use

Because the statins are the most potent drugs for lowering LDL-C, they are useful in all types of hyperlipidemia in which LDL-C is elevated, although they are less effective in homozygous LDL receptor deficiency. They are particularly useful for patients who have vascular disease or very high levels of LDL-C, such as familial hypercholesterolemia or combined hyperlipidemia, and are the drugs of choice for lowering LDL-C in secondary prevention. Several statins are approved for use in children and adolescents who have high or very high LDL-C levels.

Dosing and Efficacy

Table 3 lists the available statins, their dose ranges, and their effects on lipids. **Table 4** shows effects on LDL-C level by statin and dose. All the statins are similar in mechanism of action and side effects. They reduce LDL-C by 20% to 60%, increase HDL-C by 2% to 16%, and reduce triglycerides by 7% to 37%, depending on the drug, the dosage, and, in the case of triglycerides, baseline levels.[26] The effects also vary among patients; some may have greater and others have lesser LDL-C reductions at the same dosage. For each statin, each doubling of the dose typically produces an additional 6% further reduction of LDL-C.[27] LDL-C lowering is seen within 1 to 2 weeks after the start of therapy and is stable in about 4 to 6 weeks. Atorvastatin and rosuvastatin have long half-lives, about 14 hours and 21 hours, respectively. The other statins have half-lives of about 2 to 3 hours. Fluvastatin and lovastatin are available in extended-release preparations. Atorvastatin and fluvastatin have minimal renal clearance and may be more suitable for patients who have significant renal insufficiency.

Lovastatin is best taken with food, usually with the evening meal, but pravastatin, simvastatin, and fluvastatin can be taken without food, preferably in the evening.

Table 3
Dose ranges and efficacy of statins, ezetimibe, and bile acid sequestrants

Drug	Dose Range	Effect on LDL-C (% Decrease)	Effect on HDL-C (% Increase)	Effect on Triglycerides (% Decrease)
Statins				
Fluvastatin	20–80 mg	22–35	3–11	17–21
Pravastatin	10–80 mg	22–37	2–12	15–24
Lovastatin	10–80 mg	21–42	2–8	6–21
Simvastatin	5–80 mg	26–47	10–16	12–33
Atorvastatin	10–80 mg	39–60	5–9	19–37
Rosuvastatin	5–40 mg	45–63	8–10	10–30
Ezetimibe	10 mg	14–25	1	7–9
Bile acid sequestrants				
Cholestyramine	4–24 g	9–26	2–8	Increase 10–28
Colestipol	5–30 g (powder) 2–16 g (tablet)	10–29	3–10	Increase 7–25
Colesevelam	3.75–4.38 g (6–7 tablets)	10–25	3–10	Increase 10–25

Data from Refs. [49,50,52,55,56,66,67,89–94]

Table 4
Typical LDL-C reductions (% change from baseline) by statin dose

Drug	Reduction by Dose (% Change from Baseline)				
	5 mg	10 mg	20 mg	40 mg	80 mg
Rosuvastatin	−40	−46	−52	−55	—
Atorvastatin	—	−37	−43	−48	−51
Simvastatin	−26	−30	−38	−41	−47
Lovastatin	—	−21	−27	−31	−40
Pravastatin	—	−20	−24	−30	−36
Fluvastatin	—	—	−22	−25	−35
Ezetimibe/simvastatin	—	−45 (10/10)	−52 (10/20)	−55 (10/40)	−60 (10/80)

Data from Refs. [89–91,93–96]

Atorvastatin, rosuvastatin, and extended-release formulations of statins can be given at any time during the day. Lovastatin, simvastatin, and pravastatin are available as generic drugs in the United States. **Table 5** gives the specific features of the available statins.

Adverse Effects

The most common side effects of statins include abdominal pain, constipation, flatulence, nausea, headache, fatigue, diarrhea, and muscle complaints. Except for musculoskeletal symptoms, most side effects are infrequent, occurring in only about

Table 5
Features of individual statins

Drug	Pharmacologic Considerations	Safety Issues
Fluvastatin	Synthetic drug; minimal renal excretion	Can interact with warfarin, phenytoin, glyburide, diclofenac, fluconazole, ketoconazole
Pravastatin	Derived from fermentation product of *Aspergillus terreus*; dose reduction in renal insufficiency	Drug interaction with cyclosporine
Lovastatin	First statin marketed in United States; isolated from a strain of *Aspergillus terreus*; food intake increases absorption	Interactions with CYP3A4 substrates
Simvastatin	Synthetic derivative of fermentation product of *Aspergillus terreus*; dose reduction in severe renal insufficiency	Interactions with CYP3A4 substrates
Atorvastatin	Synthetic drug; less than 2% excreted in urine; half-life 14 hours	Interacts with CYP3A4 substrates; increases digoxin levels
Rosuvastatin	Synthetic compound; CYP450: 2C9, active metabolite	Can increase international normalized ratio (INR); monitor INR when used with warfarin

Data from Refs. [89–94,97,98]

5% of patients. The adverse effects associated with statin use correlate with drug dose.[28,29] For example, in the TNT study, atorvastatin, 80 mg, compared with 10 mg, was associated with a higher rate of premature discontinuation (7.2% versus 5.3%; $P < .001$).[15]

Although liver toxicity frequently is a concern for patients and physicians, it is not common with statin use. Hepatic aminotransferase elevation usually is mild and does not require discontinuation of the statin. It may be dose dependent, as demonstrated in the TNT study, in which persistent liver aminotransferase elevation occurred in a higher proportion of patients receiving atorvastatin, 80 mg, than in those receiving 10 mg (1.2% versus 0.2%; $P <.001$).[15] In the Expanded Clinical Evaluation of Lovastatin study, the cumulative incidence of consecutive aminotransferase elevations of greater than three times the upper limit of normal was 0.1% in both the placebo and lovastatin 20-mg/d groups, 0.9% in patients receiving lovastatin, 40 mg/d, and 1.9% in those receiving lovastatin, 80 mg/d.[30]

Thus, with the statins, only about 1% of patients have aminotransferase increases to greater than three times the upper limit of normal, and the elevation often decreases even when patients continue taking the statin.[31] A common cause of this elevation is fatty liver, which responds well to weight loss. Caution may be required in patients who have active liver infection or severe liver disease, although nonalcoholic fatty liver is not a contraindication.[32] Usual practice is to obtain baseline hepatic function tests and then to measure aminotransferases at 6 and 12 weeks. If serum aminotransferases remain elevated, it is reasonable to consider changing to a different statin or to look for other conditions or drugs that may contribute to the elevation. The routine monitoring of liver function tests in patients taking statins has been questioned, because irreversible liver damage resulting from statins is extremely rare. The Liver Expert Panel of the National Lipid Association's Statin Safety Task Force has recommended that regulatory agencies re-examine requirements for routine monitoring of liver enzymes in patients taking currently marketed statins.[32]

Muscle-related complaints occur in about 10% of patients who take statins and are the most common reason for statin discontinuation.[33,34] Patients often complain of diffuse muscle aches, soreness, or weakness that improve with discontinuation of statins. Of note, other causes of myopathy, such as hypothyroidism, vitamin D deficiency, rheumatologic conditions, or concomitant use of drugs that are metabolized through the CYP 450 system (eg, ketoconazole, itraconazole, clarithromycin, or erythromycin, among others), must be excluded.[35] Rhabdomyolysis is rare and is more likely to occur in patients who have renal insufficiency, advanced age, other coexisting acute illness, or polypharmacy.[36] (See the article by Venero and Thompson in this issue for a more detailed discussion of statin myopathy and drug interactions.)

There is no evidence that statins have direct adverse effects on renal function outside of that caused by rhabdomyolysis.[37] There has been some concern about proteinuria with rosuvastatin because of results with the 80-mg dose in early efficacy studies. Because of this concern and higher rates of myopathy with the 80-mg dose, the maximum labeled dose of rosuvastatin is 40 mg/d. Dipstick-positive proteinuria did not differ significantly among all patients taking 5 mg (0.2%), 10 mg (0.6%), or 40 mg (0.7%) of rosuvastatin or placebo (0.6%). The cause of the proteinuria is thought to be related to reduced tubular absorption rather than impaired glomerular filtration.[38] The proteinuria is transient and reversible. Studies of at least 96 weeks' duration did not reveal any deterioration in renal function regardless of the baseline glomerular filtration rate.[38]

Statins are contraindicated in pregnant women, nursing mothers, and patients who have significant hepatic dysfunction.

BILE ACID SEQUESTRANTS

BAS have been in use since the 1970s. Three BAS are on the market in the United States: cholestyramine, the first available BAS; colestipol, which became available in the early 1970s; and colesevelam, approved by the Food and Drug Administration in 2000. In randomized trials, BAS have been shown to inhibit atherogenesis and reduce cardiovascular events. The most significant outcome trial was the Lipid Research Clinics Coronary Primary Prevention Trial (LRC-CPPT), in which 3806 men age 35 to 59 years who had elevated total cholesterol levels but no evident CHD were assigned randomly to therapy with cholestyramine at its maximum dosage of 24 g/d or placebo. The primary outcome of combined CHD death and nonfatal myocardial infarction was reduced significantly, by 19%.[3,39] In other trials involving BAS alone or in combination with other agents, cholestyramine and colestipol have shown beneficial effects on coronary disease.[40–44]

Mechanism of Action

BAS are large polymers that bind negatively charged bile acids and bile salts in the small intestine. This binding interrupts the enterohepatic circulation of bile acids, leading to increased conversion of cholesterol into bile within the liver.[45,46] The resulting decreased hepatocyte cholesterol content promotes an increase in LDL receptors and increased clearance of LDL from the circulation.[47] Hepatic synthesis of cholesterol also increases, causing increased secretion of VLDL into the circulation and limiting the LDL-lowering effect of the BAS as well as raising serum triglyceride levels.[48]

Efficacy of Bile Acid Sequestrants

The major effect of the bile acid sequestrants is the reduction of LDL-C levels with a corresponding decrease of total cholesterol. The HDL-C level may increase modestly by as much as 10%.[49] As monotherapy, BAS lower LDL-C by 5% to 30% in a dose-dependent manner (see **Table 3**).[39,50–54] The effect is seen within 2 to 4 weeks of the start of therapy and generally remains stable over time.[51,53,55,56] Colestipol tablets or granules lower LDL-C by 12% at a dose of 4 g/d and by 24% at 16 g/d.[55] The dose response seen in the LRC-CPPT for cholestyramine over the dose range of 4 to 24 g/d was a decrease in LDL-C ranging from 6.6% to 28.3%.[3,39]

Because colesevelam has greater bile acid–binding capacity and affinity than cholestyramine or colestipol, it can be used at lower doses than those used for the older BAS.[49,51] LDL-C reduction usually is about 15% at a dosage of 3.8 g/d (six 625-mg tablets) and 18% at a dosage of 4.3 g/d (seven 625-mg tablets).[50,53,57]

BAS can increase cholesterol synthesis by affecting HMG-CoA reductase. Use of an HMG-CoA reductase inhibitor or statin ameliorates this effect, leading to substantial LDL-C reductions when BAS are combined with statins. The statin decreases the rise of triglyceride levels that can occur with BAS, but the BAS also may decrease the amount of triglyceride reduction that can be seen with the more potent statins.

BAS are most useful in patients in whom an elevated LDL-C level is the major lipid abnormality. They can be combined with statins or niacin to achieve greater LDL-C reductions in patients who have severe LDL-C elevation or can be used alone for initial therapy in patients at low risk or in patients who cannot tolerate statins at any dose. Cholestyramine generally is used at a dosage of 4 to 24 g/d in the powder form, provided either in a bulk container, or in single-dose, 4-g packets. Colestipol is taken either at 5 to 30 g/d in its granular form or at 2 to 16 g/d as tablets. Single-dose packets of colestipol contain 5 g of granules. Colestipol comes in 1-g tablets, which are convenient: this formulation eliminates the need for suspending the granules in a liquid, but patients may need to take up to 16 tablets daily. BAS generally are dosed once or twice per day and need to be taken close to meals. Up to 8 to 12 g can be taken as a single-dose to be effective. Colesevelam is available in 625-mg tablets with a recommended dose of six tablets per day and a maximum dose of seven tablets a day.

BAS have been reported to lower fasting blood glucose and to decrease hemoglobin A1c in patients who have diabetes.[58]

Adverse Effects

BAS are large polymers that are neither absorbed nor metabolized by the intestine and thus have essentially no systemic exposure. Therefore they are extremely safe and can be used in women of childbearing potential who are not using contraception. The most common side effects are gastrointestinal disturbances, such as constipation, nausea, bloating, abdominal pain, flatulence, and aggravation of hemorrhoids. Constipation can occur in 25% of patients and can be severe. Initiation of therapy with low doses, patient education, and use of stool softeners or psyllium can increase compliance. Cholestyramine and colestipol can affect the absorption of a wide variety of drugs, including tetracycline, phenobarbital, digoxin, levothyroxine, beta-adrenergic blocking agents, cyclosporine, warfarin, pravastatin, fluvastatin, aspirin, and thiazide diuretics, among others. When used with these two BAS, other drugs should be taken either 1 to 2 hours before or 4 to 6 hours after the BAS. Compared with cholestyramine and colestipol, colesevelam is associated with fewer side effects and fewer drug interactions.[57,59]

BAS resins are not suitable for patients who have severe constipation. BAS are contraindicated in patients who have bowel obstruction or total biliary obstruction. Cholestyramine and colestipol can cause problems in patients who have complicated drug regimens involving drugs adsorbed by these BAS. BAS can worsen hypertriglyceridemia. They are contraindicated as monotherapy in patients who have high triglyceride levels (> 400 mg/dL) and in type III hyperlipoproteinemia (dysbetalipoproteinemia). Patients who have normal baseline triglyceride levels experience minimal triglyceride increases, but those who have baseline triglyceride levels higher than 200 mg/dL may experience substantial further elevation.[55,60]

There is a theoretic concern about the absorption of fat-soluble vitamins, but only rare cases of vitamin K deficiency and bleeding have been reported.[61]

EZETIMIBE

Ezetimibe is a cholesterol absorption inhibitor that is the first of its class to become available. It is used primarily as an addition to statins to produce additional LDL-C lowering. A recently reported study comparing the effect of the combination of ezetimibe plus simvastatin versus simvastatin alone on the progression of carotid intima medial thickness (cIMT) in patients who had familial hypercholesterolemia did not show a significant difference between the two groups.[62] The study may not have been designed adequately to show a benefit in these patients who had only modestly increased cIMT at baseline because of previous statin use in 80% and failure to exclude persons who had too thin cIMT at baseline. Large clinical event trials for ezetimibe are still in progress.

Mechanism of Action

Ezetimibe selectively inhibits cholesterol absorption from the brush border of the small intestine. It acts on the enterocytes and possibly interacts with the Niemann-Pick

C1-like protein 1 transporter to inhibit cholesterol transport into enterocytes.[63] The inhibition of absorption of cholesterol in the intestine, much from biliary cholesterol, leads to decreased hepatic cholesterol levels and increased clearance of LDL-C from the plasma and consequent reduction of the plasma LDL-C level. Ezetimibe undergoes glucuronidation in the intestine and extensive enterohepatic circulation.[64]

Indications for Use

Ezetimibe produces reductions of approximately 14% to 25% in LDL-C levels (see **Table 3**).[65–67] The effect is additive with statins. Ezetimibe is used as monotherapy as well as in combination with statins or other lipid-modifying drugs. It can be useful in patients who are intolerant of statins. It is available in 10-mg tablets. Absorption is not affected by food.[64]

Adverse Effects

Side effects of ezetimibe include diarrhea and possibly myalgias. Myopathy with ezetimibe is rare and is not related clearly to the medication.[68] Ezetimibe can increase cyclosporine levels. Gemfibrozil and fenofibrate can increase ezetimibe levels, although the significance of the increase is unknown.[69] Ezetimibe monotherapy does not cause significant increases in hepatic aminotransferases; there may be a small increased incidence of aminotransferase elevations when ezetimibe is combined with a statin, but these elevations have not been related to any clinical significance.[68] There are rare reports of angioedema and allergic reactions.[64]

Ezetimibe is contraindicated in pregnancy and in severe liver dysfunction.

COMBINATION THERAPY

Combination therapy is indicated in patients who have not reached desired goals with monotherapy.[70,71] Patients who have familial hypercholesterolemia or familial combined hyperlipidemia are at particularly increased risk and may require substantial LDL-C reductions that cannot be achieved with a single agent. Target LDL-C levels of less than 70 mg/dL can be difficult to achieve with a single drug. Maximum statin doses may be associated with an increase in frequency of tolerance problems, particularly myopathy. If the highest tolerated statin dose does not achieve the target LDL-C, adding a drug from a different class may produce the desired result. Because statins, ezetimibe, and bile acid–binding resins reduce LDL-C through different mechanisms and sites of action, they can be more effective in combination than when used alone. Advantages of using combination therapy include greater efficacy, lower doses of individual drugs, and possible amelioration of tolerance problems experienced with high doses of single agents. The disadvantages of combination therapy include increased drug interactions, large number of pills, increased cost, and additive side effects. Data on clinical outcomes with combination therapy are limited.

Statin Plus Bile Acid Sequestrants

All three of the available BAS have been studied in combination with different HMG-CoA reductase inhibitors. The decreases in LDL-C range from 24% to 60% depending on the dose of BAS and of the statin.[49,50,72–75] Because BAS can provide 10% to 25% further reduction of LDL when added to statins, their use can make it possible to reach LDL-C goals in patients who cannot tolerate high statin doses. For example, colesevelam, 3.8 g/d, plus atorvastatin, 10 mg/d, lowered LDL by 48% compared with a 53% reduction achieved with atorvastatin, 80 mg, alone.[76]

The advantages of the combination of these two types of medication are that drugs from both classes have been shown to decrease CHD event rates and that substantial LDL-C reductions can be achieved. Disadvantages include the use of granules requiring suspension in liquids or large numbers of pills with the BAS and the increased side effects from older BAS. Cholestyramine and colestipol can interfere with the absorption of statins if taken simultaneously, leading to a decrease in efficacy.[75] Colesevelam does not affect statin absorption. This combination may not be ideal in patients who have high triglyceride levels but may offer an advantage in patients who have type 2 diabetes mellitus because of the reduction in blood glucose and glycated hemoglobin.[58]

Statin and Ezetimibe

The addition of ezetimibe to a given dose of a statin may produce a further LDL-C reduction of 20% or more.[77–79] In addition, it produces an additional triglyceride reduction of 7% to 13% and an increase in the HDL-C level of 1% to 5%. This effect is more pronounced with higher doses of potent statins. The combination of rosuvastatin, 40 mg/d, plus ezetimibe, 10 mg/d, led to a mean LDL-C reduction of 69.8%, allowing 79.6% of a very high-risk population to reach an LDL-C goal of less than 70 mg/dL.[78] Ezetimibe can be added to a very low dose of statins given two to three times per week to improve tolerance. A combination of simvastatin and ezetimibe exists as a commercially available pill (Vytorin, Merck/Schering-Plough). The most common side effects reflect those of the individual drugs: myalgias, gastrointestinal complaints, and transaminase elevation. The ease of use of the statin-ezetimibe combination and the usual minimal incidence of side effects make this combination a convenient approach to obtain substantial LDL-C reductions. The primary disadvantage is the lack of clinical outcomes data for ezetimibe and statin-ezetimibe combinations.

Statin Plus Niacin

Adding niacin to a statin can lower the LDL-C level by a further 10% to 20%, depending on the dose of niacin. The combination decreases LDL-C and triglyceride levels and raises the HDL-C level more than the statin alone.[80–82] The HDL-Atherosclerosis Treatment Study showed regression of atherosclerosis by coronary angiography and a decreased incidence of cardiovascular events in high-risk patients treated with simvastatin plus niacin, 2000 mg/d (with a possible dose increase to 4000 mg/d).[80] There was a 42% reduction in LDL-C level, a 36% decrease in triglyceride, and a 26% increase in HDL-C level from baseline in patients treated with this combination.

When used in combination with a statin, the maximum dose of niacin should be 2000 mg/d. Fixed-dose combinations of extended-release niacin with lovastatin (Advicor, Abbott) and simvastatin (Simcor, Abbott) are available.

The side effects of the combination of niacin with a statin are flushing, hyperglycemia, elevation of uric acid, myopathy, and hepatotoxicity. Flushing is the major side effect, can be difficult to manage, and is the most common reason for drug discontinuation. Myopathy is infrequent when the dose of niacin is 2000 mg/d or less. The effect on glycemic control usually is minimal. There may be somewhat worse glycemic control in the first few months after initiation of niacin, but it generally returns to pretreatment levels and stabilizes thereafter.[83] Hepatotoxicity can occur; liver enzymes should be monitored periodically. Nausea, fatigue, and malaise can be signs of hepatotoxicity, and patients should be encouraged to report these symptoms to providers.

About 10% of patients treated with a lovastatin/niacin combination discontinued the treatment because of flushing. Other common side effects included pruritus (16%), rash (9%), and gastrointestinal side effects (24%).[81] Similar side effect profiles were seen in patients receiving a combination of fluvastatin and niacin; flushing was the most common side effect, reported by 60.5% of patients.[84]

Niacin should be avoided in patients who have a history of uncontrolled gout, active peptic ulcer disease, or liver disease. This combination is particularly useful in patients who need increases in the HDL-C level as well as reduction of the LDL-C level.

Statin Plus Fibrate

The addition of a fibrate to a statin can produce additional LDL-C lowering in some patients. Generally, this combination is used in patients with combined triglyceride and cholesterol elevations. The combination of statin and fibrate decreases triglycerides and increases HDL-C to a level greater than achieved with either agent alone and is useful for patients who have metabolic syndrome, diabetes, and other forms of mixed dyslipidemia. In patients who have high triglyceride levels, LDL-C levels may not be lower with combination therapy than with statin therapy alone,[85] either because of the increased metabolism of VLDL and consequently higher levels of LDL-C or because of an increase in size, and thus cholesterol content, of fewer LDL particles.

The incidence of myopathy, including rhabdomyolysis, is increased with the combination of most statins with gemfibrozil, because gemfibrozil interferes with the glucuronidation of statins and leads to higher serum levels of statins and increased side effects.[35] The reported rate of rhabdomyolysis is about 15 times lower with fenofibrate combined with all other statins (0.58 per million prescriptions) than with gemfibrozil plus statin combinations (8.6 per million prescriptions).[86]

The fibrate-statin combination should be avoided in patients who have renal insufficiency, congestive heart failure, severe debility, or other conditions that may affect the metabolism of the medications. Side effects primarily include mild gastrointestinal discomfort and, less frequently, rash and pruritus. Mild aminotransferase elevation occurs in 5% of the patents and returns to normal after drug discontinuation. Rarely, myalgias and increased creatinine phosphokinase levels are reported.

Bile Acid Sequestration Plus Niacin Combination

Before the introduction of the statins, the combination of a BAS plus high doses of niacin was used to achieve substantial LDL-C reductions, particularly in high-risk patients. The Cholesterol Lowering Atherosclerosis Study used a combination of colestipol, 30 g/d, and niacin, 4.3 g/d. This combination was associated with decreased progression and increased regression of coronary artery atherosclerosis compared with placebo.[42] In the Familial Atherosclerosis Treatment Study, the combinations of lovastatin, 40 mg/d, with colestipol, 30 g/d, and niacin, 4 g/d, plus colestipol, 30 g/d, produced greater regression and decreased progression of atherosclerosis as well as fewer clinical events compared with conventional therapy (diet and colestipol).[43]

With older preparations of the BAS plus crystalline niacin, obtaining good patient compliance with therapy often was challenging. The availability of colesevelam and extended-release niacin has made this combination tolerable and useful for many patients who are unable to use statins.

Ezetimibe with Bile Acid–Binding Resins

Ezetimibe and BAS can have additive effects on LDL-C reduction. Ezetimibe inhibits cholesterol absorption, whereas bile acid–binding resins enhance cholesterol excretion via enhanced conversion to bile acids. The combination of colesevelam, 3.8 g/d, with ezetimibe, 10 mg, lowered LDL-C by 32% from baseline, whereas a 21% reduction was achieved with ezetimibe monotherapy.[87] This combination is useful for patients who do not tolerate a statin at any dose or for whom statins are contraindicated.

Statin/Resin/Niacin or Statin/Ezetimibe/Niacin Combinations

The combination of three medications can be useful in high-risk patients who have very high levels of LDL-C in order to achieve a maximum reduction of LDL-C. This approach may be necessary in patients who have familial hypercholesterolemia and baseline LDL-C levels greater than 250 mg/dL. Kane and colleagues[44] evaluated a combination of lovastatin, niacin, and colestipol versus diet alone in patients and familial hypercholesterolemia and very high LDL-C levels, studied in the University of California, San Francisco Specialized Center of Research study. Angiographic evidence of regression of atherosclerotic lesions occurred in the drug combination group compared with evidence of progression in the diet-only group.

In a study evaluating the safety and lipid-altering efficacy of the combination of ezetimibe, 10 mg, simvastatin, 20 mg, and extended-release niacin, 2 g/d, LDL-C was reduced by 58% from baseline. The HDL-C level increased by 30%, and triglycerides decreased by 42%. The main reason for discontinuation from the study was flushing.[88]

Four-Drug Combination

Occasionally four drugs may be necessary to obtain adequate LDL-C reduction in patients who have familial hypercholesterolemia. Various combinations of statin, BAS, niacin, and ezetimibe have been used in practice, but clinical studies are lacking.

SUMMARY

Elevated LDL-C is associated with increased cardiovascular mortality and morbidity. Statins, ezetimibe, and BAS resins are all effective drugs for lowering LDL-C. Statins and BAS have been shown to reduce the rates of occurrence of cardiovascular events and cardiovascular mortality and morbidity. Statins are the most potent drugs for lowering LDL-C and are well tolerated in most patients. The addition of BAS or ezetimibe to a statin produces additional LDL-C reduction, allowing many patients to reach LDL-C targets. Other combinations including niacin and fibrates may also be useful, particularly in patients who have combined lipid abnormalities.

REFERENCES

1. Kannel WB. Lipids, diabetes, and coronary heart disease: insights from the Framingham study. Am Heart J 1985;110(5):1100–7.
2. Stamler J, Vaccaro O, Neaton JD, et al. Diabetes, other risk factors, and 12-yr cardiovascular mortality for men screened in the Multiple Risk Factor Intervention trial. Diabetes Care 1993;16(2):434–44.
3. The Lipid Research Clinics Coronary Primary Prevention Trial results. I. Reduction in incidence of coronary heart disease. JAMA 1984;251(3):351–64.
4. Randomised trial of cholesterol lowering in 4444 patients with coronary heart disease: the Scandinavian Simvastatin Survival Study (4S). Lancet 1994; 344(8934):1383–9.
5. Shepherd J, Cobbe SM, Ford I, et al. Prevention of coronary heart disease with pravastatin in men with hypercholesterolemia. West of Scotland Coronary Prevention Study Group. N Engl J Med 1995;333(20):1301–7.
6. Sacks FM, Pfeffer MA, Moye LA, et al. The effect of pravastatin on coronary events after myocardial infarction in patients with average cholesterol levels.

Cholesterol and Recurrent Events Trial investigators. N Engl J Med 1996;335(14): 1001–9.

7. Downs JR, Clearfield M, Weis S, et al. Primary prevention of acute coronary events with lovastatin in men and women with average cholesterol levels: results of AFCAPS/TexCAPS. Air Force/Texas Coronary Atherosclerosis Prevention Study. JAMA 1998;279(20):1615–22.

8. Expert Panel on Detection, Evaluation and Treatment of High Blood Cholesterol in Adults. Executive summary of the third report of the National Cholesterol Education Program (NCEP) Expert Panel on Detection, Evaluation, and Treatment of High Blood Cholesterol in Adults (Adult Treatment Panel III). JAMA 2001; 285(19):2486–97.

9. Grundy SM, Cleeman JI, Merz CN, et al. Implications of recent clinical trials for the National Cholesterol Education Program Adult Treatment Panel III guidelines. Circulation 2004;110(2):227–39.

10. American Diabetes Association. Standards of medical care in diabetes–2008. Diabetes Care 2008;31:S12–54.

11. Baigent C, Keech A, Kearney PM, et al. Efficacy and safety of cholesterol-lowering treatment: prospective meta-analysis of data from 90,056 participants in 14 randomised trials of statins. Lancet 2005;366(9493):1267–78.

12. Steinberg D. Thematic review series: the pathogenesis of atherosclerosis. An interpretive history of the cholesterol controversy, part V: the discovery of the statins and the end of the controversy. J Lipid Res 2006;47(7):1339–51.

13. Heart Protection Study Collaborative Group. MRC/BHF Heart Protection Study of cholesterol lowering with simvastatin in 20,536 high-risk individuals: a randomised placebo-controlled trial. Lancet 2002;360(9326):7–22.

14. Cannon CP, Braunwald E, McCabe CH, et al. Intensive versus moderate lipid lowering with statins after acute coronary syndromes. N Engl J Med 2004; 350(15):1495–504.

15. LaRosa JC, Grundy SM, Waters DD, et al. Intensive lipid lowering with atorvastatin in patients with stable coronary disease. N Engl J Med 2005;352(14):1425–35.

16. Colhoun HM, Betteridge DJ, Durrington PN, et al. Primary prevention of cardiovascular disease with atorvastatin in type 2 diabetes in the Collaborative Atorvastatin Diabetes Study (CARDS): multicentre randomised placebo-controlled trial. Lancet 2004;364(9435):685–96.

17. Nissen SE, Nicholls SJ, Sipahi I, et al. Effect of very high-intensity statin therapy on regression of coronary atherosclerosis: the ASTEROID trial. JAMA 2006; 295(13):1556–65.

18. Nissen SE, Tuzcu EM, Schoenhagen P, et al. Effect of intensive compared with moderate lipid-lowering therapy on progression of coronary atherosclerosis: a randomized controlled trial. JAMA 2004;291(9):1071–80.

19. Endo A. The discovery and development of HMG-CoA reductase inhibitors. J Lipid Res 1992;33(11):1569–82.

20. Istvan ES, Deisenhofer J. Structural mechanism for statin inhibition of HMG-CoA reductase. Science 2001;292(5519):1160–4.

21. Bilheimer DW, Grundy SM, Brown MS, et al. Mevinolin stimulates receptor-mediated clearance of low density lipoprotein from plasma in familial hypercholesterolemia heterozygotes. Trans Assoc Am Physicians 1983;96:1–9.

22. Arad Y, Ramakrishnan R, Ginsberg HN. Lovastatin therapy reduces low density lipoprotein apoB levels in subjects with combined hyperlipidemia by reducing the production of apoB-containing lipoproteins: implications for the pathophysiology of apoB production. J Lipid Res 1990;31(4):567–82.

23. Arad Y, Ramakrishnan R, Ginsberg HN. Effects of lovastatin therapy on very-low-density lipoprotein triglyceride metabolism in subjects with combined hyperlipidemia: evidence for reduced assembly and secretion of triglyceride-rich lipoproteins. Metabolism 1992;41(5):487–93.

24. Forster LF, Stewart G, Bedford D, et al. Influence of atorvastatin and simvastatin on apolipoprotein B metabolism in moderate combined hyperlipidemic subjects with low VLDL and LDL fractional clearance rates. Atherosclerosis 2002;164(1):129–45.

25. Ooi EMM, Barrett PHR, Chan DC, et al. Dose-dependent effect of rosuvastatin on apolipoprotein B-100 kinetics in the metabolic syndrome. Atherosclerosis 2008;197(1):139–46.

26. Davidson MH, Stein EA, Dujovne CA, et al. The efficacy and six-week tolerability of simvastatin 80 and 160 mg/day. Am J Cardiol 1997;79(1):38–42.

27. Knopp RH. Drug treatment of lipid disorders. N Engl J Med 1999;341(7):498–511.

28. Bays H. Statin safety: an overview and assessment of the data—2005. Am J Cardiol 2006;97(8A):6C–26C.

29. Jacobson TA. Statin safety: lessons from new drug applications for marketed statins. Am J Cardiol 2006;97(8A):44C–51C.

30. Bradford RH, Shear CL, Chremos AN, et al. Expanded Clinical Evaluation of Lovastatin (EXCEL) study results: two-year efficacy and safety follow-up. Am J Cardiol 1994;74(7):667–73.

31. Kashani A, Phillips CO, Foody JM, et al. Risks associated with statin therapy: a systematic overview of randomized clinical trials. Circulation 2006;114(25):2788–97.

32. Cohen DE, Anania FA, Chalasani N. An assessment of statin safety by hepatologists. Am J Cardiol 2006;97(8A):77C–81C.

33. Bruckert E, Hayem G, Dejager S, et al. Mild to moderate muscular symptoms with high-dosage statin therapy in hyperlipidemic patients—the PRIMO study. Cardiovasc Drugs Ther 2005;19(6):403–14.

34. Thompson PD, Clarkson PM, Rosenson RS. An assessment of statin safety by muscle experts. Am J Cardiol 2006;97(8A):69C–76C.

35. Bottorff MB. Statin safety and drug interactions: clinical implications. Am J Cardiol 2006;97(8A):27C–31C.

36. Pasternak RC, Smith SC Jr, Bairey-Merz CN, et al. ACC/AHA/NHLBI clinical advisory on the use and safety of statins. Circulation 2002;106(8):1024–8.

37. Kasiske BL, Wanner C, O'Neill WC. National Lipid Association Statin Safety Task Force Kidney Expert Panel. An assessment of statin safety by nephrologists. Am J Cardiol 2006;97(8A):82C–5C.

38. Shepherd J, Hunninghake DB, Stein EA, et al. Safety of rosuvastatin. Am J Cardiol 2004;94(7):882–8.

39. The Lipid Research Clinics Coronary Primary Prevention Trial results. II. The relationship of reduction in incidence of coronary heart disease to cholesterol lowering. JAMA 1984;251(3):365–74.

40. Levy RI, Brensike JF, Epstein SE, et al. The influence of changes in lipid values induced by cholestyramine and diet on progression of coronary artery disease: results of NHLBI type II coronary intervention study. Circulation 1984;69(2):325–37.

41. Watts GF, Lewis B, Brunt JN, et al. Effects on coronary artery disease of lipid-lowering diet, or diet plus cholestyramine, in the St Thomas' Atherosclerosis Regression Study (STARS). Lancet 1992;339(8793):563–9.

42. Blankenhorn DH, Nessim SA, Johnson RL, et al. Beneficial effects of combined colestipol-niacin therapy on coronary atherosclerosis and coronary venous bypass grafts. JAMA 1987;257(23):3233–40.

43. Brown G, Albers JJ, Fisher LD, et al. Regression of coronary artery disease as a result of intensive lipid-lowering therapy in men with high levels of apolipoprotein B. N Engl J Med 1990;323(19):1289–98.

44. Kane JP, Malloy MJ, Ports TA, et al. Regression of coronary atherosclerosis during treatment of familial hypercholesterolemia with combined drug regimens. JAMA 1990;264(23):3007–12.

45. Grundy SM, Ahrens EH Jr, Salen G. Interruption of the enterohepatic circulation of bile acids in man: comparative effects of cholestyramine and ileal exclusion on cholesterol metabolism. J Lab Clin Med 1971;78(1):94–121.

46. Shepherd J, Packard CJ, Bicker S, et al. Cholestyramine promotes receptor-mediated low-density-lipoprotein catabolism. N Engl J Med 1980;302(22):1219–22.

47. Rudling MJ, Reihner E, Einarsson K, et al. Low density lipoprotein receptor-binding activity in human tissues: quantitative importance of hepatic receptors and evidence for regulation of their expression in vivo. Proc Nat Acad Sci USA 1990;87(9):3469–73.

48. Beil U, Crouse JR, Einarsson K, et al. Effects of interruption of the enterohepatic circulation of bile acids on the transport of very low density-lipoprotein triglycerides. Metabolism 1982;31(5):438–44.

49. Insull W Jr. Clinical utility of bile acid sequestrants in the treatment of dyslipidemia: a scientific review. South Med J 2006;99(3):257–73.

50. Aldridge MA, Ito MK. Colesevelam hydrochloride: a novel bile acid-binding resin. Ann Pharmacother 2001;35(7–8):898–907.

51. Davidson MH, Dillon MA, Gordon B, et al. Colesevelam hydrochloride (Cholestagel): a new, potent bile acid sequestrant associated with a low incidence of gastrointestinal side effects. Arch Intern Med 1999;159(16):1893–900.

52. Hunninghake DB, Bell C, Olson L. Effect of colestipol and clofibrate, singly and in combination, on plasma lipid and lipoproteins in type IIb hyperlipoproteinemia. Metabolism 1981;30(6):610–5.

53. Insull W Jr, Toth P, Mullican W, et al. Effectiveness of colesevelam hydrochloride in decreasing LDL cholesterol in patients with primary hypercholesterolemia: a 24-week randomized controlled trial. Mayo Clin Proc 2001;76(10):971–82.

54. Lyons D, Webster J, Fowler G, et al. Colestipol at varying dosage intervals in the treatment of moderate hypercholesterolaemia. Br J Clin Pharmacol 1994;37(1):59–62.

55. Insull W Jr, Davidson MH, Demke DM, et al. The effects of colestipol tablets compared with colestipol granules on plasma cholesterol and other lipids in moderately hypercholesterolemic patients. Atherosclerosis 1995;112(2):223–35.

56. Vecchio TJ, Linden CV, O'Connell MJ, et al. Comparative efficacy of colestipol and clofibrate in type IIa hyperlipoproteinemia. Arch Intern Med 1982;142(4):721–3.

57. Davidson MH, Dicklin MR, Maki KC, et al. Colesevelam hydrochloride: a non-absorbed, polymeric cholesterol-lowering agent. Expert Opin Investig Drugs 2000;9(11):2663–71.

58. Zieve FJ, Kalin MF, Schwartz SL, et al. Results of the Glucose-Lowering Effect of Welchol Study (GLOWS): a randomized, double-blind, placebo-controlled pilot study evaluating the effect of colesevelam hydrochloride on glycemic control in subjects with type 2 diabetes. Clin Ther 2007;29(1):74–83.

59. Donovan JM, Stypinski D, Stiles MR, et al. Drug interactions with colesevelam hydrochloride, a novel, potent lipid-lowering agent. Cardiovasc Drugs Ther 2000;14(6):681–90.

60. Crouse JR 3rd. Hypertriglyceridemia: a contraindication to the use of bile acid binding resins. Am J Med 1987;83(2):243–8.
61. Vroonhof K, van Rijn HJM, van Hattum J. Vitamin K deficiency and bleeding after long-term use of cholestyramine. Neth J Med 2003;61(1):19–21.
62. Kastelein JJP, Akdim F, Stroes ESG, et al. Simvastatin with or without ezetimibe in familial hypercholesterolemia. N Engl J Med 2008;358(14):1431–43.
63. Altmann SW, Davis HR Jr, Zhu LJ, et al. Niemann-Pick C1 like 1 protein is critical for intestinal cholesterol absorption. Science 2004;303(5661):1201–4.
64. Merck/Schering-Plough. Zetia (ezetimibe) U.S. prescribing information. Available at: http://www.zetia.com/zetia/shared/documents/zetia_pi.pdf. Accessed August 10, 2008.
65. Davis HR, Veltri EP. Zetia: inhibition of Niemann-Pick C1 like 1 (NPC1L1) to reduce intestinal cholesterol absorption and treat hyperlipidemia. J Atheroscler Thromb 2007;14(3):99–108.
66. Dujovne CA, Ettinger MP, McNeer JF, et al. Efficacy and safety of a potent new selective cholesterol absorption inhibitor, ezetimibe, in patients with primary hypercholesterolemia. Am J Cardiol 2002;90(10):1092–7.
67. Knopp RH, Gitter H, Truitt T, et al. Effects of ezetimibe, a new cholesterol absorption inhibitor, on plasma lipids in patients with primary hypercholesterolemia. Eur Heart J 2003;24(8):729–41.
68. Jacobson TA, Armani A, McKenney JM, et al. Safety considerations with gastro-intestinally active lipid-lowering drugs. Am J Cardiol 2007;99(6A):47C–55C.
69. Neuvonen PJ, Niemi M, Backman JT. Drug interactions with lipid-lowering drugs: mechanisms and clinical relevance. Clin Pharmacol Ther 2006;80(6):565–81.
70. Pearson TA, Laurora I, Chu H, et al. The lipid treatment assessment project (L-TAP): a multicenter survey to evaluate the percentages of dyslipidemic patients receiving lipid-lowering therapy and achieving low-density lipoprotein cholesterol goals. Arch Intern Med 2000;160(4):459–67.
71. Davidson MH, Toth PP. Combination therapy in the management of complex dyslipidemias. Curr Opin Lipidol 2004;15(4):423–31.
72. Davidson MH, Toth P, Weiss S, et al. Low-dose combination therapy with colesevelam hydrochloride and lovastatin effectively decreases low-density lipoprotein cholesterol in patients with primary hypercholesterolemia. Clin Cardiol 2001; 24(6):467–74.
73. Denke MA, Grundy SM. Efficacy of low-dose cholesterol-lowering drug therapy in men with moderate hypercholesterolemia. Arch Intern Med 1995;155(4):393–9.
74. Knapp HH, Schrott H, Ma P, et al. Efficacy and safety of combination simvastatin and colesevelam in patients with primary hypercholesterolemia. Am J Med 2001; 110(5):352–60.
75. Pan HY, DeVault AR, Swites BJ, et al. Pharmacokinetics and pharmacodynamics of pravastatin alone and with cholestyramine in hypercholesterolemia. Clin Pharmacol Ther 1990;48(2):201–7.
76. Hunninghake D, Insull W Jr, Toth P, et al. Coadministration of colesevelam hydrochloride with atorvastatin lowers LDL cholesterol additively. Atherosclerosis 2001; 158(2):407–16.
77. Ballantyne CM, Houri J, Notarbartolo A, et al. Effect of ezetimibe coadministered with atorvastatin in 628 patients with primary hypercholesterolemia: a prospective, randomized, double-blind trial. Circulation 2003;107(19):2409–15.
78. Ballantyne CM, Weiss R, Moccetti T, et al. Efficacy and safety of rosuvastatin 40 mg alone or in combination with ezetimibe in patients at high risk of cardiovascular disease (results from the EXPLORER study). Am J Cardiol 2007;99(5):673–80.

79. Goldberg AC, Sapre A, Liu J, et al. Efficacy and safety of ezetimibe coadminis-
    tered with simvastatin in patients with primary hypercholesterolemia: a random-
    ized, double-blind, placebo-controlled trial. Mayo Clin Proc 2004;79(5):620–9.
80. Brown BG, Zhao XQ, Chait A, et al. Simvastatin and niacin, antioxidant vitamins,
    or the combination for the prevention of coronary disease. N Engl J Med 2001;
    345(22):1583–92.
81. Kashyap ML, McGovern ME, Berra K, et al. Long-term safety and efficacy of
    a once-daily niacin/lovastatin formulation for patients with dyslipidemia. Am J
    Cardiol 2002;89(6):672–8.
82. McKenney JM, Jones PH, Bays HE, et al. Comparative effects on lipid levels of
    combination therapy with a statin and extended-release niacin or ezetimibe
    versus a statin alone (the COMPELL study). Atherosclerosis 2007;192(2):432–7.
83. Zhao XQ, Morse JS, Dowdy AA, et al. Safety and tolerability of simvastatin plus
    niacin in patients with coronary artery disease and low high-density lipoprotein
    cholesterol (The HDL Atherosclerosis Treatment study). Am J Cardiol 2004;
    93(3):307–12.
84. Jacobson TA, Amorosa LF. Combination therapy with fluvastatin and niacin in
    hypercholesterolemia: a preliminary report on safety. Am J Cardiol 1994;73(14):
    25D–9D.
85. Grundy SM, Vega GL, Yuan Z, et al. Effectiveness and tolerability of simvastatin
    plus fenofibrate for combined hyperlipidemia (the SAFARI trial). Am J Cardiol
    2005;95(4):462–8.
86. Jones PH, Davidson MH. Reporting rate of rhabdomyolysis with fenofibrate +
    statin versus gemfibrozil + any statin. Am J Cardiol 2005;95(1):120–2.
87. Bays H, Rhyne J, Abby S, et al. Lipid-lowering effects of colesevelam HCl in
    combination with ezetimibe. Curr Med Res Opin 2006;22(11):2191–200.
88. Guyton JR, Brown BG, Fazio S, et al. Lipid-altering efficacy and safety of ezeti-
    mibe/simvastatin coadministered with extended-release niacin in patients with
    type IIa or type IIb hyperlipidemia. J Am Coll Cardiol 2008;51(16):1564–72.
89. Merck. MEVACOR U.S. prescribing information. Available at: http://www.merck.
    com/product/usa/pi_circulars/m/mevacor/mevacor_pi.pdf. Accessed August 10, 2008.
90. Merck. ZOCOR (simvastatin): US prescribing information. Available at: http://
    www.merck.com/product/usa/pi_circulars/z/zocor/zocor_pi.pdf. Accessed August
    10, 2008.
91. Pfizer. Lipitor (atorvastatin calcium): US prescribing information. Available at: http://
    media.pfizer.com/files/products/uspi_lipitor.pdf. Accessed August 10, 2008.
92. Bristol-Myers-Squibb. PRAVACHOL (pravastatin sodium): US prescribing informa-
    tion. Available at: http://packageinserts.bms.com/pi/pi_pravachol.pdf. Accessed
    August 10, 2008.
93. Novartis. Lescol, Lescol XL, (fluvastatin sodium) prescribing information. Available
    at: http://www.pharma.us.novartis.com/product/pi/pdf/Lescol.pdf. Accessed August
    10, 2008.
94. AstraZeneca, CRESTOR (rosuvastatin calcium): US prescribing information.
    Available at: http://www1.astrazeneca-us.com/pi/crestor.pdf. Accessed August
    10, 2008.
95. Merck/Schering-Plough, U.S. prescribing information for Vytorin. Available at: http://
    www.vytorin.com/vytorin/shared/documents/vytorin_pi.pdf. Accessed August 14,
    2008.
96. Jones PH, Davidson MH, Stein EA, et al. Comparison of the efficacy and safety of
    rosuvastatin versus atorvastatin, simvastatin, and pravastatin across doses
    (STELLAR* Trial). Am J Cardiol 2003;92(2):152–60.

97. Bellosta S, Paoletti R, Corsini A. Safety of statins: focus on clinical pharmacokinetics and drug interactions. Circulation 2004;109(23):III50–7.
98. Jacobson TA. Comparative pharmacokinetic interaction profiles of pravastatin, simvastatin, and atorvastatin when coadministered with cytochrome P450 inhibitors. Am J Cardiol 2004;94(9):1140–6.

Other Therapies for Reducing Low-Density Lipoprotein Cholesterol: Medications in Development

Evan A. Stein, MD, PhD[a,b,]*

KEYWORDS

- LDL cholesterol • Apo B antisense • MTP inhibitors
- Squalene synthase inhibitors • PCSK9 inhibitors

It has been more than 2 decades since lovastatin (Mevacor), the first of the 3-hydroxy-3-methylglutaryl coenzyme A (HMG-CoA) reductase inhibitors (statins), was approved on September 1, 1987, for general use for lowering of low-density lipoprotein cholesterol (LDL-C). Since that time, the statins repeatedly have been shown to significantly and substantially reduce all forms of atherosclerotic disease, especially coronary heart disease (CHD) and stroke, no matter what the starting levels of LDL-C and the underlying absolute risk for CHD was in the population in the trial.[1–4] Over the past 20 years there have been more effective statins developed and approved and higher doses of the original statins[5–7] used, such that with the most effective of these agents at their highest dose, an average reduction in LDL-C of close to 55% from baseline is achievable.[7] The efficacy and safety of this class of compounds has resulted in their becoming the largest therapeutic class of medications used today and in history.

Despite the success of the statins, a second class of agents, cholesterol absorption transport inhibitors, also has been developed and approved in the past decade for LDL-C lowering, although there is only one representative, ezetimibe, currently available.[8] This agent also has excellent tolerability and safety along with moderate reductions in LDL-C of approximately 18%, given alone or added to a statin. Thus,

[a] Metabolic and Atherosclerosis Research Center, 4685 Forest Avenue, Cincinnati, OH, USA
[b] Pathology and Laboratory Medicine, University of Cincinnati, Cincinnati, OH 45267, USA
* Metabolic and Atherosclerosis Research Center, 4685 Forest Avenue, Cincinnati, OH, USA
E-mail address: esteinmrl@aol.com

Endocrinol Metab Clin N Am 38 (2009) 99–119
doi:10.1016/j.ecl.2008.11.011
0889-8529/08/$ – see front matter © 2009 Elsevier Inc. All rights reserved.

there is a potential for achieving average LDL-C reductions of up to 65% with combination therapy.[9]

Why, therefore, would there be a need for additional LDL-lowering agents?

1. Many clinical endpoint trials have confirmed that more LDL-C reduction results in more cardiovascular disease risk reduction.[10–12]
2. Clinical practice guidelines[13–15] from the National Cholesterol Education Program, American Heart Association, and American College of Cardiology and European guidelines continue to lower LDL-C goals for high-risk and even lower-risk patients who have CHD, with target goals in patients who have existing CHD and additional risk factors now set at less than 70 mg/dL in the United States and less than 2 mmol/L in Europe and Asia. Recent studies have shown that even with current therapies, many patients, especially those considered at high and very high risk, are not achieving these goals.[16]
3. Special populations, such as those with familial hypercholesterolemia (FH) and other forms of severe hypercholesterolemia, do not achieve even old goals and often require significantly greater LDL-C reductions than the 65% achievable by combining the highest dose of the most effective statin, rosuvastatin (40 mg), and ezetimibe.[9]
4. Perhaps the largest need, however, is for the growing number of patients who are statin adverse,[17] for whom there are limited alternatives to achieving significant LDL-C reductions if even low-dose statin cannot be tolerated.[18] Although in the first 2 decades of statin development and general use the focus on statin toxicity was rare, severe and life-threatening rhabdomyolysis, mild nonspecific myalgias, and other muscle-related side effects (MRSEs) have become major impediments to instituting successful lipid-lowering therapy in everyday medical practice. The magnitude of the problem recently has been evaluated (**Table 1**),[17] demonstrating an approximate prevalence of 5% to 10% of patients affected by MRSEs. Thus, with more than 20 million patients requiring more than 35% LDL-C reduction, there are a projected 1 to 2 million patients who are unable to tolerate statins and need effective LDL-C lowering currently unachievable with nonstatin therapy.

There remains, therefore, a medical need for new, effective, and safe medications to reduce LDL-C.

Table 1
PRIMO: risk for muscular symptoms with individual statins

Statin	Dosage	Patients who have Muscular Symptoms[a]	Odds Ratio (95% CI)[b]	P Value[c]
Pravastatin	40 mg/d	10.9%	—	—
Atorvastatin	40–80 mg/d	14.9%	1.421 (1.171–1.723)	<0.001
Simvastatin	40–80 mg/d	18.2%	1.812 (1.463–2.245)	<0.001
Fluvastatin	80 mg/d	5.1%	0.437 (0.352–0.542)	<0.001

[a] Percentage values relative to the total number of patients who had or did not have muscular symptoms.
[b] Odds ratios were calculated using pravastatin as the reference.
[c] P values were determined by Pearson's chi-square test.
From Bruckert E, Hayem G, Dejager S, et al. Mild to moderate muscular symptoms with high-dosage statin therapy in hyperlipidemic patients—the PRIMO study. Cardiovasc Drugs Ther 2005;19:403–14; with permission.

LOW-DENSITY LIPOPROTEIN CHOLESTEROL–LOWERING AGENTS IN DEVELOPMENT
Apolipoprotein B Antisense

The statins, cholesterol absorption transport inhibitors, and bile acid sequestrants reduce intracellular cholesterol directly or indirectly, mainly in the liver, thus decreasing circulating LDL-C by up-regulation of the LDL receptor (LDLR) (**Fig. 1**). An alternative approach to increasing LDL-C removal via the LDLR is to decrease apolipoprotein (Apo) B–containing lipoprotein formation or release from the liver or the intestines (see **Fig. 1**). This decrease in turn results in reduced chylomicrons, remnants, very low-density lipoprotein (VLDL), intermediate-density lipoprotein (IDL), and LDL entering the circulation. The two current approaches to achieving this are inhibition of the enzyme, microsomal triglyceride transport protein (MTP) (discussed later), and inhibition of Apo B production. A basic and major difference between these two approaches, however (discussed later), is that Apo B antisense inhibits only production of Apo B100–containing lipoproteins, which are found in the liver, whereas MTP inhibitors (MTPi) generally reduce hepatic Apo B100–containing lipoproteins and intestinally produced Apo B48 lipoproteins, which transport dietary fat via chylomicrons.

The mechanisms for inhibiting Apo B production is shown in **Fig. 2**. As a brief overview, this process[19] starts with a master blueprint for Apo B production encoded in DNA. DNA consists of two strands, one representing the "sense" genetic code sequence, whereas the other strand, containing complementary base pairs, is the "antisense" coding. During transcription, the sense and antisense strands separate and the antisense strand serves as a template for the next step, which is to produce a single-stranded mRNA, a type of working blueprint. This mRNA has a base pairing matching the DNA antisense and also is termed, sense. On reaching the cytosol, ribosomes translate the mRNA to produce proteins, in this case Apo B. It has been shown that it is possible to develop agents with RNase activity, called antisense, that degrades a specific mRNA, impairing its translation of the downstream protein (see **Fig. 2**). Thus, these antisense agents essentially shoot the messenger.

A potential advantage of antisense drugs is their increased specificity for the liver; thus, they are best used to inhibit proteins predominantly made in the liver, such as

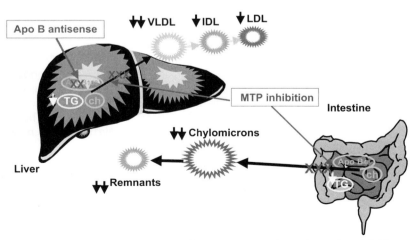

Fig. 1. Reducing plasma Apo B–containing lipoprotein entry into plasma by inhibiting Apo B production or lipidation of Apo B.

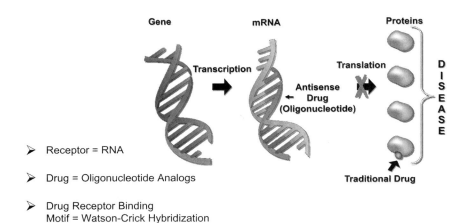

> Receptor = RNA

> Drug = Oligonucleotide Analogs

> Drug Receptor Binding
  Motif = Watson-Crick Hybridization

> Post Receptor Binding
  Events = Degradation/Inhibition of Receptor

Fig. 2. Antisense drugs.

Apo B, and several other proteins important in lipid metabolism, such as Apo CIII, lipoprotein(a) (Lp[a]), and proprotein convertase subtilisin/kexin type 9 (PCSK9) (discussed later).

Initial development of antisense drugs demonstrated that they had predictable sites of accumulation with the major organs being liver, kidney, fat, and the reticular endothelium system.[19] All antisense drugs developed to date are of single-strand antisense nucleotide sequences that are complementary to mRNA, called antisense oligonucleotides (ASOs). The tissue levels are predictable from plasma concentrations, where they are 90% protein bound, and correlate well with the pharmacology of ASOs. They disappear from the bloodstream rapidly but remain in tissue for prolonged periods, often months.

ASOs generally are 20 base pairs long and behave stably and predictably irrespective of sequence.[19] Mipomersen (ISIS 301012)[20] is the nonadecasodium salt of a 20-base (20-mer) phosphorothioate oligonucleotide. Each of the 19 inter-nucleotide linkages is a $3'$-O to $5'$-O phosphorothioate diester. Ten of the 20 sugar residues are 2-deoxy-D-ribose; the remaining 10 are $2'$ methoxyethyl ($2'$ MOE)-D-ribose. The residues are arranged such that five MOE nucleosides at the $5'$ and $3'$ ends of the molecule flank a gap of 10 $2'$ deoxynucleosides (**Fig. 3**). Each of the nine cytosine bases is methylated at the 5-position. The $2'$ MOE-5-methyluridine nucleosides also are designated $2'$ MOE ribothymidine, termed second-generation ASOs. The molecular formula of mipomersen is $C_{230}H_{305}N_{67}O_{122}P_{19}S_{19}Na_{19}$ and the molecular weight is 7594.9 amu.

The only Apo B antisense drug in clinical development is mipomersen, a second-generation ASO (see **Fig. 3**), which has several advantages over first-generation ASOs in that it has increased affinity for mRNA, seems better tolerated, and, because of the use of $2'$ MOE modification, has increased resistance to nuclease activity and a prolonged half-life. ASOs are metabolized by nucleases, endonucleases and exonucleases; for example, as mipomersen is broken down by nucleases, the fragments are excreted in the urine. Mipomersen binds by Watson–Crick base pairing and is complementary to a 20-nucleotide segment of the coding region for the mRNA for Apo B. This

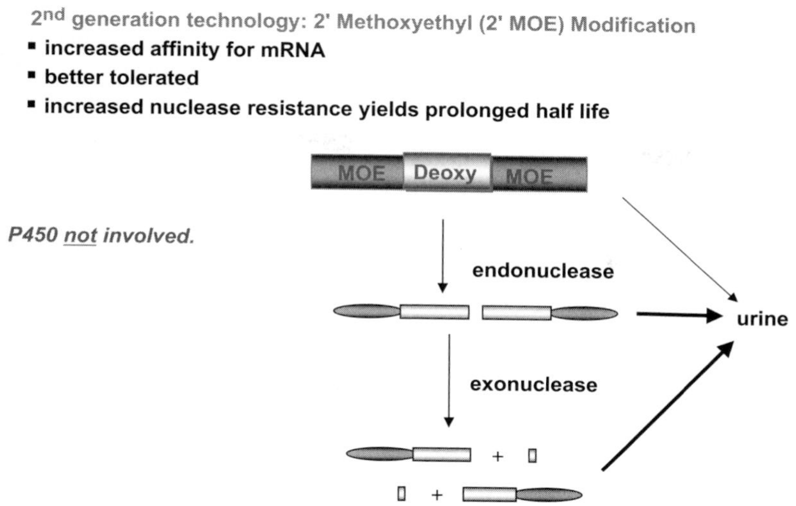

2nd generation technology: 2' Methoxyethyl (2' MOE) Modification
- **increased affinity for mRNA**
- **better tolerated**
- **increased nuclease resistance yields prolonged half life**

P450 not involved.

Fig. 3. Second-generation antisense technology: mipomersen (ISIS 301012).

selective hybridization/binding to its cognate mRNA results in the RNase H-mediated degradation of the Apo B message, thus inhibiting translation of the Apo B protein (see **Fig. 2**).[21]

There also is no cytochrome P450 metabolism, and potential drug-drug interaction is anticipated to be minimal. Early studies have shown no interactions with simvastatin or ezetimibe.[22]

Side effects seen so far in clinical trials seem related mostly to the ASOs, not to the target mRNA sequence to Apo B, and relate predominantly to injection-site reactions and liver enzyme elevation,[22] although the latter could be a consequence of the mechanism of action.

Apo B100 is a critical protein required for the release and transport of atherogenic lipoproteins, VLDL, IDL, LDL, and likely Lp(a). Preclinical studies in animals showed that mipomersen not only reduces Apo B100 but also reduces decreased atherosclerotic plaques. As mipomersen is specific for Apo B100 and accumulates minimally in the intestinal tract, it would not be expected to affect B48 and chylomicrons or fat absorption.

Because of the structure of current ASOs, they are poorly absorbed[19] and need to be given parenterally. Initial administration in humans was intravenous to achieve faster hepatic concentrations and proof of efficacy in the limited time associated with phase 1 trials. As the drug has advanced in longer-term studies, however, supported by longer animal toxicology, it has been given subcutaneously, approximately once a week.[23] Mipomersen has been assessed in several phase 2 trials in a variety of patient phenotypes initially as monotherapy, followed by combinations with lower-dose statins and then high-dose statins and other lipid-lowering agents.[22–25]

Unlike traditional dose-ranging trials of small-molecule, lipid-altering agents in which maximal and stable effects on the major lipid fractions can be seen in 4 to 6 weeks, it is estimated that it will take up to 6 months for mipomersen to achieve steady state. Thus, it is likely that initial phase 2 trials of 6 to 12 weeks provide an underestimation of the final achievable reductions in LDL-C and other Apo B–related lipoproteins. The initial dose-ranging study[22] was performed in patients who had moderately elevated LDL-C on diet alone and involved 50 subjects, 10 on placebo and 8 each on mipomersen (50, 100, 200, 300, and 400 mg), administered weekly for 12 weeks and then monitored for a further 90 days. The results (shown in **Fig. 4**) demonstrate a progressive dose response–related reduction in LDL-C and Apo B, reaching nearly 70% at the 400 mg per week dose after 12 weeks. In many of the patients treated with the 400-mg dose, their LDL-C and Apo B reached barely detectable levels. The sustained reduction in LDL-C and Apo B did not return to pretreatment values, even 90 days after cessation of treatment.

A second dose-ranging phase 2 trial,[23] performed in patients already on stable doses of simvastatin or atorvastatin and who had LDL-C greater than 100 mg/dL, was performed on 62 subjects who had similar doses of 50, 100, 200, 300, and 400 mg given for 4 weeks. Similar to the monotherapy results, a dose-dependent reduction in LDL-C and Apo B was seen, which reached approximately 50% at the two highest doses. Again the effect was maintained during the 30-day monitoring period after stopping the drug.

Additional studies have been performed in patients who had heterozygous FH (HeFH)[24] and homozygous FH (HoFH).[25] In these trials, mipomersen was added to their current and maximal lipid therapy, which included the highest doses of simvastatin, atorvastatin, or rosuvastatin, usually combined with ezetimibe and in some patients resins and niacin. The HeFH trial was double blind with a placebo control group, and the doses assessed were 50 to 300 mg given for 6 weeks, with one group given 300 mg for 13 weeks.[25] Results (**Table 2**) show significant reductions in LDL-C of 36% and 46%, seen with the 300-mg weekly dose after 6 and 13 weeks, respectively.

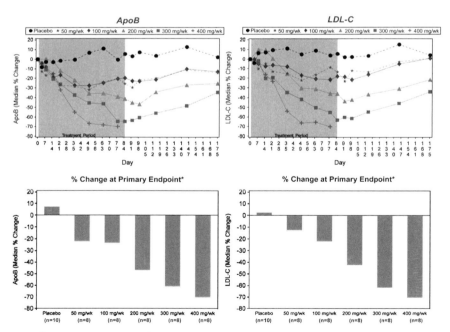

*Primary endpoint analysis was 14 days post last dose, Day 99 for 50-300 mg/week cohorts, Day 78 for 400mg/week

Fig. 4. ISIS 301012 monotherapy. Dose-dependent Apo B and LDL-C reduction. (*Data from* Kastelein JJ, Wedel MK, Baker BF, et al. Potent reduction of apolipoprotein B and low-density lipoprotein cholesterol by short-term administration of an antisense inhibitor of apolipoprotein B. Circulation 2006;114:1729–35.)

Table 2
Mipomersen heterozygous familial hypercholesterolemia study; mean percent changes from baseline[a]

	Placebo N = 10[b]	50 mg/wk N = 7	100 mg/wk N = 8	200 mg/wk N = 9	300 mg/wk N = 8 (6 wk)	300 mg/wk N = 8 (13 wk)
Apo B	−6%	−9%	−9%	−20%[c]	−33%[d]	−43%[c]
LDL-C	−5%	−12%	−11%	−20%[c]	−36%[d]	−46%[c]
Triglyceride	−17%	5%	6%	−25%	−27%	−24%
Non–HDL-C	−6%	−10%	−6%	−26%	−30%[c]	−39%[d]
HDL-C	11%	−7%	−1%	−4%	10%	5%
Apo A1	−1%	−1%	0%	−5%	1%	−2%
Lp(a)	−3%	0%	−19%	−17%	−25%	−37%

Three patients at 300 mg/wk had ALT >3 × upper limit of normal.
[a] Day 43 for 6-week treatment; day 99 for 13-week treatment.
[b] Eight for 6 weeks; two for 13 weeks.
[c] P<.02 versus placebo.
[d] P<.01 versus placebo.
Data from Kastelein J, Trip M, Davidson M, et al. Safety and activity of ISIS 301012 in heterozygous familial hypercholesterolemia [abstract 341]. Presented at Drugs Affecting Lipid Metabolism. Journal of Clinical Lipidology 2007;1(5):475.

Robust dose- and time-related reductions in Apo B, triglycerides, non–high-density lipoprotein cholesterol (HDL-C), and Lp(a) also were noted (see **Table 2**). No significant change in HDL-C or Apo A1 was seen at any dose.

A pilot study[26] of HoFH was conducted in an open-label manner with three to four patients in each dose group, starting at 50 mg and progressing to 100, 200, and 300 mg given for 12 weeks, provided prior dose already administered seemed safe. At the highest dose tested (300 mg) in the three patients on maximal drug therapy (**Table 3**) but not on LDL apheresis, dramatic and consistent reductions in LDL-C and Apo B were seen, ranging from 45% to 51% and 43% to 54%, respectively. In one subject, mipomersen, in combination with atorvastatin (80 mg), ezetimibe (10 mg), colesevelam (3.75 g), and niacin-ER (1000 mg daily), a LDL-C less than 100 mg/dL was achieved (see **Table 3**). The reductions in Lp(a) noted in the HeFH study also were seen in the patients who had HoFH, and HDL-C, which generally is low in HoFH, seemed to increase. Orphan drug status for mipomersen for treatment of HoFH has been granted by the Food and Drug Administration (FDA).[26]

As with all new and effective lipid-lowering agents, long-term viability often hinges on safety and tolerability. For mipomersen, the most common side effect seen so far (**Table 4**) is injection site reactions (ISRs). More than 90% of subjects experience ISRs, which usually are mild, painless, slightly erythematous, and transient. Histologically they consist of activated polymorphonuclear leucocytes and macrophages. The incidence seems related to the ASO and not the specific antisense and there is no anamnestic response. In treating more than 300 subjects with mipomersen, only one subject has dropped out of trials because of an ISR.

The major long-term safety concerns center around potential liver toxicity, given prior data from drugs that inhibit assembly and release of Apo B–containing lipoproteins, such as the MTPi (discussed later). Liver function data from approximately 150 subjects from phase 2 and the blinded HeFH trials show that only at the very highest dose tested (400 mg) did significant numbers of patients have sustained increases of more than 3 times the upper limit of normal of alanine aminotransferase (ALT), with many of these subjects having undetectable levels of LDL-C. Even in patients who had

Table 3
Mipomersen in homozygous familial hypercholesterolemia

	Patient 1 (1010)			Patient 2 (1011)			Patient 3 (1013)		
Concurrent therapies	80-mg atorvastatin (1 y)			80-mg atorvastatin (10 y) + 10-mg ezetimibe + 3.75 g colesevelam + 1 g niacin			40-mg rosuvastatin (4 y) + 10-mg ezetimibe		
Age (years)	23			48			32		
Lipids	Baseline	Day 99	Percent change	Baseline	Day 99	Percent change	Baseline	Day 99	Percent change
Apo B	369	171	−54%	180	103	−43%	283	156	−45%
LDL-C	651	318	−51%	197	99	−50%	445	246	−45%
VLDL-C	18	10	−44%	33	24	−26%	30	20	−33%
Non-HDL	669	328	−51%	230	123	−46%	475	266	−44%
HDL-C	27	35	32%	29	28	−2%	27	31	15%
Apo A1	86	92	7%	109	109	0%	89	90	2%
TC	695	363	−48%	258	151	−41%	502	297	−41%
TG	90	49	−45%	163	118	−28%	151	99	−34%
Lp(a)	104	36	−65%	140	128	−9%	108	54	−50%

Baseline values and interim results of 300-mg dose.
Data from Stein EA. High LDL cholesterol on three drugs. Presented at American College of Cardiology Annual Scientific Meeting. New Orleans, March 27.

Table 4
Mipomersen (ISIS 301012)—phase 2 integrated safety analysis: adverse experiences

	Placebo	ISIS 301012	Blinded
Number of patients (exposures)	19	86	42
Injection site reactions	4 (21%)	81 (94%)	33 (79%)
Headache	10 (53%)	28 (33%)	8 (19%)
Nasopharyngitis	4 (21%)	20 (23%)	8 (19%)
Influenza-like illness	1 (5%)	12 (14%)	2 (5%)
Fatigue	0 (0%)	10 (12%)	4 (10%)
Pyrexia	0 (0%)	10 (12%)	2 (5%)
Back pain	2 (11%)	9 (11%)	4 (10%)
Diarrhea	2 (11%)	6 (7%)	2 (5%)
Abdominal discomfort	2 (11%)	1 (1%)	0 (0%)
Neck pain	2 (11%)	0 (0%)	0 (0%)

In approximately 134 patients treated (data currently available for 128 treated or blinded patients and 19 placebo patients) with ISIS 301012 in four phase 2 trials, including the ongoing, blinded HeFH study, these adverse experiences occurred with >10% incidence.
Courtesy of Isis Pharmaceuticals, Inc., Carlsbad, CA; with permission

HoFH and were treated with a 300-mg dose, in addition to all existing lipid-lowering therapy, other than a temporary and slight increase in ALT associated with unusual alcohol intake during the holidays, no significant increases in hepatic enzymes were seen. The dose selected for further development (200 mg) was associated with minimal sustained transaminase elevations greater than 3 times the upper limit of normal. No cases of concomitant increases in bilirubin were reported in these early trials.

It is likely that provided the safety and efficacy seen in the early studies are maintained throughout phase 3 development, mipomersen could be approved for use within a few years, at least in patients who have HoFH. A recent announcement from ISIS Pharmaceuticals, however, indicates that the FDA has requested a clinical cardiovascular endpoint trial to demonstrate that reduction in LDL-C by this mechanism will result in improved outcomes before the drug is approved for treatment in other hypercholesterolemic patients.[26]

Microsomal Triglyceride Transfer Protein Inhibitors

MTP is a heterodimeric lipid transfer protein that is localized in the endoplasmatic reticulum of hepatocytes and enterocytes and plays a critical role in lipoprotein lipidation of Apo B (**Fig. 5**). This is vital to the formation of chylomicrons, VLDL, and their downstream lipoproteins, including remnants, IDL, and LDL (see **Fig. 1**).

Ever since the discovery in 1992 by Wetterau and colleagues[27] of MTP deficiency as the cause of a rare inherited disorder associated with very low levels of LDL-C, called abetalipoproteinemia, this enzyme has been a target of lipid-lowering drug development. Abetalipoproteinemia also is characterized by fat malabsorption, steatorrhea, and hepatic steatosis.[28] Before the development and treatment with water-soluble forms of vitamin E, the disorder also was associated with several serious neurologic disorders resulting from malabsorption of vitamin E and an inability to transport this lipid-soluble vitamin to the periphery and central nervous system as a result of the very low levels of Apo B–containing lipoproteins, which transport it and other lipid-soluble vitamins.[29]

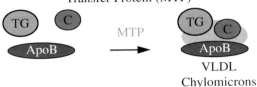

Fig. 5. Molecular mechanism of MTPi. (*From* Wetterau JR, Aggerbeck LP, Bouma ME, et al. Absence of microsomal triglyceride transfer protein in individuals with abetalipoproteinemia. Science 1992;258:999–1001; with permission.)

Systemic microsomal triglyceride transfer protein inhibitors

Experimental animal and human studies starting in the mid-1990s confirmed that MTP inhibition reduces hepatic secretion of VLDL and intestinal secretion of chylomicrons.[30–33] Initial MTPi compounds were systemically active and inhibited the enzyme in the liver and intestine; although there may be some modest differences in the various agents as to where they exert their maximal effect, all have an impact on Apo B100 and B48 lipoprotein formation. The first MTPi to enter humans, implitapide (BAY 13-9952), demonstrated significant effects on hepatic and intestinal within 10 days of exposure.[31] By the early 2000s, there were three systemic compounds in development, implitapide from Bayer,[30] BMS-201038 from Bristol-Myers Squibb,[34] and CP-346086 from Pfizer.[35]

In 2001, Farnier and colleagues[36] reported a large, 399-patient, phase 2, dose-ranging, 4-week, double-blind, placebo-controlled, and parallel-group design study, MISTRAL, comparing the efficacy and the safety of four dosages of implitapide (20, 40, 80, and 160 mg per day), placebo, and cerivastatin (0.3 mg per day) in patients who had primary hypercholesterolemia. LDL-C reductions with implitapide ranged from −8.2% with 20 mg to −55.1% with 160 mg ($P<.001$ compared with placebo). These reductions were compared with −33.3% with 0.3-mg cerivastatin and −0.2% with placebo. In addition, dose-related reductions were seen in other Apo B–related lipids, from −6.4% with 20 mg to −44.8% with 160 mg in total cholesterol, from −5.7% to −49% in Apo B, and from −1.3% to −29% in triglycerides. Lp(a) did not follow the same dose-dependent response. Reductions in HDL-C, however, from −1.8% to −17.9%, and in Apo A1, from −2% to −22.3%, were found across the dose range. The percentage of adverse experiences increased with the dose of implitapide with an unacceptable high incidence of digestive adverse experiences (mainly diarrhea) in the 80-mg and 160-mg groups. The percentages of patients who had elevations in hepatic transaminases greater than 3 times the upper limit of normal were 8%, 8%, 27%, and 25% for ALT in groups receiving, respectively, 20, 40, 80, and 160 mg of implitapide compared with 0% in the placebo and cerivastatin groups.[36] After these results Bayer abandoned further development of the compound given the high rate of liver function abnormalities even at a marginally effective and commercially viable dose.

BMS-201038 was reported in a 7-day multiple ascending-dose, phase 1 study to produce large reductions in LDL-C, ranging from 54% to 86% with doses of 25 to 100 mg.[35] A high rate of hepatosteatosis and gastrointestinal adverse experiences, however, were encountered, although the 25-mg dose was further studied in a longer phase 2 trial. Neither the Bristol-Myers Squibb nor Pfizer compounds have had phase 2 data reported but both compounds were not carried into further development for similar reasons. An observation from these trials is that, unlike statins, where after the starting dose the additional LDL-C reduction on doubling the dose of the statin is relatively flat at approximately 5% to 7%,[37] the dose response with MTPi seemed steep.

After being abandoned by major pharmaceutical companies, implitapide and BMS-201038 were given to individual academic investigators, and small studies to develop them for HoFH and severe HeFH were continued.[38,39] In 2005, BMS-201038 was licensed to a small start-up company, Aegerion, and renamed AEGR-733, and in 2006 the same company obtained implitapide and renamed it AEGR-427.[40] AEGR-733 entered new phase 2 trials at significantly lower dosages (5, 7.5, and 10 mg daily) than the 25-mg dose originally tested by Bristol-Myers Squibb.[40] Each dose was administered for 4 weeks in a dose-escalating study with two other arms, ezetimibe only and a combination of ezetimibe and AEGR-733 where the dose of AEGR-733 was similarly escalated every 4 weeks.

The results of these latest studies recently were reported.[40,41] The reductions in Apo B and LDL-C were dose related and robust. Specifically, LDL-C decreased 19%, 26%, and 30%; triglyceride reductions, however, were modest at 1%, 7%, and 10% at 5, 7.5, and 10 mg, respectively. In addition, clinically and statistically significant reductions, ranging from 6.5% to 9.2% in HDL-C and 9% to 11% in Apo A1, were seen with all doses, given alone or in combination with ezetimibe, and were sustained over the 12-week trial.[40] In the AEGR-733 monotherapy group, 32% of patients discontinued the trial, mainly for gastrointestinal side effects, which were experienced by 64% of subjects in this group. Elevated transaminases in 18% of the 56 patients treated with AEGR-733, alone or in combination with ezetimibe, resulted in their stopping the drug in the 12-week trial.[40,41]

A small pilot trial of BMS-201038/AEGR-733 also has been reported in patients who had HoFH,[39] in which all lipid-lowering therapy was washed out and doses of 0.03, 0.1, 0.3, and 1 mg/kg (equivalent to 1.5–2.4, 5.5–8, 15–24, and 55–80 mg per day, with the mean doses at each of the four titration steps 2.0, 6.7, 20.1, and 67.0 mg per day) force-titrated every 4 weeks. Significant reductions in LDL-C were seen at the higher doses reaching approximately 50% at the 55- to 80-mg dose. Again, significant elevations of the hepatic transaminase, ALT, were seen in more than half the subjects starting at the lower doses. Hepatic MRI showed hepatic fat accumulation in nearly all patients, with substantial increases seen in some, again starting before administration of the highest and most effective dose. **Box 1** compares and contrasts the MTPi and Apo B antisense approaches.

Based on the past and recent results reported for systemic MTPi, their future looks uncertain as the tolerability, transaminase elevations, and probable hepatic steatosis present substantial regulatory and commercial hurdles. These problems are compounded by the sustained and significant negative impact on Apo A1 and HDL-C. Even if development continues into phase 3, with these safety concerns approval of any MTPi for general use is extremely unlikely without a clinical endpoint trial. Unlike mipomersen, given the more modest additional reductions in LDL-C and the negative effects on HDL-C, the size of such a trial for an MTPi, such as AEGR-733, would be anticipated to be substantially larger or longer and the outcome far less certain.

Intestinal microsomal triglyceride transfer protein inhibitors
Recently, Surface Logix described a MTPi, SLx-4090, that was minimally or not absorbed, works only in the intestinal tract, and was tested in humans.[42] SLx-4090 is

> **Box 1**
> **Differences between apolipoprotein B antisense and microsomal triglyceride transfer protein inhibitor drugs**
>
> - Apo B antisense reduces hepatic Apo B$_{100}$–containing lipoproteins whereas MTPi reduce both hepatic Apo B$_{100}$ and intestinal Apo B$_{48}$
> - MTPi are administered orally on a daily basis whereas Apo B antisense requires refrigeration of the drug and parenteral, usually subcutaneous, administration on a weekly basis and produces ISRs.
> - Large and sustained reductions in LDL-C, up to 50%, are seen with Apo B antisense without significant increases in hepatic transaminases or hepatic fat accumulation
> - Large decreases in Lp(a) have been reported with Apo B antisense but not MTPi.
> - Uniform reductions in HDL-C of 6% to 10% have been reported with MTPi at all doses, as monotherapy or in combination with statins. Effect on HDL-C with Apo B antisense is neutral or slightly increased.
> - MTPi, as a result of inhibition of intestinal fat transport, produces loose stools, which increases with dose.

a first-in-class inhibitor of enterocytic MTP, designed to overcome or reduce the gastrointestinal and especially the hepatic transaminase and fat accumulation problems inherent in systemic MTP inhibition (described previously). By inhibiting only MTP in enterocytes, the drug reduces triglycerides and cholesterol transport into the lymphatic circulation and subsequent delivery to the liver.

Early results with SLx-4090 hold promise that the drug may be effective not only in dyslipidemia but also as a weight loss agent.[42] In preclinical studies, a systemically available MTPi was used as a control and animal studies were used to look at the effects of acute and chronic dosing on postprandial and fasting triglyceride levels, respectively. SLx-4090 had similar efficacy to the positive control with significant reductions in postprandial and fasting triglyceride levels. Even at efficacious doses, however, the drug was unable to be detected in plasma after 6 weeks of treatment. More importantly, and using a systemic MTPi as a control, there was no buildup of fat in the liver and no increase in hepatic transaminase levels. In a recently completed, small, 24-patient, double-blind, placebo-controlled, dose-ranging phase 2a study of 14-day duration, SLx-4090 was reported to show reductions in LDL-C and postprandial triglycerides.[42] The drug also was reported well tolerated with no apparent effect on liver function testing. This longer duration study also confirmed that the compound was undetectable in the systemic circulation. The company announced in late 2008 plans to initiate a larger phase 2b study of SLx-4090 late in 2008. If indeed SLx-4090 proves a nonsystemically available inhibitor of MTPi that can reduce LDL-C, even indirectly, in a manner similar to ezetimibe by reducing cholesterol absorption and avoids toxicities in the liver associated with systemic MTPi, this could prove a much more promising and viable approach.

Squalene Synthase Inhibitors

For several decades, drugs that were known to inhibit any of the many steps involved in the cholesterol synthetic pathway (**Fig. 6**) generally were avoided as targets for lipid-lowering therapy. This was because of a scandal with a drug, called triparanol (MER 29), marketed in 1959 by Merrell Pharmaceutical Company of Cincinnati, that inhibited the final step in cholesterol synthesis, desmosterol to cholesterol.[43,44] This nonrecyclable compound proved toxic in humans, leading to baldness, cataracts, and

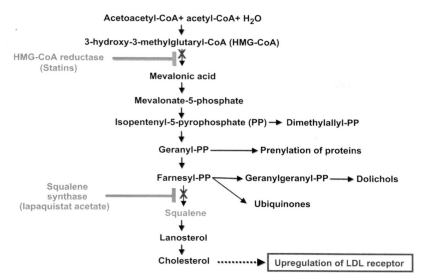

Fig. 6. Cholesterol pathway.

impotence. The drug was withdrawn in 1962 after an investigation by the FDA, which found that the company had falsified the preclinical data submitted to the agency, which led to its approval. The company and three officials responsible later pleaded no contest, were fined, and entered into settlement with those exposed to the drug.[44] It took nearly 2 decades after this disaster, until the Nobel Prize–winning researchers Brown and Goldstein discovered the major rate-limiting enzyme, HMG-CoA reductase, which controlled intracellular cholesterol content, which in turn regulated the LDLR activity and uptake of circulating LDL-C,[45] and to develop another drug that inhibited cholesterol synthesis. Furthermore, extensive studies were required to show that inhibition of HMG-CoA reductase with statins and the resultant accumulation of 4-hydroxy, 3-methoxy HMG-CoA was water soluble, recyclable, and nontoxic to animals and humans.

Other potential opportunities for inhibition in the cholesterol synthetic pathway exist after HMG-CoA reductase, but these have to occur before the cyclization and formation of squalene, a nonrecyclable compound.

One of these synthetic enzymes, squalene synthase, has been a desired target since the 1970s. Interest lagged, however, until after the successful development of the statins, and in the 1990s several pharmaceutical companies announced compounds in early development.[46–53] Only one compound, however, lapaquistat (TAK-475) from Takeda Pharmaceuticals, has ever entered advanced development.[46]

In addition to lowering plasma LDL-C by up-regulation of the LDLR similar to statins, squalene synthase inhibitors (SSIs) may have the potential to overcome, or reduce, one of the major side effects that have emerged with statin therapy, myalgias, and other MRSEs. This potential to reduce MRSEs with SSIs is related to their inhibiting the synthetic pathway further downstream after formation of several key mevalonate-derived compounds involved in intracellular energy, especially ubiquinone.[54] Ubiquinone, also called coenzyme Q10, is a prenylated protein that is part of the electron chain, which functions as an antioxidant in mitochondrial and other lipid membranes and is of importance in the normal functioning of skeletal muscle.[55] The impairment of ubiquinone synthesis with statins and the potential to produce MRSEs was seriously considered in the late 1980s during early statin development with the addition of the coenzyme to the statin patented at the time by Merck, the developers of lovastatin.[56] Although several recent trials have attempted to assess the potential effect of ubiquinone co-administration in patients who have MRSEs and are on statins, the results have been variable and disappointing.[57]

Inhibition of squalene synthase results in accumulation of farnesyl pyrophosphate, the last water-soluble intermediate in cholesterol synthetic pathway. Although farnesyl pyrophosphate has known routes for metabolism, it most likely is excreted via urine as dicarboxylic acid.[58] These farnesyl-derived dicarboxylic acids have the potential to result in toxic acidosis and were increased sufficiently in animal studies using several SSIs, especially the zaragozic acids,[59] resulting in their termination from further development prior to exposure in humans. Preclinical studies with lapaquistat demonstrated no toxic acidosis although there was a mild increase in urinary levels of dicarboxylic acids,[46] but not sufficient to prevent the drug from entering into human studies where no significant acidosis was seen.

Pharmacologically, lapaquistat undergoes rapid gastrointestinal absorption with a time to maximal blood levels (T_{max}) of approximately 3.5 hours and has high first-pass clearance by the liver where it is converted to two active metabolites, MI and MII, which are excreted in the bile and subsequently the feces with minimal, 0.2%, renal excretion.[46] Although significantly metabolized via the cytochrome P450 3A4 system, lapaquistat seems not to have significant drug interactions with statins, such as simvastatin and atorvastatin, which are metabolized through the same cytochrome P450 3A4 system. Lapaquistat has been studied extensively in a large multi-year, phase 3, global development program involving more than 4000 patients exposed to the drug, mainly at 100 mg daily for up to 3 years.

The population groups in these trials included a variety of hypercholesterolemic patients, including those who had severe HoFH and those who had HeFH; lapaquistat (100 mg) was added to maximal dose statin and, in many FH patients, those also taking ezetimibe and even bile acid sequestrants and niacin. Although peer-reviewed publications are few at this time, a robust phase 2, dose-ranging trial of more than 200 patients with approximately 60 patients per treatment arm (placebo, lapaquistat [25, 50, and 100 mg] and atorvastatin [10 mg]) evaluating the drug as monotherapy has been presented at an international meeting.[60] Compared with placebo, significant dose-related reductions in LDL-C of 16%, 18%, and 26% were seen with a 36% LDL-C reduction with atorvastatin (10 mg). Similar reductions were seen in Apo B, total cholesterol, and triglycerides, with modest increases in HDL-C.[60] When added to stable doses of atorvastatin, an additional 20% decrease in LDL-C was found.[61]

Initial safety and tolerability seemed good with the 100-mg dose, even in combination with the highest dose of the most efficacious statins. One, and possibly two, patients, however, developed a sustained increase in ALT/aspartate aminotransferase of greater than 3 times the upper normal range and an increase in total bilirubin 2 times that of the upper limit of normal. This combination of liver abnormalities, known as Hy's law,[62] is viewed seriously by the FDA as an indirect indication of drug-associated hepatitis with the potential to lead to liver failure in approximately 10% of patients.

Thus, the hurdles for approval by the FDA were increased to the point where the Takeda Company terminated their development program in early 2008.[63] Whether or not the cause of the liver findings can be determined, and if they were related directly to the compound and can be overcome, or whether or not other SSIs will enter future clinical development remains to be seen. Lapaquistat demonstrated, however, that inhibition of squalene synthase can achieve significant additional LDL-C reductions in the order of 20% when added to the highest dose of rosuvastatin and atorvastatin even when they are combined with ezetimibe. This indicates that there is further capacity to up-regulate the LDLR and achieve meaningful reductions in plasma LDL-C.

Proprotein Convertase Subtilisin/Kexin Type 9 Inhibitors

In 2003 Abifadel and colleagues[64] described a new form of autosomal dominant hypercholesterolemia, which was not associated with mutations in the genes coding for the LDLR or its ligand, Apo B. They reported two mutations in the gene encoding PCSK9 that were responsible for this new form of FH. PCSK9 is a member of nuclear protease family involved in degradation of the LDLR/Apo B receptor (**Fig. 7**). The mechanism by which PCSK9 leads to increased proteolysis of the LDLR originally was belived to be via some type of enzymatic degradation. The mechanism recently has been elucidated by Horton and colleagues,[65] however, who demonstrated a more complicated pathway. The interaction between the LDLR and PCSK9 is over-viewed briefly (see **Fig. 7**). The LDLR is responsible for transporting cholesterol into hepatocytes and maintaining the pool of cholesterol in the endoplasmic reticulum. If the pool is depleted, for example, from increased use, reduced endogenous synthesis, or reduced delivery from the gut, there is activation of key transcription factors, called sterol regulatory element-binding proteins, which lead to increased levels of mRNA and increased synthesis of the LDLR. At the same time there seems to be concomitant increased synthesis of PCSK9.[66] As PCSK9 results in degradation of LDLRs, this action mostly likely is a counterregulatory mechanism designed to prevent excessive uptake of cholesterol into cells.

Although mutations leading to increased PCSK9 activity, called gain of function, have been associated with increased levels of LDL-C, as found in autosomal dominant hypercholesterolemia, mutations that lead to loss of function result in lower levels of LDL-C. These mutations and reduced LDL-C levels also are associated with reduced risk for cardiovascular disease. In the Atherosclerosis Risk in Communities Study,[67] African Americans who had a loss-of-function PCSK9 mutation leading to 40-mg/dL lower LDL-C had a 90% reduction in coronary events in their middle years, from ages 40 to 55. White subjects who had another loss-of-function PCSK9 mutation, leading to 20-mg/dL lower LDL-C, had a 50% reduction in coronary events at the

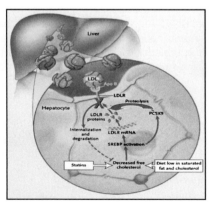
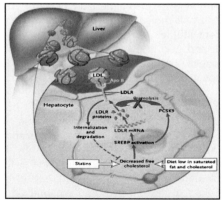

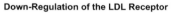

Down-Regulation of the LDL Receptor   Up-Regulation of the LDL Receptor

Fig. 7. PCSK9 and its regulation of the LDLR. (*Adapted from* Tall A. Protease variants, LDL, and coronary heart disease. N Engl J Med 2006;354:1310–2; with permission. Copyright © 2006, Massachusetts Medical Society.)

same ages. In addition to these experiments of nature, creation of animal models that overexpress PCSK9 have almost no LDLR activity and resemble FH, whereas the opposite, animal knockout models of PCSK9 have shown increased LDLR activity and lower plasma LDL-C.

These exciting findings have generated considerable interest because reduction in PCSK9 has no apparent negative clinical associations and thus appears an ideal target for therapeutic intervention. Furthermore, by increasing LDLR longevity with down-regulation of PCSK9, there may be added benefit to combination use with statins and other drugs that up-regulate LDLR synthesis. This is because statins have been shown to increase PCSK9 levels as measured by plasma levels.[68]

Although a small molecule that is safe and effective and that targets PCSK9 would be optimal as a therapeutic agent, this is likely to prove difficult for several reasons. Studies by Horton and colleagues show that mutations or changes in PCSK9 that alter its functional ability or even its binding domain to the LDLR do not reduce its ability to redirect the receptor toward a path of increased catabolism.

Thus, the small molecule approach could take several pathways such as: (1) such molecules could prevent the autocatalytic process that results in the mature PCSK9 being formed; this would have to be very specific to PCSK9 and also not result in possible toxicity from the resultant alternative forms of PCSK9 that may be formed; or (2) small molecules could block the ability of PCSK9 to bind to the LDLR.

An alternative approach, however, using the same antisense technology (described previously) for Apo B already has been successfully demonstrated in an animal model,[69] where a second-generation antisense ASO directed at murine PCKS9 reduced PCSK9 expression and decreased LDL-C by 38% in 6 weeks. This study also showed that along with inhibition of PCSK9 expression there was a twofold increase in hepatic LDLR protein levels. Based on the promise shown in these animal experiments combined with the human experience with the Apo B ASO, mipomersen, in May 2007, ISIS Pharmaceuticals and Bristol-Myers Squibb announced a collaboration[70] to "discover, develop and commercialize novel antisense drugs targeting proprotein convertase subtilisin kexin 9 (PCSK9) for the prevention and treatment of cardiovascular disease." It is believed that the first of these will enter human trials sometime in 2009 and open another exciting era in LDL-lowering therapy.

Several other companies[71] recently have announced preclinical results of drugs targeting PCSK9, also aimed at RNA interference using a somewhat different approach with small molecules, called small interfering RNA. Anlylam presented data from rodent studies targeting PCSK9 using RNA interference that significantly reduced LDL and Apo B levels. After a single injection the effect was rapid and lasted up to 3 weeks. GlaxoSmithKline and Santaris Pharma are other companies with similar drugs in early development for PCSK9.[71]

Cholesterol Absorption Inhibitors

Inhibition of cholesterol absorption has been a validated mechanism for reducing plasma LDL-C and one such agent, ezetimibe, has been successfully demonstrated to achieve reductions of approximately 18%, as monotherapy or added to other lipid-lowering agents, such as statins or fibrates.[8] Ezetimibe, the first in the class of cholesterol absorption inhibitors, had a mechanism of action poorly understood at the time of its approval and was initially discovered as part of a program to find compounds that inhibited the enzyme, acyl COA: cholesterol acyl transferase.[8] More recent discoveries, however, have provided a mechanism of action that is consistent with the binding to and blockade of a sterol transporter on the brush border membrane of intestinal epithelial cells, a Niemann-Pick C1 Like 1 protein transporter.[72]

Through inhibition of intestinal cholesterol absorption, ezetimibe effectively results in net cholesterol excretion because two thirds of cholesterol absorbed via the gut is recycled self-synthesized cholesterol, not just dietary. In addition, by reducing delivery of cholesterol to the liver via Apo B48 lipoproteins, chylomicrons, and its remnants, there is a resultant increase in hepatocyte LDLR expression, which increases removal of LDL-C.

Despite the approval and marketing of ezetimibe for more than 5 years there has been no additional cholesterol absorption transport inhibitors successfully developed although several are, or have been, in early phase 2 development.[73–75] These include compounds from AstraZeneca (AZD4121),[73] Microbia Pharmaceuticals (MCP 201),[74] and Sanofi (AVE 5530),[75] with only the latter now entering further development. The initial AVE 5530 randomized, double-blind, parallel-group, placebo-controlled, ezetimibe-calibrated, 4-week phase 2 multicenter study was conducted in Eastern Europe, Korea, South Africa, and Latin and South America and has not been reported as this time. AVE 5530 is now in widespread global phase 3 clinical development as monotherapy and in combination with statins, targeting a wide array of dyslipidemic patients.[76]

SUMMARY

Although the past 30 years have been the most fruitful and productive in lipid research, from basic science to drug development to demonstration of clinical benefit, cardiovascular disease remains the major cause of mortality and morbidity in industrialized societies. With the rapid industrialization of countries, such as India and China, countries that have nearly half the world's population, cardiovascular disease is rapidly becoming the leading cause of all global death and disability. It is fortunate that most of the most effective lipid-lowering drugs, the statins, have become generic and inexpensive. There remains a large unmet medical need, however, for new and effective agents that are safe. Hopefully, some of those discussed in this article will fill that need.

REFERENCES

1. Randomised trial of cholesterol lowering in 4444 patients with coronary heart disease: the Scandinavian Simvastatin Survival Study (4S). Lancet 1994; 344(8934):1383–9.
2. Sacks FM, Pfeffer MA, Moye LA, et al. The effect of pravastatin on coronary events after myocardial infarction in patients with average cholesterol levels. Cholesterol and Recurrent Events Trial Investigators. N Engl J Med 1996;335: 1001–9.
3. Shepherd J, Cobbe SM, Ford I, et al. West of Scotland Coronary Prevention Study Group. Prevention of coronary heart disease with pravastatin in men with hypercholesterolemia. N Engl J Med 1995;333:1301–7.
4. Heart Protection Study Collaborative Group. MRC/BHF Heart Protection Study of cholesterol lowering with simvastatin in 20 536 high-risk individuals: a randomised placebo-controlled trial. Lancet 2002;360:7–22.
5. Nawrocki JW, Weiss SR, Davidson MH, et al. Reduction of LDL cholesterol by 25–60% in patients with primary hypercholesterolemia by atorvastatin, a new HMG-CoA reductase inhibitor. Arterioscler Thromb Vasc Biol 1995;15:678–82.
6. Davidson MH, Stein E, Hunninghake DB, et al. Lipid-altering efficacy and safety of simvastatin 80 mg/day: worldwide long-term experience in patients with hypercholesterolemia. Nutr Metab Cardiovasc Dis 2000;10:253–63.

7. Jones PH, Davidson MH, Stein EA, et al. STELLAR Study Group. Comparison of efficacy and safety of rosuvastatin versus atorvastatin, simvastatin, and pravastatin across doses (STELLAR Trial). Am J Cardiol 2003;92:152–60.

8. Davidson MH, Ballantyne CM, Kerzner B, et al. Ezetimibe Study Group. Efficacy and safety of ezetimibe coadministered with statins: randomised, placebo-controlled, blinded experience in 2382 patients with primary hypercholesterolemia. Int J Clin Pract 2004;58:746–55.

9. Stein EA, Ose L, Retterstol K, et al. Further reductions in low-density lipoprotein cholesterol and C-reactive protein with the addition of ezetimibe to maximum dose rosuvastatin in patients with severe hypercholesterolemia. J Clin Lipidol 2007;1:280–6.

10. LaRosa JC, Grundy SM, Waters DD, et al. Treating to New Targets (TNT) Investigators. Intensive lipid lowering with atorvastatin in patients with stable coronary disease. N Engl J Med 2005;352:1425–35.

11. Pedersen TR, Faergeman O, Kastelein JJ, et al. Incremental Decrease on End Points Through Aggressive Lipid Lowering (IDEAL) Study Group. JAMA 2005; 294:2437–45.

12. Cannon CP, Braunwald E, McCabe CH, et al. Pravastatin or Atorvastatin Evaluation and Infection Therapy-Thrombolysis In Myocardial Infarction 22 Investigators. Intensive versus moderate lipid lowering with statins after acute coronary syndromes. N Engl J Med 2004;350:1495–504.

13. Grundy SM, Cleeman JI, Merz CN, et al. National Heart, Lung, and Blood Institute, American College of Cardiology Foundation, American Heart Association. Implications of recent clinical trials for the National Cholesterol Education Program Adult Treatment Panel III guidelines. Circulation 2004;110:227–39.

14. Smith SC Jr, Allen J, Blair SN, et al. AHA/ACC, National Heart, Lung, and Blood Institute. AHA/ACC guidelines for secondary prevention for patients with coronary and other atherosclerotic vascular disease: 2006 update: endorsed by the National Heart, Lung, and Blood Institute. Circulation 2006;113:2363–72.

15. Ian Graham I, Atar D, Borch-Johnsen K, et al. for the Task Force. European guidelines on cardiovascular disease prevention in clinical practice: executive summary. Atherosclerosis 2007;194:1–45.

16. Davidson MH, Maki KC, Pearson TA, et al. Results of the National Cholesterol Education (NCEP) Program Evaluation ProjecT Utilizing Novel E-Technology (NEPTUNE) II survey and implications for treatment under the recent NCEP Writing Group recommendations. Am J Cardiol 2005;96:556–63.

17. Bruckert E, Hayem G, Dejager S, et al. Mild to moderate muscular symptoms with high-dosage statin therapy in hyperlipidemic patients—the PRIMO study. Cardiovasc Drugs Ther 2005;19:403–14.

18. Stein EA, Ballantyne CM, Windler E, et al. Efficacy and tolerability of fluvastatin XL 80 mg alone, ezetimibe alone and the combination of fluvastatin XL 80 mg with ezetimibe in patients with a history of muscle-related side effects with other statins: a randomized, double-blind, double-dummy trial. Am J Cardiol 2008;101:490–6.

19. Crooke ST, editor. Antisense drug technology. Principles, strategies and applications. 2nd edition. New York: Marcel Dekker, Inc; 2008.

20. Crooke RM, Graham MJ, Lemonidis KM, et al. An apolipoprotein B antisense oligonucleotide lowers LDL cholesterol in hyperlipidemic mice without causing hepatic steatosis. J Lipid Res 2005;46:872–84.

21. Monia BP, Lesnik EA, Gonzalez C, et al. Evaluation of 2'-modified oligonucleotides containing 2'-deoxy gaps as antisense inhibitors of gene expression. J Biol Chem 1993;268:14514–22.

22. Kastelein JJ, Wedel MK, Baker BF, et al. Potent reduction of apolipoprotein B and low-density lipoprotein cholesterol by short-term administration of an antisense inhibitor of apolipoprotein B. Circulation 2006;114:1729–35.
23. Isis reports new data for mipomersen in routine high cholesterol patients and provides cumulative safety summary [press release]. Newswire. November 13, 2007. Accessed February 12, 2008.
24. Kastelein J, Trip M, Davidson M, et al. Safety and activity of ISIS 301012 in heterozygous familial hypercholesterolemia [abstract 341]. Presented at Drugs Affecting Lipid Metabolism. Journal of Clinical Lipidology 2007;1(5):475.
25. Stein EA. High LDL-C on three drugs. Presented at ACC National Meeting. New Orleans, March 26, 2007.
26. Princeton, N.J. and CARLSBAD, Calif., May 9, 2007/PRNewswire-FirstCall via COMTEX News Network/–Bristol-Myers Squibb Company (NYSE: BMY) and Isis Pharmaceuticals, Inc. (Nasdaq: ISIS). Accessed May 20, 2008.
27. Wetterau JR, Aggerbeck LP, Bouma ME, et al. Absence of microsomal triglyceride transfer protein in individuals with abetalipoproteinemia. Science 1992; 258:999–1001.
28. Scriver CR, Beaudet AL, Sly WS, Valle D, Childs B, Kinzler KW, Vogelstein B, editors. The metabolic and molecular bases of inherited disease. 8th Edition. New York: McGraw-Hill Professional; 2000.
29. Rader DJ, Brewer HB Jr. Abetalipoproteinemia: new insights into lipoprotein assembly and vitamin E metabolism from a rare genetic disease. JAMA 1993;270:865–9.
30. Stein EA, Isaacsohn JL, Mazzu A, et al. Effect of BAY 13-9952, a microsomal triglyceride transfer protein inhibitor on lipids and lipoproteins in dyslipoproteinemic patients [abstract 1342]. Circulation 1999;100(18 Suppl 1).
31. Stein EA, Ames SA, Moore LJ, et al. Inhibition of post-prandial fat absorption with the MTP inhibitor BAY 13-9952 [abstract 2193]. Circulation 2000;102(18, Suppl II):II-601 (presented at AHA national meeting, New Orleans [LA], November 12–15, 2000).
32. Zaiss S, Gruetzmann R, Ulrich M. BAY 13-9952, an inhibitor of the microsomal triglyceride transfer protein (MTP), dose-dependently blocks the formation of atherosclerotic plaques and renders them more stable in apoE knockout mice [abstract 1343]. Circulation 1999;100(18 Suppl 1).
33. Bischoff H, Denzer D, Gruetzmann R, et al. BAY 13-9952 (implitapide): pharmacodynamic effects of a new and highly active inhibitor of the microsomal-triglyceride-transfer-protein (MTP) [abstract TuP9:W16]. Eur Heart J 2000;21(Suppl).
34. Wetterau JR, Gregg RE, Harrity TW, et al. An MTP inhibitor that normalizes atherogenic lipoprotein levels in WHHL rabbits. Science 1999;282:751–4.
35. Chandler CE, Wilder DE, Pettini JL, et al. CP-346086: an MTP inhibitor that lowers plasma total, VLDL, and LDL cholesterol and triglycerides by up to 70% in experimental animals and in humans. J Lipid Res 2003;44:1887–901.
36. Farnier M, Stein E, Megnien S, et al. Efficacy and safety of implitapide, a microsomal triglyceride transfer protein inhibitor in patients with primary hypercholesterolemia. Abstract Book of the XIV International Symposium on Drugs Affecting Lipid Metabolism in New York, September 9–12, 2001:46.
37. Roberts WC. The rule of 5 and the rule of 7 in lipid-lowering by statin drugs. Am J Cardiol 1997;80:106–7.
38. Available at: http://www.clinicaltrials.gov/ct/show/NCT00079859. Accessed February 12, 2008.
39. Cuchel M, Bloedon LT, Szapary PO, et al. Inhibition of microsomal triglyceride transfer protein in familial hypercholesterolemia. N Engl J Med 2007;356: 148–56.

40. Common stock registration statement. AMENDMENT NO. 3 to FORM S-1; May 25, 2007. Washington, DC: Aegerion Pharmaceuticals, Inc., United States Securities and Exchange Commission; 2007. Available at: www.sec.gov/Archives/edgar/data/1338042/000119312507123502/ds1a.htm. Accessed June 16, 2007.

41. Samaha FF, McKenney J, Bloedon LT, et al. Inhibition of microsomal triglyceride transfer protein alone or with ezetimibe in patients with moderate hypercholesterolemia. Nat Clin Pract Cardiovasc Med 2008;5:497–505.

42. Surface Logix Achieves objectives with SLx-4090 in phase 2a clinical trial. Available at: http://www.surfacelogix.com/news/news_080129.htm. Accessed January 29, 2008.

43. Steinberg D, Avigan J, Feigelson EB. Effects of triparanol (mer-29) on cholesterol biosynthesis and on blood sterol levels in man. J Clin Invest 1961;40(5):884–93.

44. Triparanol side effects. Time Magazine. April 3, 1964.

45. Brown MS, Goldstein JL. A receptor-mediated pathway for cholesterol homeostasis. Science 1986;232:34–47.

46. Amano Y, Nishimoto T, Tozawa R, et al. Lipid-lowering effects of TAK-475, a squalene synthase inhibitor, in animal models of familial hypercholesterolemia. Eur J Pharmacol 2003;466:155–61.

47. Baxter A, Fitzgerald BJ, Hutson JL, et al. Squalestatin 1, a potent inhibitor of squalene synthase, which lowers serum cholesterol in vivo. J Biol Chem 1992;267:11705–8.

48. Ciosek CP Jr, Magnin DR, Harrity TW, et al. Lipophilic 1,1-bisphosphonates are potent squalene synthase inhibitors and orally active cholesterol lowering agents in vivo. J Biol Chem 1993;268(33):24832–7.

49. Dufresne C, Wilson KE, Singh SB, et al. Zaragozic acids D and D2: potent inhibitors of squalene synthase and of Ras farnesyl-protein transferase. J Nat Prod 1993;56(11):1923–9.

50. Amin D, Rutledge RZ, Needle SN, et al. RPR 107393, a potent squalene synthase inhibitor and orally effective cholesterol-lowering agent: comparison with inhibitors of HMG-CoA reductase. J Pharmacol Exp Ther 1997;281:746–52.

51. Hiyoshi H, Yanagimachi M, Ito M, et al. Effect of ER-27856, a novel squalene synthase inhibitor, on plasma cholesterol in rhesus monkeys: comparison with 3-hydroxy-3-methylglutaryl-CoA reductase inhibitors. J Lipid Res 2000;41:1136–44.

52. Ugawa T, Kakuta H, Moritani H, et al. YM-53601, a novel squalene synthase inhibitor, reduces plasma cholesterol and triglyceride levels in several animal species. Br J Pharmacol 2000;131:63–70.

53. Watanabe S, Hirai H, Kambara T, et al. CJ-13981 and CJ-13982, new squalene synthase inhibitors. J Antibiot (Tokyo) 2001;54(12):1025–30.

54. Folkers K, Langsjoen P, Willis R, et al. Lovastatin decreases coenzyme Q levels in humans. Proc Natl Acad Sci U S A 1990;87:8931–4.

55. Ghirlanda G, Oradei A, Manto A, et al. Evidence of plasma CoQ10-lowering effect by HMG-CoA reductase inhibitors: a double-blind, placebo-controlled study. J Clin Pharmacol 1993;(33):226–9.

56. US Patent 4 933 165. Coenzyme Q.sub.10 with HMG-CoA reductase inhibitors. A pharmaceutical composition and method of counteracting HMG-CoA reductase inhibitor-associated myopathy is disclosed. The method comprises the adjunct administration of an effective amount of an HMG-CoA reductase inhibitor and an effective amount of coenzyme Q.sub.10. Rahway (NJ): Inventors: Brown MS (Dallas, TX). Assignee: Merck & Co Inc.; June 12, 1990.

57. Marcoff L, Thompson PD. The role of coenzyme Q10 in statin-associated myopathy. J Am Coll Cardiol 2007;49:2231–7.

58. Bostedor RG, Karkas JD, Arison BH, et al. Farnesol- derived dicarboxylic acids in the urine of animals treated with zaragozic acid A or with farnesol. J Biol Chem 1997;272:9197–203.
59. Vaidya S, Bostedor R, Kurtz MM, et al. Massive production of farnesol-derived dicarboxylic acids in mice treated with the squalene synthase inhibitor zaragozic acid A. Arch Biochem Biophys 1998;355:84–92.
60. Piper E, Price G, Chen Y. TAK-475, a squalene synthase inhibitor improves lipid profle in hyperlipidemic subjects [abstract 1493]. Circulation 2006;114(18 Suppl):II-288.
61. Piper E, Price G, Munsaka M, et al. TAK-475, a squalene synthase inhibitor, coadministered with atorvastatin: a pharmacokinetic study [abstract]. American Society for Clinical Pharmacology and Therapeutics Annual Meeting March 21–24, 2007 Anaheim, CA (PI-75). Clin Pharmacol Ther 2007;91(Suppl 1):S37.
62. Clinical white paper. CDER-PHRMA-AASLD Conference 2000. Available at: http://www.fda.gov/Cder/livertox/clinical.pdf; November 2000. Accessed April 18, 2008.
63. Discontinuation of development of TAK-475, a compound for treatment of hyper-cholesterolemia. Available at: http://www.takeda.com/press/article_29153.html. Accessed March 28, 2008.
64. Abifadel M, Varret M, Rabès JP, et al. Mutations in PCSK9 cause autosomal dominant hypercholesterolemia. Nat Genet 2003;34:154–6.
65. McNutt MC, Lagace TA, Horton JD. Catalytic activity is not required for secreted PCSK9 to reduce low density lipoprotein receptors in HepG2 cells. J Biol Chem 2007;282:20799–803.
66. Alborn WE, Cao G, Careskey HE, et al. Serum proprotein convertase subtilisin kexin type 9 is correlated directly with serum LDL cholesterol. Clin Chem 2007;53:1814–9.
67. Cohen JC, Boerwinkle E, Mosley TH Jr, et al. Sequence variations in PCSK9, low LDL, and protection against coronary heart disease. N Engl J Med 2006;354:1264–72.
68. Dubuc G, Chamberland A, Wassef H, et al. Statins upregulate PCSK9, the gene encoding the proprotein convertase neural apoptosis regulated convertase-1 implicated in familial hypercholesterolemia. Arterioscler Thromb Vasc Biol 2004;24:1454–9.
69. Graham MJ, Lemonidis KM, Whipple CP, et al. Antisense inhibition of proprotein convertase subtilisin/kexin type 9 reduces serum LDL in hyperlipidemic mice. J Lipid Res 2007;48:763–7.
70. Bristol-Myers Squibb selects Isis drug targeting PCSK9 as development candidate for prevention and treatment of cardiovascular disease. Carlsbad (CA): PRNewswire-FirstCall; April 8, 2008.
71. Available at: http://www.myfatdog.com/. Accessed August 3, 2008.
72. Altmann SW, Davis HR Jr, Zhu LJ, et al. Niemann-Pick C1 Like 1 protein is critical for intestinal cholesterol absorption. Science 2004;303:1201–4.
73. AstraZeneca AZD4121. Available at: http://www.myfatdog.com/phase_ii_pipe line. Accessed August 3, 2008.
74. Microbia MD-0727/MCP 201. Available at: http://www.microbia.com/pdfs/MicrobiaFinancing030107.pdf. Accessed August 3, 2008.
75. Kramer W, Girbig F, Corsiero D, et al. Aminopeptidase N (CD13) is a molecular target of the cholesterol absorption inhibitor Ezetimibe in the enterocyte brush border membrane. J Biol Chem 2005;280(2):1306–20.
76. Chew P. Presented at Cowen - 28th Annual Health Care Conference. Boston, March 18, 2008. Available at: http://en.sanofi-aventis.com/Default.aspx. Accessed January 16, 2009.

Managing Statin Myopathy

Carmelo V. Venero, MD[a], Paul D. Thompson, MD[a,b],*

KEYWORDS

• Statin • Myopathy • Skeletal muscle • Myalgia
• Cholesterol • Creatine kinase

3-Hydroxy-3-methyl-glutaryl coenzyme A (HMG-CoA) reductase inhibitors (statins) are the most effective and frequently used medications to lower low-density lipoprotein cholesterol (LDL-C) levels, and many studies have documented that statins also reduce cardiovascular events.[1–4] Statins are well tolerated by most patients but 3[5] to 10%[6] of patients develop myalgia with these drugs and fatal rhabdomyolysis has been estimated to occur in approximately 1.5 in 10 million statin prescriptions.[7] Statins can produce a variety of myopathic complaints including myalgia, muscle cramps, weakness, elevated creatine kinase (CK) levels with or without symptoms, and, rarely, frank rhabdomyolysis with renal compromise. The present review examines the symptoms of statin myalgia and suggests clinical approaches to its management.

DEFINITION OF TERMS

Different groups have offered different definitions for the symptoms and findings of statin myopathy. The American College of Cardiology/American Heart Association/National Heart, Lung, and Blood Institute (ACC/AHA/NHLBI) Clinical Advisory on statins defined myopathy as any muscle disease; myalgia as muscle ache or weakness without increased serum CK levels; myositis as muscle symptoms with elevated CK levels; and rhabdomyolysis as muscle symptoms with marked CK elevations (>10 times upper limit of normal [ULN]) plus an elevated serum creatinine.[8] The Food and Drug Administration (FDA) defines rhabdomyolysis as organ damage, typically renal

No funding was received for this report.

Carmelo V. Venero, MD, is a Cardiovascular Disease Fellow at the University of Tennessee Medical Center Knoxville, Tennessee. Paul D. Thompson received research support from Merck/Pfizer/Astra Zenica/B.Braun; is a consultant for Astra Zenica/Merck; is on the Speaker's Bureau for Merck/Pfizer/Abbott/AstraZenica/ScheringPlough; is a stock shareholder of Schering Plough/Merck/Illumina/Zoll; and receives occasional speaking honoraria from Merck/Pfizer/Abbott/AstraZenica/ScheringPlough.

[a] The Henry Low Heart Center, Hartford Hospital, 80 Seymour Street, Hartford, CT 06102, USA
[b] University of Connecticut School of Medicine, 263 Farmington Avenue, Farmington, CT 06030-1912, USA
* Corresponding author. The Henry Low Heart Center, Hartford Hospital, 80 Seymour Street, Hartford, CT 06102.
E-mail address: pthomps@harthosp.org (P.D. Thompson).

Endocrinol Metab Clin N Am 38 (2009) 121–136
doi:10.1016/j.ecl.2008.11.002
0889-8529/08/$ – see front matter © 2009 Elsevier Inc. All rights reserved.

insufficiency, with a CK level greater than 10,000 IU/L.[9] The A-to-Z Trial, a large international randomized double-blind trial, defined rhabdomyolysis as a serum CK level greater than 50 times ULN (10,000 IU/L) with or without renal failure.[10] Such marked increases in CK are unusual in clinical trials, and because such definitions ignore the more frequent smaller CK elevations, they limit the ability to compare the frequency of statin-associated CK elevations among the available statins.

The National Lipid Association's (NLA) Muscle Safety Expert Panel[11] has proposed a classification of rhabdomyolysis based solely on the presence and magnitude of the CK increase (**Box 1**). This assumes that any increase in CK levels is associated with some injury and leakage of the sarcolemma.[12] Rhabdomyolysis in this schema is divided into mild (CK levels are <10 times ULN), moderate (CK $\geq$10 but <50 times ULN), and marked (CK $\geq$50 times ULN). This approach has not been widely adopted, but would increase the number of reported adverse events during statin studies and might increase the probability of differentiating muscle toxicity among the various agents.

THE INCIDENCE OF STATIN-RELATED MYOPATHY

It is difficult to discern the incidence of statin myopathy for a variety of reasons. Severe rhabdomyolysis is extremely rare and, as discussed, lower levels of CK increases are rarely reported in clinical trials. Few early studies elicited myopathic complaints in the absence of CK increases, and most studies have avoided recruiting subjects with risk factors for myopathy. Muscle strength has not been tested in any clinical trials. There also seems to be a gap between the low incidence of myopathic complaints reported in clinical trials and the experience of practicing clinicians. This could be due to the factors mentioned above or to over-reporting of myalgia in clinically managed patients. It is even more difficult to compare the incidence of myopathy among

---

Box 1
Myopathy terminology

1. ACC/AHA/NHLBI Clinical Advisory on Statins

    a. Myopathy—general term for any disease of muscle

    b. Myalgia—muscle ache or weakness without CK elevation

    c. Myositis—muscle symptoms with increased CK levels

    d. Rhabdomyolysis—muscle symptoms with marked CK levels (typically >10× ULN) and with creatinine elevation

2. NLA Muscle Safety Expert Panel suggested terminology

    a. Myopathy—general term for every potential muscle problem

        i. Asymptomatic myopathy: serum CK elevation without myalgia or weakness

        ii. Symptomatic myopathy: presence of myalgia, weakness or cramps

    b. Rhabdomyolysis—evidence of muscle cell injury evidenced by an increase in serum CK levels

        i. Mild CK increase: CK levels > normal but < 10× ULN

        ii. Moderate CK increase: CK levels $\geq$10 × ULN, but < 50× ULN

        iii. Marked CK Increase: CK levels $\geq$ 50× ULN

different statins because there are few studies using two or more statins for a prolonged period that have carefully examined myopathic complaints.

Fatal rhabdomyolysis has been estimated using the FDA Adverse Event Reports System (AERS) and a national prescription auditing system at 1.5 deaths per 10 million prescriptions.[7] Deaths associated with cerivastatin were 21-fold more frequent than for the class in total, but these data are suspect because the FDA AERS depends on the voluntary reporting of events.

Rhabdomyolysis is rare in statin clinical trials. Among more than 80,000 subjects randomized to statin or placebo in 30 clinical trials lasting 0.2 to 5.4 years and reported before 2003, there were only seven cases of rhabdomyolysis, defined as CK values greater than 10× ULN in the statin, and five cases in the placebo groups.[5] Law and Rudnicka calculated a clinical trial incidence of rhabdomyolysis, defined as CK greater than or equal to 10× ULN or to 2,000 U/L, of 4.4 versus 2.8 per 100,000 person-years in the statin and placebo groups respectively, a nonsignificant difference.[13]

Rhabdomyolysis is also rare in clinical practice. A combined analysis of two clinical cohort studies, from the United States[14] and the United Kingdom,[15] in which rhabdomyolysis was identified by physician diagnosis, hospital admission, muscle symptoms, and a serum CK level greater than 10,000 U/L, reported only 3.4 cases of rhabdomyolysis per 100,000 person-years in patients treated with statins other than cerivastatin. The rate was 10-fold higher when these statins were combined with gemfibrozil, 13-fold higher for cerivastatin and greater than 3000-fold higher for the combination of cerivastatin and gemfibrozil.[13] For obvious reasons, cerivastatin has been withdrawn from the market.

Myositis is also rare in clinical trials. Myositis, defined either by the study investigators or as a CK greater than 10× ULN, occurred in 49 participants treated with statins and 44 persons with placebo among 42,323 and 41,435 clinical trial subjects, respectively.[5]

Minor muscle complaints are more frequent, but also relatively rare in clinical trials, and do not differ between treatment group and placebo groups. Among 68,629 participants in 12 clinical trials, muscle pain, tenderness, or weakness sufficient to consult a physician or to stop taking the treatment tablets occurred in 97 statin and 92 placebo subjects per 100,000 person-years of treatment.[13] The largest trial examining myalgias is the Heart Protection Study.[16] This study allocated 10,269 patients to 40 mg of simvastatin and 10,267 to placebo for a median of 5 years. At least one episode of unexplained muscle pain or weakness occurred in 32.9% of the simvastatin and 33.2% of the placebo group, but only 0.5% in each group stopped treatment because of such complaints.

In contrast to these controlled clinical trials, the PRIMO (Prediction of Muscular Risk in Observational conditions) study reported muscular complaints in 10.5% of 7924 unselected patients treated with fluvastatin 80, atorvastatin 40–80, pravastatin 40, or simvastatin 40–80 mg for at least 3 months.[6] There are limitations to this report in that subjects were not blinded and data were obtained by questionnaire, but these results may more closely represent the experience of physicians prescribing higher-dose statins.

THE RISK FACTORS FOR STATIN MYOPATHY

Most of the information on factors that increase the risk of statin myopathy is based on studies examining the incidence of clinically important rhabdomyolysis and myositis. Few studies have examined risk factors for the more minor myopathic symptoms including myalgia, CK increases less than 10 fold, and muscle cramps. It is generally assumed, but unproven, that the same risk factors contribute to all myopathic symptoms.

Factors that increase the risk of statin myopathy include conditions that increase statin serum and muscle concentration, drugs that affect statin metabolism, and factors that increase muscle susceptibility to injury (**Box 2**). Statin myopathy is a class effect and can occur with all available agents. Nevertheless, the experience with cerivastatin illustrates that the statin itself affects the frequency of statin myopathy although this may be mediated via differences in statin catabolism.

Statin concentration increases with drug dose, advanced age, debilitation, reduced body size, female gender, decreased renal and hepatic function, hypothyroidism, and concomitant medications.[17] Statin serum concentration can be affected by other compounds that affect statin hepatic or intestinal catabolism. The cytochrome P-450 system is responsible for the conversion of fat- to water-soluble compounds for clearance.[18] CYP3A4 is the major cytochrome P-450 isoenzyme in the liver and intestinal wall.[18] Lovastatin, simvastatin and atorvastatin are catabolized primarily by CYP3A4 (**Table 1**)[19] so that other medications also catabolized by this enzyme can occupy catalytic sites and increase statin concentrations. Drugs known to increase statin concentrations in part because of their catabolism by the CYP3A4 system include itraconazole, verapamil, cyclosporine, macrolide antibiotics, diltiazem, amiodarone, protease inhibitors and antidepressants such as the tricyclic antidepressants, nefazodone, venlaflaxine, fluvoxamine, fluoxetine, and sertraline (**Table 2**).[19,20]

Box 2
Risk factors associated with statin-induced myopathy

1. Factors related to an increase in statin serum level

    a. Statin dose

    b. Small body frame

    c. Decreased statin metabolism and excretion

        i. Drug–drug interactions

        ii. Grapefruit juice (possibly also pomegranate & starfruit)

        iii. Hypothyroidism and diabetes mellitus[9]

        iv. Advanced age

        v. Liver disease

        vi. Renal disease

2. Factors related to muscle predisposition

    a. Alcohol consumption

    b. Drug abuse (cocaine, amphetamines, heroin)

    c. Heavy exercise

    d. Baseline muscular disease:

        i. Multisystemic diseases: diabetes mellitus, hypothyroidism

        ii. Inflammatory or inherited metabolic muscle defects

Table 1
Pharmacokinetic characteristics of statins

Statin	Absorption (%)	Bioavailability (%)	Lipophilicity	Primary Metabolic Pathways	Elimination Half-Life (h)	Urinary Excretion (%)	Fecal Excretion (%)
Atorvastatin	30	12	Yes	CYP3A4	15–30	2	98
Fluvastatin XL	95	6	Yes	CYP2C9	4.7	5	95
Lovastatin[a]	30	5[b]	Yes	CYP3A4	2.9	10	83
Pravastatin	34	18	No	Sulfation	1.3–2.8	20	71
Rosuvastatin	50	20	No	Minimal hepatic metabolism[c]	20.8	10	90
Simvastatin[a]	60–80	5	Yes	CYP3A4	2–3	13	58

[a] Administered as inactive prodrug requiring activation by liver metabolism.
[b] Immediate-release lovastatin should be administered with food to increase bioavailability.
[c] <10% metabolism by CYP2C9 and CYP2C19.

Data from Ballantyne CM, Corsini A, Davidson MH, et al. Risk for myopathy with statin therapy in high-risk patients. Arch Intern Med 2003;163:553–64; and Harper CR, Jacobson TA. The broad spectrum of statin myopathy: from myalgia to rhabdomyolysis. Curr Opin Lipidol 2007;18(4):401–8.

Table 2
Drugs affecting statin metabolism

Drug(s)	Statin(s) Affected	Comments
Glucuronidation inhibitor		
Gemfibrozil	All	Fenofibrate preferred fibrate to combine with statin, especially when statin used beyond its starting dose
CYP3A4 Inhibitors		
Itraconazole, ketoconazole	Atorvastatin, lovastatin, simvastatin	Avoid concomitant use if possible
Macrolide antibiotics	Atorvastatin, lovastatin, simvastatin, pravastatin	Avoid concomitant use if possible
Protease inhibitors	Lovastatin, simvastatin affected more than atorvastatin	Pravastatin and fluvastatin can be used at usual doses Atorvastatin may be use at lowest possible dose
	Rosuvastatin	Rosuvastatin should be limited to 10 mg/day in patients using lopinavir/ritonavir
Verapamil, diltiazem	Simvastatin, lovastatin, atorvastatin	Recommended maximal dose of simvastatin 20 mg/day and lovastatin 40 mg/day when used in patients receiving concomitant verapamil
Amiodarone	Simvastatin, lovastatin, atorvastatin	Recommended maximal dose of simvastatin 20 mg/day and lovastatin 40 mg/day
CYP2C9 Inhibitors		
Fluconazole, ketoconazole	Fluvastatin, rosuvastatin	Avoid concomitant use if possible
Various Mechanisms		
Cyclosporine	All except fluvastatin	Fluvastatin has no drug interaction with cyclosporine Rosuvastatin does not increase cyclosporine level but highest dose should be 5 mg/day Other statins require lowest possible dose with monitoring of cyclosporine levels
Colchicine	Lovastatin, simvastatin affected more than atorvastatin Pravastatin, fluvastatin	Fluvastatin, pravastatin, rosuvastatin, and atorvastatin are less likely to interact with colchicine

All patients treated with statin and above mentioned drugs are at increased risk for myotoxicity and should be monitored for myopathy.

Fluvastatin, and to a lesser degree rosuvastatin, are metabolized by CYP2C9, so their concentrations may be affected by interactions with fluconazole and ketoconazole.[19,20] Pravastatin is the only statin not metabolized by the cytochrome P-450 system.[19] For these reasons fluvastatin, rosuvastatin, and pravastatin are less likely to interact with other medications. Different individuals are affected differently by these drug interactions, however, because there is up to a 10-fold variation in specific cytochrome P-450 isoenzymes activity among different individuals due to genetic variants in these enzymes.[20]

An interaction with the intestinal CYP3A4 may also explain the ability of certain tropical juices such as grapefruit, starfruit, and pomegranate to increase statin levels and the risk of muscle injury.[21] These juices contain an irreversible or "suicide" inhibitor of intestinal CYP3A4 producing increased bioavailability of atorvastatin, lovastatin, and simvastatin.[22] Grapefruit juice reduces CYP3A4 activity by 50% within 4 hours and by 30% for as long as 24 hours after ingestion.[22] This effect of grapefruit juice disappears over 3–7 days.[22] Several studies document that 600 mL of double strength grapefruit juice for 3 days produces a >10-fold increase in the area under the curve (AUC) of simvastatin and lovastatin, but only a 2.5-fold increase in atorvastatin's AUC. Grapefruit juice, 240–600 mL of regular-strength for 3 days, raises the AUC 1.4- and 1.94-fold for atorvastatin and lovastatin respectively.[23] Consequently, even this modest intake significantly increases statin levels. An intake of > 1 quart/day has been selected as the amount for concern,[8] but it is likely that the continued daily intake of even small quantities of certain tropical juices can increase statin availability because of the irreversible inhibition of intestinal CYP3A4. This is generally not an important clinical problem and should be considered only when prescribing high statin doses to high-risk patients or when unexplained rhabdomyolysis occurs. Tropical juices should not affect metabolism of statins not metabolized by CYP3A4, but pomegranate juice has been associated with rhabdomyolysis in at least one patient taking rosuvastatin and ezetimibe.[21]

The CYP system does not explain all drug interactions with statins. Gemfibrozil is the concomitant medication most frequently associated with rhabdomyolysis, but has limited interaction via the CYP system involved in the catabolism of currently available statins.[24] Statins undergo glucuronidation as part of their phase II metabolism.[25] Gemfibrozil appears to increase statin concentration by competitively inhibiting statin glucuronidation, and this inhibition is most marked in vitro with cerivastatin.[25] Gemfibrozil increases the hydroxyl acid statin AUC by 5.6-fold when given simultaneously with cerivastatin, by 2- to 3-fold with simvastatin, lovastatin, and pravastatin, and by 1- to 1.5-fold with rosuvastatin and atorvastatin, whereas such interaction has not been observed when combined with fluvastatin.[25] Gemfibrozil also inhibits CYP2C8, an additional cerivastatin catabolism pathway.[24] Gemfibrozil's inhibition of both cerivastatin glucuronidation and CYP catabolism probably explains the markedly higher risk for rhabdomyolysis when gemfibrozil and cerivastatin were used together.[26] In contrast, fenofibrate does not appear to affect glucuronidation of statins, and appears to be safer when used with statins.[24]

The elimination route of statins also affects their plasma concentration. The statins are primarily excreted via bile into feces,[27] therefore patients with biliary tract disease are at increased risk for statin myotoxicity. Atorvastatin and fluvastatin have less than 6% urine excretion,[19] which makes them useful in chronic kidney disease. Only 10% of rosuvastatin is eliminated in the urine,[19] but it should be used cautiously in patients with decreased renal function because its long half-life can increase serum concentrations in such patients.

Considerable marketing attention has been given to the differences in statin hydrophilicity. Muscle, in contrast to liver, has no active statin transport system so that the statin must transverse the lipid-rich sarcolemma to gain entry into the muscle.[5] More water-soluble compounds such as pravastatin and rosuvastatin may be less likely to gain access and to cause myopathic complaints. Although theoretically attractive, there is no conclusive evidence that statin water solubility is a major factor in determining myopathic risk since rhabdomyolysis has occurred with all available agents regardless of hydrophilicity.

Other drugs and individual susceptibility also increase the risk of statin myopathy. Alcohol is a direct muscle toxin and may increase the risk of myopathy.[28] Colchicine is also a muscle toxin and has been associated with statin myopathy.[29–34] This has generally been attributed to colchicine's metabolism via the CYP3A4 pathway and the presence of renal failure in most cases,[31–34] but myopathy has also been reported with colchicine and fluvastatin[30] or pravastatin,[29] agents not catabolized by CYP3A4.

Skeletal muscle genetic metabolic variants probably also increase the risk of myopathy.[28] These patients may present with increased CK levels before statin therapy or persistent CK elevations 2–3 months after stopping the statin. Among 110 patients with presumed statin myopathy, 10% were found to be heterozygous or homozygous for mutations causing myophosphorylase deficiency or Mc Ardle's disease, carnitine palmitoyltransferase II deficiency or myoadenylate deaminase deficiency.[35] Other genetic variants linked to increased risk for statin myotoxicity include polymorphism in the CYP2D6 enzyme, which decreases the catabolism of statins;[36] CoQ2 gene variants, which reduces the production of coenzyme Q10 (CoQ10), a mitochondrial transport protein;[37] and serotonin receptors HTR38 and HTR7 genes variants, which cause individual differences in pain perception.[38]

Physical activity has been associated with increased CK levels[39] and symptoms[6] during statin treatment. Exercise itself can increase CK levels, especially exercise in which the muscle contracts while lengthening such as downhill locomotion or lowering a weight. CK levels were 62% and 77% higher 24 and 48 hours after downhill treadmill exercise in patients treated with lovastatin compared with placebo patients, and some patients increased their CK levels 10- to 20-fold higher the day after exercise.[39] In the PRIMO study, patients who participated in some "intense form of sport" reported muscle symptoms during statin therapy 38% more frequently than patients performing less vigorous activities.[6]

THE PATHOPHYSIOLOGICAL MECHANISMS OF STATIN-INDUCED MYOPATHY

The cause of statin-induced myopathy is unknown and it is not certain that the same metabolic changes produce the entire spectrum of statin complaints. Statins block cholesterol synthesis early in its metabolic pathway at a step that not only reduces cholesterol synthesis but also the production of other important metabolites including ubiquinone or coenzyme Q10, dolichols and other prenylated isoprenoids required for normal functioning of the skeletal myocyte (**Fig. 1**). Consequently, most theories on the cause of statin myopathy involve changes in one of these end products.

Decreased cholesterol production could produce several metabolic alterations associated with statin myopathy. Cholesterol participates in the regulation of cell membrane fluidity and small changes in the cholesterol:phospholipid ratio can modify membrane excitability, primarily driven by affecting sodium, potassium, and especially chloride channels.[40] Treatment of rabbit and rat muscle with statins has induced membrane hyperexcitability similar to myopathies associated with chloride transport impairment.[40] Lowering cholesterol production could decrease sarcolemmal cholesterol altering the membrane's stability, but this seems unlikely since myopathy does not appear directly related to cholesterol levels during treatment. Alternatively, increased muscle cell LDL receptor activity, produced by reduced intracellular cholesterol levels, could facilitate the uptake of LDL and very low density lipoprotein (VLDL) particles leading to a "fat myopathy."[41] Increased intramuscular fat content has been

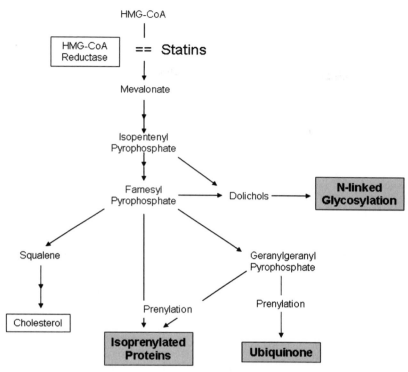

Fig. 1. The mevalonate pathway. Statins block the conversion of HMG-CoA to mevalonate by inhibiting HMG-CoA reductase, decreasing cholesterol production but also suppressing formation of isoprenoids required for the normal function of the muscle. (*Data from* Thompson PD, Clarkson P, Karas RH. Statin-associated myopathy. JAMA 2003;289:1681–90, and Baker SK. Molecular clues into the pathogenesis of statin-mediated muscle toxicity. Muscle Nerve 2005;31:572–80.)

demonstrated in some patients with statin myopathy.[42] Increased LDL receptor activity could also increase the uptake of plant sterols and increased muscle sitosterol levels have been detected in subjects with statin myopathy treated with simvastatin 80 mg for 8 weeks.[41] An increased skeletal muscle plant sterol level could promote statin myopathy by inhibiting cellular growth, de novo cholesterol and deoxyribonucleic acid synthesis, and induction of apoptosis.[41]

The observation that squalene synthase inhibitors, which reduce cholesterol production without decreasing isoprenylated metabolites, produce a 50-fold decrease in in vitro myotoxicity compared with atorvastatin and simvastatin[43] supports the concept that decreases in some noncholesterol product of the mevalonate pathway produces statin myopathy. A reduction of the isopentenylation of selenocysteine tRNA, the isoprenoids dolichols and ubiquinone, and the guanosine triphosphate (GTP)-binding proteins Rho, Ras, and Rac affect processes such as N-linked glycosylation, electron-transport in the mitochondrial membrane and intracellular trafficking of membrane-associated proteins essential for myogenesis and myoregeneration.[44] The isoprenylated GTP-binding proteins Ras, Rac, and Rho promote cell maintenance and growth, and inhibit apoptosis.[5] Apoptosis occurs in human muscle cells acutely exposed to statins in vitro.[45] Addition of mevalonate prevents the statin-induced apoptosis suggesting that products distal to mevalonate are responsible for the skeletal cell apoptosis.[45] Isoprenylation, farnesylation and geranylgeranylation regulate the activity of the GTP-binding proteins. Statins decrease these proteins' geranylgeranylation and farnesylation with subsequent increase in cytosolic calcium and activation of mitochondria-mediated apoptosis.[45] Moreover, these GTP-binding proteins regulate the recuperation of muscle fibers after exercise possibly explaining the synergistic myopathic effect of exercise and statins.[5]

Perhaps the most popular theory for statin myopathy is depletion of intramuscular ubiquinone producing mitochondrial dysfunction. Ubiquinone is an essential component of the mitochondrial respiratory chain and is involved in mitochondrial electron transport. Serum ubiquinone levels decrease during statin therapy, but ubiquinone is transported in lower density lipoprotein particles and its decrease is commensurate with decreases in blood cholesterol.[46] This suggests that the decrease in serum ubiquinone is due to reduction in the transport particles.[46] Muscle biopsies studies have failed to detect consistent reductions in muscle ubiquinone levels[46] although one study in statin-naive subjects found reductions of 30% in intramuscular ubiquinone levels in subjects treated with simvastatin 80 mg for 8 weeks.[41] Muscle ubiquinone levels remained, however, within the low normal range.[41] Physical inactivity decreases muscle mitochondria, raising the possibility that reduced physical activity produced by the myopathy decreases mitochondrial volume, thereby reducing intramuscular ubiquinone levels and not that the decrease in ubiquinone produces the myopathy.

Several studies have suggested that changes in the ubiquitin proteasome pathway (UPP) may contribute to statin myopathy. The UPP system is responsible for the recognition and degradation of many skeletal muscle proteins and is involved in conditions involving muscle mass loss such as cancer cachexia, diabetes, uremia, and sepsis. Urso and colleagues[47] demonstrated increased transcription of members of the UPP system in an exercise-injury model of statin myopathy. Atrogin-1, a component of the UPP system, is induced early in the atrophy process. Urso reported marked reductions in Atrogin transcription in their model. In contrast, Hanai and colleagues[48] found increases in atrogin-1 expression in human skeletal muscle in patients with statin myopathy, and animal cells lacking atrogin-1 were resistant to statin myotoxicity. Both studies suggest a critical role for atrogin-1 and the UPP system in statin-induced myotoxicity, although the direction and significance of change are not clear.

Differences in pain perception may also affect the frequency of statin myalgia. The serotonergic system has been related to myalgic syndromes such as fibromyalgia,[49] and polymorphisms in genes encoding for the serotonin receptors HTR33 and HTR7 are statistically related to myalgias in statin-treated patients.[38] In the PRIMO study, patients with a background of fibromyalgia-like symptoms were three times more likely to have muscular symptoms with statins, whereas patients treated with antidepressants had a 50% risk reduction of muscular symptoms (OR 0.51, 95% CI 0.35–0.74, $P = .0004$).[6]

THE MANAGEMENT OF STATIN MYOPATHY

The management of statin myopathy includes preventing symptoms in the first place, monitoring patients with symptoms or CK elevations, using novel strategies to lower lipids in statin intolerant patients, and constantly evaluating the risk and benefits of these agents in individual patients (**Box 3**).

Muscle complaints and frank rhabdomyolysis generally increase with increasing statin doses so that patients should be treated with the lowest dose necessary to

---

Box 3
Statin-related myopathy management recommendations

1. Asymptomatic patients

   a. Routine surveillance of CK levels is not required except in high-risk patients

   b. If CK measured

      i. CK < 5× ULN: reassurance

      ii. CK ≥5 - <10× ULN: monitor for symptoms and periodical CK determination

      iii. CK ≥10× ULN: stop statin and reconsider risks and benefits of statin treatment

2. Symptomatic patients

   a. Reconsider risks and benefits of statin treatment

   b. Tolerable symptoms

      i. Follow recommendations per CK guidelines mentioned above

      ii. May try tonic water or coenzyme Q10 supplementation

   c. Intolerable symptoms or serum CK values ≥ 10× ULN, stop statin

      i. Patients with associated acute renal failure or CK > 10,000 U/L

         1. Once recovered, benefit-risk of statin therapy needs to be reconsidered. Careful use of alternative lipid lowering agent is recommended

      ii. Other patients, once symptoms and CK returned to baseline can:

         1. Rechallenge same statin and dose to evaluate reproducibility of symptoms

         2. Switch to statin containing regimen tried in patients intolerant to daily statin

            a. Fluvastatin XL 80 mg and EZT 10 mg/day

            b. Atorvastatin 10 mg BIW and EZT 10 mg/day

            c. Rosuvastatin (2.5–10 mg) 2 or 3 times/week

            d. Atorvastatin (10–40 mg) 3 times a week

         3. Try coenzyme Q10 supplementation

         4. Unable to tolerate or unwilling to retry statins requires use of alternative lipid lowering agents (including red yeast rice) or LDL apheresis for qualified patients

When CK increased search for causes of CK elevation, such as increased physical activity, trauma/falls, infections, hypothyroidism, alcohol, or cocaine use.
Abbreviations: BIW, twice a week; EZT, ezetimibe.

---

achieve their therapeutic goal. Concomitant therapy with gemfibrozil should be avoided, although its use is sometimes unavoidable in patients with financial constraints because gemfibrozil is off-patent. In these instances the dose of statin should be reduced and patients monitored for myopathy. We tend to select atorvastatin, pravastatin, or fluvastatin for therapy in patients at high risk for myopathy because of age or concomitant medications since these agents appear well-tolerated.[7]

Patients should be gently warned about the symptoms of myotoxicity, and physicians should not ignore unexplained systemic complaints in patients on high-dose statin therapy. The diagnosis of rhabdomyolysis may be delayed because patients report a flu-like illness. We recommend discontinuing statins for 5 days before extreme exertion such as marathon running given the magnified muscle injury produced by exercise during statin therapy. We also discontinue statins when patients develop rhabdomyolysis from other causes such as vascular injury, and before major surgery such as aortic aneurysm repair. This latter recommendation is controversial but based on the belief that the risk for muscle hypoperfusion is increased during such surgery, and that the risk of continued statin therapy outweighs the small risk of their discontinuation.

Creatine Kinase Measurment

Baseline CK measurements before statin therapy are useful and recommended by the National Cholesterol Education Program–Adult Treatment Panel III (NCEP–ATP III). Many patients have baseline CK elevations and a baseline level helps differentiate statin from endogenous CK increases. Routine surveillance of CK levels is not required except for patients at high risk for myopathy such as those with hepatic or renal disease or on medications that could interfere with statin metabolism.

Increases in CK levels are common during statin therapy and may be due to other factors, most notably unusual physical activity. Consequently, asymptomatic increases in CK should prompt a query about recent exercise and a search for other muscle toxins such as alcohol or cocaine use and hypothyroidism. Once other causes of increased CK are excluded, we recommend that patients with asymptomatic CK increases less than 5× ULN be reassured and asked to report symptoms, that patients with asymptomatic CK increase greater than or equal to 5×, but less than 10× ULN be monitored for symptoms and have periodic CK determinations monthly or bimonthly, and that asymptomatic patients with CK greater than or equal to 10× ULN have the statin stopped or carefully evaluated for the risks and benefits of further treatment.

Symptomatic Patients

We continue symptomatic patients on the statin if therapy is justified by a risk/benefit analysis, if the patient deems the symptoms tolerable, and using the CK guidelines above. If the symptoms are intolerable, we stop the statin until the patient feels normal. This can take up to 2 months.[11] We then restart the statin at a lower dose or try a different statin. If the patient can only tolerate a lower dose, we add ezetimibe to achieve the LDL goal. If no statin is tolerated, we use another lipid-lowering class of medication or LDL apheresis for qualified patients.[50]

We have also had apparent clinical success with atypical treatment regimens although only some of these are published in peer-reviewed journals. Some patients deemed intolerant of statins can successfully use over-the-counter red yeast rice, which has lovastatin among its active ingredients.[51] Two 600 mg tablets with the evening meal can reduce LDL-C 22%–26%.[51,52] We are uncertain why "statin intolerant" patients can tolerate this regimen, but suspect it is due to some patients' concern about standard pharmaceutical products. We have also used atorvastatin or rosuvastatin every other day[53,54] or rosuvastatin twice weekly[55] in statin-intolerant patients with good tolerance and LDL reductions. Fluvastatin XL with or without ezetimibe,[56] and twice-a-week atorvastatin combined with daily ezetimibe[57] are also effective. Some statin intolerant patients can tolerate statins for brief periods of time, for example, 4 weeks. If these patients definitely require statin therapy, we treat them using what we call "pulse therapy," meaning that we treat them until they are 1–2 weeks away from the usual start of their pain. We then give them a week or two off therapy before restarting treatment. This approach is based on the belief that some time with lower cholesterol levels is more beneficial than consistently higher levels.

We have had apparent clinical success advising patients with statin-related leg cramps to consume 12 ounces of tonic water, which contains quinine, at bedtime. We also occasionally use coenzyme Q10 supplements, and some patients appear to benefit. We do not know whether this represents a placebo effect or the fact that some patients actually benefit physiologically. CoQ10 supplementation has produced variable results in treating statin myopathy.[46,58,59] Nevertheless, given the lack of known risks to CoQ10, it can be tried in patients with statin myalgias unable to be treated with other agents.

SUMMARY

Statins are extremely well tolerated, but approximately 10% of patients in clinical practice experience some form of muscle-related side effects. These can range from asymptomatic CK elevation, to muscle pain, weakness, and its most severe form, rhabdomyolysis. Higher-risk patients for statin myopathy are those older than 80, with a small body frame, on higher statin doses, on other medications, or with other systemic diseases including hepatic or renal diseases, diabetes mellitus, or hypothyroidism. The cause of statin myopathy has not been defined. In symptomatic patients, the symptoms and CK levels determine whether statin therapy can be continued or must be stopped. Several novel strategies may be useful in managing statin-related muscle symptoms.

REFERENCES

1. Randomised trial of cholesterol lowering in 4444 patients with coronary heart disease: the scandinavian simvastatin survival study (4S). Lancet 1994; 344(8934):1383–9.
2. Downs JR, Clearfield M, Weis S, et al. Primary prevention of acute coronary events with lovastatin in men and women with average cholesterol levels: results of AFCAPS/TexCAPS. Air Force/Texas Coronary Atherosclerosis Prevention Study. JAMA 1998;279(20):1615–22.
3. Sacks FM, Pfeffer MA, Moye LA, et al. The effect of pravastatin on coronary events after myocardial infarction in patients with average cholesterol levels. Cholesterol and recurrent events trial investigators. N Engl J Med 1996;335(14): 1001–9.
4. Shepherd J, Cobbe SM, Ford I, et al. Prevention of coronary heart disease with pravastatin in men with hypercholesterolemia. West of Scotland Coronary Prevention Study Group. N Engl J Med 1995;333(20):1301–7.
5. Thompson PD, Clarkson P, Karas RH. Statin-associated myopathy. JAMA 2003; 289(13):1681–90.
6. Bruckert E, Hayem G, Dejager S, et al. Mild to moderate muscular symptoms with high-dosage statin therapy in hyperlipidemic patients–the PRIMO study. Cardiovasc Drugs Ther 2005;19(6):403–14.
7. Staffa JA, Chang J, Green L. Cerivastatin and reports of fatal rhabdomyolysis. N Engl J Med 2002;346(7):539–40.
8. Pasternak RC, Smith SC Jr, Bairey-Merz CN, et al. ACC/AHA/NHLBI clinical advisory on the use and safety of statins. J Am Coll Cardiol 2002;40(3):567–72.
9. Ballantyne CM, Corsini A, Davidson MH, et al. Risk for myopathy with statin therapy in high-risk patients. Arch Intern Med 2003;163(5):553–64.
10. de Lemos JA, Blazing MA, Wiviott SD, et al. Early intensive vs a delayed conservative simvastatin strategy in patients with acute coronary syndromes: phase Z of the A to Z trial. JAMA 2004;292(11):1307–16.

11. Thompson PD, Clarkson PM, Rosenson RS. An assessment of statin safety by muscle experts. Am J Cardiol 2006;97(8A):69C–76C.
12. Poels PJ, Gabreels FJ. Rhabdomyolysis: a review of the literature. Clin Neurol Neurosurg 1993;95(3):175–92.
13. Law M, Rudnicka AR. Statin safety: a systematic review. Am J Cardiol 2006; 97(8A):52C–60C.
14. Graham DJ, Staffa JA, Shatin D, et al. Incidence of hospitalized rhabdomyolysis in patients treated with lipid-lowering drugs. JAMA 2004;292(21):2585–90.
15. Black C, Jick H. Etiology and frequency of rhabdomyolysis. Pharmacotherapy 2002;22(12):1524–6.
16. Heart Protection Study Collaborative Group. MRC/BHF Heart Protection Study of cholesterol lowering with simvastatin in 20,536 high-risk individuals: a randomised placebo-controlled trial. Lancet 2002;360(9326):7–22.
17. Sewright KA, Clarkson PM, Thompson PD. Statin myopathy: incidence, risk factors, and pathophysiology. Curr Atheroscler Rep 2007;9(5):389–96.
18. Bottorff MB. Statin safety and drug interactions: clinical implications. Am J Cardiol 2006;97(8A):27C–31C.
19. Bellosta S, Paoletti R, Corsini A. Safety of statins: focus on clinical pharmacokinetics and drug interactions. Circulation 2004;109(23 Suppl 1):III50–7.
20. Bolego C, Baetta R, Bellosta S, et al. Safety considerations for statins. Curr Opin Lipidol 2002;13(6):637–44.
21. Sorokin AV, Duncan B, Panetta R, et al. Rhabdomyolysis associated with pomegranate juice consumption. Am J Cardiol 2006;98(5):705–6.
22. Kiani J, Imam SZ. Medicinal importance of grapefruit juice and its interaction with various drugs. Nutr J 2007;6:33.
23. Saito M, Hirata-Koizumi M, Matsumoto M, et al. Undesirable effects of citrus juice on the pharmacokinetics of drugs: focus on recent studies. Drug Saf 2005;28(8): 677–94.
24. Prueksaritanont T, Tang C, Qiu Y, et al. Effects of fibrates on metabolism of statins in human hepatocytes. Drug Metab Dispos 2002;30(11):1280–7.
25. Goosen TC, Bauman JN, Davis JA, et al. Atorvastatin glucuronidation is minimally and nonselectively inhibited by the fibrates gemfibrozil, fenofibrate, and fenofibric acid. Drug Metab Dispos 2007;35(8):1315–24.
26. Prueksaritanont T, Zhao JJ, Ma B, et al. Mechanistic studies on metabolic interactions between gemfibrozil and statins. J Pharmacol Exp Ther 2002;301(3): 1042–51.
27. Corsini A, Bellosta S, Baetta R, et al. New insights into the pharmacodynamic and pharmacokinetic properties of statins. Pharmacol Ther 1999;84(3):413–28.
28. Harper CR, Jacobson TA. The broad spectrum of statin myopathy: from myalgia to rhabdomyolysis. Curr Opin Lipidol 2007;18(4):401–8.
29. Alayli G, Cengiz K, Canturk F, et al. Acute myopathy in a patient with concomitant use of pravastatin and colchicine. Ann Pharmacother 2005;39(7–8):1358–61.
30. Atasoyu EM, Evrenkaya TR, Solmazgul E. Possible colchicine rhabdomyolysis in a fluvastatin-treated patient. Ann Pharmacother 2005;39(7–8):1368–9.
31. Hsu WC, Chen WH, Chang MT, et al. Colchicine-induced acute myopathy in a patient with concomitant use of simvastatin. Clin Neuropharmacol 2002;25(5):266–8.
32. Justiniano M, Dold S, Espinoza LR. Rapid onset of muscle weakness (rhabdomyolysis) associated with the combined use of simvastatin and colchicine. J Clin Rheumatol 2007;13(5):266–8.
33. Torgovnick J, Sethi N, Arsura E. Colchicine and HMG Co-A reductase inhibitors induced myopathy–a case report. Neurotoxicology 2006;27(6):1126–7.

34. Tufan A, Dede DS, Cavus S, et al. Rhabdomyolysis in a patient treated with colchicine and atorvastatin. Ann Pharmacother 2006;40(7–8):1466–9.

35. Vladutiu GD, Simmons Z, Isackson PJ, et al. Genetic risk factors associated with lipid-lowering drug-induced myopathies. Muscle Nerve 2006;34(2):153–62.

36. Frudakis TN, Thomas MJ, Ginjupalli SN, et al. CYP2D6*4 polymorphism is associated with statin-induced muscle effects. Pharmacogenet Genomics 2007;17(9):695–707.

37. Oh J, Ban MR, Miskie BA, et al. Genetic determinants of statin intolerance. Lipids Health Dis 2007;6:7.

38. Ruano G, Thompson PD, Windemuth A, et al. Physiogenomic association of statin-related myalgia to serotonin receptors. Muscle Nerve 2007;36(3):329–35.

39. Thompson PD, Zmuda JM, Domalik LJ, et al. Lovastatin increases exercise-induced skeletal muscle injury. Metabolism 1997;46(10):1206–10.

40. Sirvent P, Mercier J, Lacampagne A. New insights into mechanisms of statin-associated myotoxicity. Curr Opin Pharmacol 2008;8:1–6.

41. Paiva H, Thelen KM, Van Coster R, et al. High-dose statins and skeletal muscle metabolism in humans: a randomized, controlled trial. Clin Pharmacol Ther 2005;78(1):60–8.

42. Phillips PS, Haas RH, Bannykh S, et al. Statin-associated myopathy with normal creatine kinase levels. Ann Intern Med 2002;137(7):581–5.

43. Nishimoto T, Tozawa R, Amano Y, et al. Comparing myotoxic effects of squalene synthase inhibitor, T-91485, and 3-hydroxy-3-methylglutaryl coenzyme A (HMG-CoA) reductase inhibitors in human myocytes. Biochem Pharmacol 2003; 66(11):2133–9.

44. Baker SK. Molecular clues into the pathogenesis of statin-mediated muscle toxicity. Muscle Nerve 2005;31(5):572–80.

45. Dirks AJ, Jones KM. Statin-induced apoptosis and skeletal myopathy. Am J Physiol Cell Physiol 2006;291(6):C1208–12.

46. Marcoff L, Thompson PD. The role of coenzyme Q10 in statin-associated myopathy: a systematic review. J Am Coll Cardiol 2007;49(23):2231–7.

47. Urso ML, Clarkson PM, Hittel D, et al. Changes in ubiquitin proteasome pathway gene expression in skeletal muscle with exercise and statins. Arterioscler Thromb Vasc Biol 2005;25(12):2560–6.

48. Hanai J, Cao P, Tanksale P, et al. The muscle-specific ubiquitin ligase atrogin-1/MAFbx mediates statin-induced muscle toxicity. J Clin Invest 2007;117(12): 3940–51.

49. Koeppe C, Schneider C, Thieme K, et al. The influence of the 5-HT3 receptor antagonist tropisetron on pain in fibromyalgia: a functional magnetic resonance imaging pilot study. Scand J Rheumatol Suppl 2004;33(119):24–7.

50. Thompsen J, Thompson PD. A systematic review of LDL apheresis in the treatment of cardiovascular disease. Atherosclerosis 2006;189(1):31–8.

51. Liu J, Zhang J, Shi Y, et al. Chinese red yeast rice (Monascus purpureus) for primary hyperlipidemia: a meta-analysis of randomized controlled trials. Chinas Med 2006;1:4.

52. Huang CF, Li TC, Lin CC, et al. Efficacy of Monascus purpureus Went rice on lowering lipid ratios in hypercholesterolemic patients. Eur J Cardiovasc Prev Rehabil 2007;14(3):438–40.

53. Juszczyk MA, Seip RL, Thompson PD. Decreasing LDL cholesterol and medication cost with every-other-day statin therapy. Prev Cardiol 2005;8(4):197–9.

54. Backes JM, Venero CV, Gibson CA, et al. Effectiveness and tolerability of every-other-day rosuvastatin dosing in patients with prior statin intolerance. Ann Pharmacother 2008;42:341–6.

55. Gadarla M, Kearns A, Thompson PD. Efficacy of rosuvastatin (5 mg and 10 mg) twice a week in patients intolerant to daily statins. Am J Cardiol 2008;10(12): 1747–8.
56. Stein EA, Ballantyne CM, Windler E, et al. Efficacy and tolerability of fluvastatin XL 80 mg alone, ezetimibe alone, and the combination of fluvastatin XL 80 mg with ezetimibe in patients with a history of muscle-related side effects with other statins. Am J Cardiol 2008;101(4):490–6.
57. Athyros VG, Tziomalos K, Kakafika AI, et al. Effectiveness of ezetimibe alone or in combination with twice a week atorvastatin (10 mg) for statin intolerant high-risk patients. Am J Cardiol 2008;101(4):483–5.
58. Caso G, Kelly P, McNurlan MA, et al. Effect of coenzyme q10 on myopathic symptoms in patients treated with statins. Am J Cardiol 2007;99(10):1409–12.
59. Young JM, Florkowski CM, Molyneux SL, et al. Effect of coenzyme Q(10) supplementation on simvastatin-induced myalgia. Am J Cardiol 2007;100(9):1400–3.

Hypertriglyceridemia: Impact and Treatment

Ira J. Goldberg, MD

KEYWORDS

- Chylomicrons • VLDL • Lipolysis • Pancreatitis • Fatty acids
- Metabolic syndrome

In many ways transport of triglyceride seems to be one of the most primitive systems developed to allow movement of lipids within organisms. Triglyceride, a molecule created by addition of three fatty acids to a 3-carbon glycerol backbone, is the major form of stored and circulating energy. In human blood the amount of potential energy from fat is more than twice that of glucose. The fatty acids circulate in two forms: so-called "free fatty acids" that are associated with plasma proteins, primarily albumin, and esterified fatty acids within triglyceride and phospholipids that are a component of lipoproteins. Because triglycerides are nonpolar, they are not soluble in plasma. A detergent-like surface composed of phospholipids and proteins surrounds the triglyceride in circulating lipoproteins. Triglyceride from the diet and that synthesized in the liver are delivered to peripheral (nonhepatic) tissues where the triglyceride is used as energy or stored.

CHYLOMICRON METABOLISM

Chylomicrons are the transported form of dietary triglycerides and other hydrophobic lipids such as cholesteryl esters and retinyl esters (vitamin A). Chylomicrons are assembled within intestinal epithelial cells. The center or core of these spherical particles is a fat droplet containing primarily triglycerides and other hydrophobic lipids. The surface is composed of phospholipid, free cholesterol, and apolipoproteins (apos). The largest protein is apoB48, so denoted because it is 48% of full-length liver apoB, termed "apoB100." ApoAl, apoCs, apoAIV, and apoE also are found on the chylomicron surface. Aside from the need for lipid and proteins, assembly of chylomicrons requires the actions of microsomal triglyceride transfer protein (MTP). MTP deficiency leads to abetalipoproteinemia. The small intestine secretes chylomicrons into the lymphatics, chylomicrons enter the circulation via the thoracic duct, and surface apoproteins then are exchanged; apoAIV moves to high-density lipoprotein (HDL), whereas more apoC and apoE shift to chylomicrons.

Division of Preventive Medicine and Nutrition, Department of Medicine, Columbia University College of Physicians and Surgeons, 630 West 168th Street, New York, NY10032, USA
E-mail address: ijg3@columbia.edu

Endocrinol Metab Clin N Am 38 (2009) 137–149
doi:10.1016/j.ecl.2008.11.005
0889-8529/08/$ – see front matter © 2009 Elsevier Inc. All rights reserved.

Lipoprotein lipase (LpL) clearly is needed for most plasma triglyceride hydrolysis. This enzyme was discovered by the serendipitous observation that the use of heparin to prevent blood coagulation also "cleared" the blood of dietary chylomicrons.[1] Patients who had severe fasting chylomicronemia usually presenting in childhood were shown to be incapable of producing postheparin plasma that could hydrolyze chylomicron triglyceride.[2] LpL expression allows the physiologic regulation of triglyceride delivery, and its expression is most robust in the tissues that most avidly obtain triglyceride from the bloodstream: cardiac and skeletal muscle and adipose tissue. LpL is regulated by feeding/fasting; during feeding its activity is increased in adipose tissue to facilitate fat storage; during fasting it is activated in skeletal muscle to allow use of non-glucose energy. Aside from its expression, LpL is regulated by angiopoietin-like proteins 3 and 4 that may convert the active dimeric enzyme into inactive monomers,[3] activated by apoCII—the required cofactor that is contained in triglyceride-rich lipoproteins and HDL[4]—and inhibited by apoCIII.[5] LpL is associated with the luminal surface of endothelial cells in LpL-expressing tissues. Several factors might affect the interaction of LpL with circulating triglyceride-rich lipoproteins: apoA5 is a newly described heparin-binding apoprotein, and GPIHBP is an endothelial protein thought to affect LpL and chylomicron association with the capillary surface.[6] Genetic variations of many of these factors have been found to track with triglyceride levels in humans.[7]

A basic tenet of lipid metabolism is that triglycerides do not cross cell membranes. Rather, triglycerides enter cells either in conjunction with the uptake of a non-metabolized lipoprotein or after their lipolysis to free fatty acids. There is controversy about whether fatty acid entry into cells is caused by a biophysical process in which the fatty acids dissolve in the membrane and then are associated with intracellular binding proteins (a process termed "flip flop") or by a membrane transporter, the best studied of which is CD36. Both animals[8] and humans[9] with CD36 deficiency have marked reduction in fatty acid uptake, especially in the heart and skeletal muscle. Esterification of the fatty acids to coenzyme A, akin to the phosphorylation of glucose, seems to trap the fatty acids within the cell. In addition, intracellular fatty acid–binding proteins, conversion of fatty acids to triglyceride, and oxidation all effectively create a fatty acid gradient across the cell membrane.

Because both chylomicrons and very-low-density lipoproteins (VLDLs) require an LpL-mediated step to begin their plasma catabolism, it is not surprising that these two plasma sources of triglyceride can compete for lipolysis. Chylomicrons are larger, are more apt to collide with the endothelial surface,[10] and are cleared more rapidly from the bloodstream in normal humans. Saturation of LpL occurs at approximately 5 mM triglyceride, equal to $0 \sim 440$ mg/dL. The human in vivo data are consistent with this value; when plasma triglyceride levels exceed approximately 500 mg/dL, chylomicron as well as VLDL clearance is retarded.[11]

Energy-requiring tissues like the heart and exercising skeletal muscle use fatty acids as their primary source of energy. An alternative use of fatty acids is for these tissues and others such as adipose tissues to convert the fatty acids back to stored triglyceride. During fasting, stored adipose triglyceride is released into the bloodstream via the actions of adipose triglyceride lipase and hormone-sensitive lipase. Activation of adipose triglyceride lipase and hormone-sensitive lipase occurs in concert with reduced LpL activity and, therefore, reduced uptake of circulating fatty acids. Skeletal muscle uptake of plasma triglyceride and LpL activity are in the opposite direction, greatest during fasting and least postprandially. Chronic exercise increases skeletal muscle LpL and allows greater uptake and oxidation of fatty acids.

Aside from supplying dietary fatty acids, chylomicrons also are the route of entry of several fatty soluble vitamins. The best studied is vitamin A, the retinoids. Because they are hydrophobic, retinyl esters and also cholesteryl esters are included in the core (center) of chylomicrons. Some vitamin A is delivered to tissues during lipolysis; most retinyl esters enter the liver along with chylomicron remnants. Retinol is re-secreted from the liver and circulates while associated with retinol-binding protein. This protein recently has been implicated in insulin resistance and diabetes.[12]

Most chylomicron remnants and their accompanying triglycerides are destined for the liver.[13] Chylomicrons contain apoB48, the shortened form of apoB that does not contain the low-density lipoprotein (LDL) receptor-binding domain. Within the hepatic space of Disse, proteoglycans capture remnants. Cell surface receptors such as the LDL receptor and/or the LDL receptor–related protein interact with remnant apoE allowing receptor-mediated lipoprotein uptake. Other hepatic receptors such as scavenger receptor BI also may mediate liver acquisition of remnants. Defects in liver uptake of remnants lead to dysbetalipoproteinemia, as discussed later.

VERY-LOW-DENSITY LIPOPROTEIN METABOLISM

Both the number and size of VLDL particles affect the plasma triglyceride concentration. VLDLs are the primary source of triglyceride in the plasma of fasting non-hypertriglyceridemic humans. Factors that control liver production of triglyceride and apoB100 have been studied intensively. Liver triglycerides are assembled either from albumin-associated fatty acids or from lipoprotein-triglyceride returning to the liver. In addition, the liver is a site of active fatty acid synthesis from excess carbohydrate. Hepatic triglyceride along with some cholesterol combines with apoB100 and phospholipids to form VLDL, a step that also requires MTP. Most of the mass of the VLDL (55%–85% by weight) comes from triglyceride. Larger VLDLs contain more triglyceride and have a lower density that sometimes approaches that of small chylomicrons. Caloric excess, diabetes mellitus, and alcohol consumption lead to greater triglyceride secretion from the liver. Like chylomicrons, VLDLs contain apoCI, CII, CIII, and E.

Interaction and the partial metabolism of VLDL within the plasma allows for two fates. Small VLDL particles or VLDL remnants, also sometimes referred to as "intermediate density lipoproteins," are removed from the plasma via their interaction with cell surface lipoprotein receptors. Both apoB100 and apoE allow hepatic and cellular uptake via the LDL receptor. Other VLDLs, especially those initially secreted as smaller particles, undergo plasma remodeling by lipid transfer proteins and hepatic lipase leading to the production of the atherogenic lipoprotein LDL. Hepatic lipase is a member of the lipase gene family but does not require apoCII for its activity.

CAUSES AND CLINICAL CONSEQUENCES OF HYPERTRIGLYCERIDEMIA
Hyperchylomicronemia

Clinical presentation
The most dramatic example of severe hypertriglyceridemia is that of fasting hyperchylomicronemia. Fasting hyperchylomicronemia can result from a primary defect in chylomicron metabolism or can be secondary to increased VLDL and saturation of LpL; this situation occurs when triglyceride levels exceed ~500 mg/dL. Thus, familial hypertriglyceridemia, familial combined hyperlipidemia, and dysbetalipoproteinemia can present with fasting hyperchylomicronemia. One common cause of such exacerbations is diabetes that is not controlled, leading to increased adipose intracellular lipolysis, the return of fatty acids to the liver, greater secretion of VLDL triglyceride, and saturation of LpL. Several dietary and environmental factors also modulate triglyceride production. The most dramatic is alcohol, a major substrate for triglyceride

production. In addition, diets that are rich in free carbohydrates and especially free sugars induce triglyceride production. In laboratory animals, fructose increases de novo production of lipids in the liver, including both cholesterol and triglyceride, depending on the species.

Defective clearance of plasma lipids is a major cause of fasting hyperchylomicronemia. Genetic defects in LpL prevent chylomicron clearance. LpL deficiency usually, but not always, presents in childhood. The symptoms vary from difficulty feeding young infants to frank pancreatitis, which sometimes is mistaken for appendicitis. The plasma often is milky, and whole blood may have a pinkish "cream of tomato" hue. The trigger level of triglyceride elevation leading to pancreatitis is variable; patients sometimes have triglyceride levels in excess of 10,000 mg/dL with no symptoms, whereas others develop pancreatitis at much lower triglyceride levels (but usually in excess of 2000 mg/dL).

The pathophysiology of the relationship between hyperchylomicronemia and pancreatitis is unknown. One theory is that the lipid-rich blood sludges leading to pancreatic ischemia. Another possibility is that the small amount of lipases that normally leak from the acinar cells lead to exuberant local lipolysis, the creation of toxic local concentrations of free fatty acids and lysolecithin, and further acinar cell damage to adjacent cells. Additional insults to the acinar cells such as that provided by alcohol, can fan this process.

Although most patients who have severe hyperchylomicronemia but who do not develop pancreatitis are asymptomatic, a few with extreme levels above 10,000 mg/dL develop the hyperchylomicronemia syndrome.[14] Presumably this syndrome is caused by reduced blood flow or defective oxygen delivery. These patients have dyspnea and confusion that may be indistinguishable from early dementia.

The marked increase in blood triglyceride can lead to the accumulation of triglycerides in several organs and can be observed in the blood. The increase in blood is appreciated best either by examining the blood directly, allowing the red cells to settle and observing a creamy layer on the plasma, or by noting the pinkish discoloration of the blood on ophthalmic examination, lipemia retinalis. Eruptive xanthomas are 2- to 5-mm papules with a yellow center surrounded by erythema and are caused by triglyceride-enriched skin macrophages. These lesions sometimes are confused with acne or folliculitis. For unclear reasons, eruptive xanthomas are found most commonly on the buttocks and extensor surfaces of the arms and the back. Enlargement of the liver and spleen is common and is thought to be caused by triglyceride engorgement of these organs.

Aside from the severe hypertriglyceridemia, other laboratory indices sometimes are abnormal. Plasma sodium is reduced; liver functions are sometimes elevated. Often the clinical laboratory will defer making several measurements and note the severe lipemia. If these other measurements are required, plasma can be centrifuged, the chylomicron layer removed, and the remaining plasma examined.

Causes

Several genetic defects lead to fasting chylomicronemia and severe hypertriglyceridemia. These defects include defective production and mutations of the LpL gene and apoCII. It is estimated that these account for approximately 50% of the primary severe hypertriglyceridemias. It is likely that other defects such as that in the *GPIHBP* gene found in mice[6] occur in humans. Autoimmune conditions can be associated with defective triglyceride catabolism caused by inhibition of LpL, apoCII, or heparin. Antibodies against heparin are thought to prevent normal LpL association with the endothelial surface.

Although genetic LpL deficiency has been reported to present in adulthood, most cases of severe hyperchylomicronemia in adulthood are associated with partial LpL deficiency or other causes. In adults, the most important cause is type 2 diabetes and obesity: increased dietary intake associated with defective clearance of lipoproteins. Postprandial lipemia is a prominent feature of diabetes.[15] A thorough history of triglyceride-raising medications should be taken, as discussed later.

Diagnostic evaluation

Genetic LpL deficiency is diagnosed both by the clinical setting and biochemical deficiency of LpL activity in the postheparin blood; LpL deficiency typically is associated with younger age of onset, especially childhood. A family history of low HDL is the most common lipid abnormality in the heterozygous carriers.[16] LpL variants also are a determinant of HDL levels within the general population. A family history of French Canadian ancestry is suggestive.

Although a presumptive diagnosis can be made on clinical grounds, it sometimes is useful for genetic reasons and treatment approach to confirm the diagnosis of LpL deficiency. More than 100 mutations of the LpL gene have been described,[17] and for this reason biochemical rather than genetic evaluation still is performed. Fasting patients are given an intravenous injection of 60 units/kg of heparin, releasing the LpL into the bloodstream.[18] Ten minutes later a sample of postheparin blood is obtained and stored on ice. The plasma is frozen and sent to a lipid specialty laboratory for analysis (such as at Columbia, the University of Washington, Washington University, and several other academic and nonacademic lipid specialty laboratories). Heparins are calibrated by their anticoagulant activity and their ability to release LpL into the plasma varies. Hepatic lipase (as discussed later) also is measured routinely in these samples. Postheparin samples should not clot. If they do, it may be an indicator of a defective injection or antibodies to heparin (eg, in the setting of an autoimmune disease). Postheparin plasma usually is not obtained during an acute episode. Patients who have a history of bleeding disorders or recent use of anticoagulant or antiplatelet drugs should be studied with caution, if at all.

ApoCII, the LpL activator, and inhibitors of LpL such as antibodies[19] can be detected by mixing the patient's serum with a standard human or bovine source of LpL and then assessing activity.

Acute therapies

All causes of severe acute hypertriglyceridemia are alleviated by removing the major source of triglycerides, that is, dietary fat. Triglycerides in the level of several thousand usually plummet to below 1000 within a day or two when the patient is fasting. In the setting of pancreatitis, there is theoretic support for the infusion of insulin with or without glucose as a means to reduce free fatty acid flux to the liver and to stimulate LpL activity. Plasmapheresis also has been performed, although it rarely is required.

Acute hypertriglyceridemia requires attention to factors that might have provoked the marked elevation in chylomicrons. The evaluation must include a careful search for triglyceride-raising drugs (**Box 1**), poor glycemic control, recent dietary fat "binges," and assessment for autoimmune and thyroid diseases.

Chronic therapies

Chronic treatments are aimed at reducing triglyceride levels and preventing recurrent pancreatitis. The goal of therapy is to maintain triglyceride levels below 500 mg/dL. The primary treatment of hyperchylomicronemia is dietary. Even in the setting of genetic LpL deficiency, patients who rigorously adhere to a low-fat diet maintain

---

Box 1
Hypertriglyceridemia

Hyperchylomicronemia: triglyceride levels >1000 mg/dL

Defective lipolysis

    Lipoprotein lipase deficiency

    ApoCII deficiency

Defective lipolysis and increased triglyceride production

    Heterozygous lipoprotein lipase deficiency and pregnancy, estrogen, diabetes, alcohol

Triglyceride overproduction and lipoprotein lipase saturation

    Familial hypertriglyceridemia

    Dysbetalipoproteinemia

    Familial hypertriglyceridemia

Fasting hypertriglyceridemia: triglyceride level 150–500 mg/dL (includes high and moderately high levels of ATP3)

Increased very-low-density lipoprotein

    Associated diseases

        Diabetes mellitus type 2, obesity, glycogen storage disease, lipodystrophy, alcohol, renal failure, nephrotic syndrome, stress, sepsis, Cushing syndrome, pregnancy, acromegaly, hepatitis

Drugs

    Hormones: estrogen, tamoxifen, glucocorticoids

    Anti-hypertensives: thiazides, β-blockers

    Bile acid–binding resins (cholestyramine, colesevelam)

    HIV: protease inhibitors

    Retinoids

    Rapamycin

    Antipsychotics/selective serotonin reuptake inhibitors

Increased intermediate-density lipoproteins

ApoE2/E2

Hepatic lipase deficiency

Hypothyroidism

Autoimmune disease

---

plasma levels of triglycerides that are below 1000 mg/dL; triglyceride levels below 200 mg/dL and increases of HDL to within the normal range do not occur. Although simple carbohydrates increase liver production of triglycerides and are an important approach in patients who have moderate hypertriglyceridemia, the primary dietary approach for treating fasting hyperchylomicronemia is the reduction of fat in the diet. This diet is not complicated; most patients can reduce their intake of fried foods, meats, and whole-fat dairy products readily. Medium-chain triglyceride oils are sold by several manufacturers who advertise on the Internet. These fatty acids are thought to pass through the intestinal lining and combine directly with albumin. Medium-chain triglyceride oils can be used for cooking and in salad dressings. In occasional cases in which dietary compliance is difficult, treatment with the fat-absorption inhibitor orlistat (Xenical or OTC Alli) may be useful.[20] This drug blocks the active site of pancreatic lipase leading to fat malabsorption. Although primarily used as a weight-loss drug, it effectively produces the equivalent of a low-fat diet. Patients should be warned of diarrhea.

Responses to reduction in alcohol intake (if causative) and control of hyperglycemia often are dramatic, indicating the secondary nature of the hyperchylomicronemia in many patients. In all patients who have pancreatitis, alcohol intake should be totally prohibited. Weight loss and improved diabetes control are essential.

Traditional triglyceride-lowering agents have some role; these agents are more effective in patients who do not have genetic LpL deficiency. Omega-3 fatty acids in high doses from over-the-counter sources or in the more concentrated prescribed ethyl ester form (Lovaza) are useful in all cases of hypertriglyceridemia. Omega-3 fatty acids are useful in patients who have genetic LpL deficiency[21] but should not be given along with orlistat, which blocks their absorption. Both niacin and fibric acid drugs are useful but probably are most beneficial in non–LpL-deficient patients.

Fasting hypertriglyceridemia

Triglyceride levels of 150 to 500 mg/dL are considered abnormal, but their pathologic importance is uncertain. The National Cholesterol Education Program (NCEP) categorizes triglyceride levels of 200 to 499 mg/dL as high and levels of 150 to 199 mg/dL as borderline high.[22] Several different clinical conditions lead to fasting hypertriglyceridemia. Familial combined hyperlipidemia (FCHL) is associated with increased apoB production and, at different times and in different family members, can present with hypertriglyceridemia (increased VLDL), increased cholesterol (LDL), or both. FCHL is associated with greater risk of vascular disease.[23] The concomitant obesity, insulin resistance, and/or overt diabetes in many hypertriglyceridemic patients often makes it difficult to isolate one specific cause of this metabolic disturbance.

Dysbetalipoproteinemia (type 3 hyperlipoproteinemia) is caused by a homozygous mutation in apoE, apoE2/E2, leading to defective clearance of chylomicron remnants. Its prevalence is 1 in 10,000 population. These patients present with elevated triglyceride and cholesterol levels resulting from defective lipid clearance of remnant lipoproteins. Patients who have dysbetalipoproteinemia sometimes have tuberous and palmar xanthomas and a propensity to peripheral vascular disease.

Heterozygous LpL deficiency is relatively common in some populations. As these individuals age, or when the LpL deficiency is superimposed on other conditions that tend to elevate triglycerides, hypertriglyceridemia can result.

A variety of other clinical conditions and drugs can elevate triglycerides (see **Box 1**). Diabetes, obesity, and renal disease are common causes of fasting hypertriglyceridemia. The most common drugs associated with hypertriglyceridemia are estrogen-like compounds, thiazides, beta-blockers, protease inhibitors, steroids, immunosuppressive drugs, retinoids (isotretinoin, Accutane), bile acid–binding resins, and newer antipsychotic medications.

Genetic hypoalphalipoproteinemia syndromes—lecithin cholesterol acyltransferase deficiency, Tangier disease, and apoAI Milano—are associated invariably with moderate hypertriglyceridemia. Because mice defective in apoAI production show a similar tendency to hypertriglyceridemia,[24] it is assumed that the reduced apoCII reservoir on HDL is responsible.

Diagnosis

The association of other disorders, medication use, and dietary choices often uncovers the culprits that lead to hypertriglyceridemia associated with some genetic predisposition. When both triglyceride and cholesterol levels are elevated, a search for the underlying lipoprotein disorder sometimes is useful. By ultracentrifugation, the diagnosis of dysbetalipoproteinemia caused by the presence of cholesterol-enriched VLDL can be differentiated from that of FCHL. The usual ratio of VLDL triglyceride to cholesterol of ~5 is reduced to 3 or less. ApoE genotyping also is useful. Cholesterol-enriched VLDL also is found in patients who have hypothyroidism, renal failure, and hepatic lipase deficiency.

Cardiac risk

Despite decades of epidemiologic correlation data, the relationship between triglyceride levels and vascular disease still is in dispute (see the review by Jacobson and colleagues)[25] Recent studies implicate the postprandial triglyceride level as a stronger risk factor than the fasting triglyceride level.[26,27] Moreover, the lack of clear-cut intervention data proving that reductions in triglyceride are beneficial for cardiovascular health make treatment of these disorders a murky area. Nonetheless, the most recent NCEP guidelines recommending treatment of elevated non-HDL cholesterol levels endorse reduction in VLDL when the VLDL level is associated with cholesterol levels higher than 30 mg/dL (ie, whenever the triglyceride level exceeds 150 mg/dL).[22]

The analysis of cardiovascular risk is confounded further by the reduction in HDL that almost uniformly accompanies hypertriglyceridemia caused by the cholesteryl ester transfer protein reaction. This relationship is not found in the setting of alcohol and estrogen.

Cholesterol, not triglyceride, is the hallmark of atherosclerosis and is the cause of foam cell development. Although some patients who have severe hypertriglyceridemia and coronary artery disease have been reported,[28] and mice with a similar defect develop small lesions with advanced age,[29] these findings do not dispel the widely held belief that larger, very triglyceride-enriched lipoproteins are nonatherosclerotic because they cannot penetrate the artery wall.[30] LpL deficiency is not the cause of most hypertriglyceridemia, however, and multiple in vitro experiments have implicated remnant lipoproteins and the lipolysis products, free fatty acids, and lysolecithin, as vasculotoxins.

How can the potential vascular risk be assessed in hypertriglyceridemic patients? This question remains unanswered. Family history seems to be useful. Some have argued that the presence of small, dense LDL particles, an almost universal finding with hypertriglyceridemia in the presence of normal cholesteryl ester transfer protein, is such a marker. Perhaps C-reactive protein measurements are helpful here. The measurement of arterial wall calcium might separate patients who have disease from others whose triglyceride levels are less atherogenic.[31]

Treatment

Dietary and lifestyle changes—weight loss, management of diabetes, and increased exercise—are the initial treatment approach. Alcohol reduces fatty acid oxidation and provides a substrate for greater triglyceride synthesis.[32] Free carbohydrate-rich foods are converted to triglycerides rapidly; fructose, in particular, increases the expression of the fatty acid–regulating transcription factor SREBP-1c.[33] Fish oils are a good dietary addition and seem to have few drawbacks. Stress has been associated with increases in triglyceride levels, perhaps because of catecholamine induction of adipose tissue lipolysis.

Several standard lipid-lowering agents are used in moderate hypertriglyceridemia. Niacin and fibric acids reduce fasting triglyceride levels by 40% to 50%. These medications also reduce non-HDL cholesterol.

Niacin Niacin, or nicotinic acid, inhibits the mobilization of free fatty acids from peripheral tissues but also may have poorly understood effects in reducing hepatic synthesis of triglycerides and secretion of VLDL. Nicotinic acid also is the most effective drug for treating HDL elevation. Like all triglyceride-reducing agents, niacin causes a shift from small, dense LDL particles to large, buoyant LDL particles. Nicotinic acid at a dosage of 2 to 2.5 g/d can decrease the triglyceride level by 45%. Sustained-release niacin, marketed as Niaspan, reduces triglyceride to a similar extent as nonprescription niacin.

Niacin, even slower-release niacin, often is difficult for many patients to tolerate; persistence, encouragement, and patience by both the patients and physicians often are required. Flushing of the skin, which is more akin to sunburn than a "hot flash," is most common. Although some patients have generalized cutaneous erythema, others complain primarily of itching. With Niaspan taken at night, the symptoms often occur during sleep. Over time most patients develop tachyphylaxis to this side effect. Ingestion of alcohol, spicy foods, hot showers before bedtime, and an empty stomach encourage the niacin flush. Taking aspirin or ibuprofen 30 to 60 minutes before each dose of nicotinic acid may reduce flushing in some patients. As detailed in other articles in this issue, the biology of the flushing and agents to block it are being investigated currently. In many patients niacin augments glucose intolerance, leading to the need for diabetic drugs in some patients who have metabolic syndrome or alterations in current diabetic regimens. Non–slow-release forms of niacin, which can be obtained over the counter, are less expensive, and are similarly effective for lipid management, increase plasma uric acid by blocking its excretion, and may precipitate or exacerbate gout. Gastrointestinal symptoms such as diarrhea and bloating occur. Occasional patients develop hepatitis, which often is preceded by a dramatic reduction in plasma cholesterol that is outside the normal response to the drugs. This author has seen several niacin-treated patients who developed hives (a process that must be distinguished from the transient flushing) that required discontinuation of the drugs.

Fibric acids Two fibric acid medications are available in the United States: gemfibrozil (Lopid) and fenofibrate (Tricor, Lofibra, Antara). Other agents are available in Europe. Peroxisomal proliferator activated receptor (PPAR) α is a transcription factor that induces the expression of genes needed for fatty acid oxidation in tissues, including liver and muscles.[34] This action includes induction of LpL in multiple tissues, including the liver. Fibric acids bind to a sequence in the promoter of apoCIII and reduce its gene transcription,[35] possibly leading to more rapid turnover of plasma VLDL. Fibrate treatment reduces plasma triglyceride levels by 25% to 40% and also reduces postprandial triglyceride levels. These drugs do not affect insulin actions. Increases in LDL levels sometimes are seen with fibrates because more VLDL are converted to LDL. Fibrates are especially effective in dysbetalipoproteinemia,[36] and a dramatic response to these drugs might assist in making the diagnosis.

Some proof of beneficial clinical outcome in patients who have moderate hypertriglyceridemia treated with fibric acid drugs is available. Gemfibrozil was beneficial in the Helsinki Heart Study, especially among subjects who had higher triglyceride levels (see the review by Gotto[37]). This drug also reduced cardiac events in the Veterans Affairs High-Density Lipoprotein Cholesterol Intervention Trial,[38] an effect that might be related to increases in HDL level, reduced triglyceride level, or other effects of this drug.[39]

Fenofibrate has become the more commonly used fibrate in the United States, in part because it seems to have less interaction with statins and reduced risk of myositis.[40] This difference suggests that the two drugs are not totally interchangeable and might have different clinical effects. Although both gemfibrozil and fenofibrate reduce triglyceride levels to a similar degree, fenofibrate is a more effective LDL-reducing agent: LDL cholesterol reductions of up to 20% have been reported.[36] In the Fenofibrate Intervention and Event Lowering in Diabetes study, despite a reduction in cardiac events, fenofibrate treatment was not associated with a reduction in total or cardiac mortality.[41]

Omega-3 fatty acids In high doses, intake of over-the-counter omega-3 fatty acids reduces triglyceride levels; lower doses of the purified fatty ethyl ester compound Lovaza are required.[42] These compounds decrease the production of triglyceride. The mechanism is not completely clear, but a recent study suggested that greater oxidation of these double-bond–rich lipids increased degradation of apoB.[43] Other studies using artificial chylomicron-like particles found that lipid emulsions enriched with omega-3 were cleared more rapidly from the circulation.[44]

The major advantage of fish oils is that they are a natural product, seem to have very few drug interactions, and are relatively free of side effects. The over-the-counter forms are less expensive than prescription medications. Approximately 3 g/d of eicosapentaenoic acid (EPA)/ docosahexaenoic acid (DHA) are necessary to reduce hypertriglyceridemia effectively. To see an effect within a few months thus requires taking 10 to 12 caplets containing 300 mg EPA/DHA each day; less than half this number of caplets is needed for the more purified prescription forms containing more than 800 mg EPA/DHA per caplet. Aside from the discomfort of taking so many pills, patients sometime complain of eructation and a "fishy" aftertaste. In patients who had heart disease, lower doses of fish oil ($\sim$ 800 mg EPA/DHA) were associated with reduced mortality,[45] an effect that might indicate an anti-arrhythmic property of these oils.

Statins Statins can be the initial therapy in moderate hypertriglyceridemia but are not indicated in severe hypertriglyceridemia. Up-regulation of the LDL receptor and, in FCHL, reduced VLDL secretion[46] can lead to a triglyceride reduction of 10% to 20%. There are data for the use of these drugs in children. Moreover, the LDL reduction that occurs might be more important than any ancillary triglyceride reduction.

Anti-diabetic drugs In patients who have type 2 diabetes or metabolic syndrome, weight loss, exercise, and glucose-lowering agents are central to triglyceride reduction. Without improved glucose control, hypertriglyceridemia often persists despite medications. Metformin, the most commonly prescribed medication for type 2 diabetes, sometimes is used even without overt diabetes because this medication sometimes can lead to reduced appetite and also reduces triglyceride levels.

Pioglitazone and rosiglitazone, PPARγ agonists that increase insulin sensitivity, reduce triglyceride levels through increased clearance of plasma triglyceride.[47] In a comparative study,[48] pioglitazone did not change LDL cholesterol levels, whereas rosiglitazone, like many agents that increase VLDL conversion to LDL, increased LDL cholesterol levels by 8% to 16%. Pioglitazone led to a modest 14% to 26%

decrease in triglyceride levels in various studies. It is possible that the difference in these two drugs might be that pioglitazone has partial PPARα agonist effects.

SUMMARY

Hypertriglyceridemia is best viewed as two distinct clinical syndromes, even though their presentations are similar. Fasting chylomicronemia causes pancreatitis and requires draconian dietary changes and medications to prevent recurrence of this potentially fatal complication. Moderate hypertriglyceridemia (triglyceride levels < 500 mg/dL) often is associated with or is a harbinger of metabolic syndrome and type 2 diabetes. Its independent role as a cardiac risk factor is not completely resolved. Nonetheless, either to normalize this laboratory value or to comply with the NCEP Adult Treatment Panel III guideline to reduce non-HDL cholesterol levels, treatment of moderate hypertriglyceridemia is generally accepted clinical practice.

REFERENCES

1. Hahn PF. Abolishment of alimentary lipemia following injection of heparin. Science 1943;98:19–20.
2. Havel RJ, Gordon RSJ. Idiopathic hyperlipidemia: metabolic studies in an affected family. J Clin Invest 1960;39:1777–90.
3. Sukonina V, Lookene A, Olivecrona T, et al. Angiopoietin-like protein 4 converts lipoprotein lipase to inactive monomers and modulates lipase activity in adipose tissue. Proc Natl Acad Sci U S A 2006;103:17450–5.
4. LaRosa JC, Levy RI, Herbert P, et al. A specific apoprotein activator for lipoprotein lipase. Biochem Biophys Res Commun 1970;41:57–62.
5. Brown WV, Baginsky ML. Inhibition of lipoprotein lipase by an apoprotein of human very low density lipoprotein. Biochem Biophys Res Commun 1972;46:375–81.
6. Beigneux AP, Davies BS, Gin P, et al. Glycosylphosphatidylinositol-anchored high-density lipoprotein-binding protein 1 plays a critical role in the lipolytic processing of chylomicrons. Cell Metab 2007;5:279–91.
7. Kathiresan S, Musunuru K, Orho-Melander M, et al. Defining the spectrum of alleles that contribute to blood lipid concentrations in humans. Curr Opin Lipidol 2008;19:122–7.
8. Coburn CT, Knapp FF Jr, Febbraio M, et al. Defective uptake and utilization of long chain fatty acids in muscle and adipose tissues of CD36 knockout mice. J Biol Chem 2000;275:32523–9.
9. Fukuchi K, Nozaki S, Yoshizumi T, et al. Enhanced myocardial glucose use in patients with a deficiency in long-chain fatty acid transport (CD36 deficiency). J Nucl Med 1999;40:239–43.
10. Goldberg IJ. Lipoprotein lipase and lipolysis: central roles in lipoprotein metabolism and atherogenesis. J Lipid Res 1996;37(4):693–707.
11. Brunzell JD, Hazzard WR, Porte D Jr, et al. Evidence for a common, saturable, triglyceride removal mechanism for chylomicrons and very low density lipoproteins in man. J Clin Invest 1973;52:1578–85.
12. Hammarstedt A, Pihlajamaki J, Graham TE, et al. High circulating levels of RBP4 and mRNA levels of aP2, PGC-1alpha and UCP-2 predict improvement in insulin sensitivity following pioglitazone treatment of drug-naive type 2 diabetic subjects. J Intern Med 2008;263:440–9.
13. Savonen R, Nordstoga K, Christophersen B, et al. Chylomicron metabolism in an animal model for hyperlipoproteinemia type I. J Lipid Res 1999;40:1336–46.

14. Chait A, Brunzell JD. Chylomicronemia syndrome. Adv Intern Med 1992;37: 249–73.

15. Ginsberg HN. Diabetic dyslipidemia: basic mechanisms underlying the common hypertriglyceridemia and low HDL cholesterol levels. Diabetes 1996;45(Suppl 3): S27–30.

16. Wilson DE, Emi M, Iverius PH, et al. Phenotypic expression of heterozygous lipoprotein lipase deficiency in the extended pedigree of a proband homozygous for a missense mutation. J Clin Invest 1990;86:735–50.

17. Goldberg IJ, Merkel M. Lipoprotein lipase: physiology, biochemistry, and molecular biology. Front Biosci 2001;6:D388–405.

18. Krauss RM, Levy RI, Fredrickson DS, et al. Selective measurement of two lipase activities in postheparin plasma from normal subjects and patients with hyperlipoproteinemia. J Clin Invest 1974;54:1107–24.

19. Brunzell JD, Miller NE, Alaupovic P, et al. Familial chylomicronemia due to a circulating inhibitor of lipoprotein lipase activity. J Lipid Res 1983;24:12–9.

20. Tolentino MC, Ferenczi A, Ronen L, et al. Combination of gemfibrozil and orlistat for treatment of combined hyperlipidemia with predominant hypertriglyceridemia. Endocr Pract 2002;8:208–12.

21. Rouis M, Dugi KA, Previato L, et al. Therapeutic response to medium-chain triglycerides and omega-3 fatty acids in a patient with the familial chylomicrone- mia syndrome. Arterioscler Thromb Vasc Biol 1997;17:1400–6.

22. Third Report of the National Cholesterol Education Program (NCEP) Expert Panel on Detection, Evaluation, and Treatment of High Blood Cholesterol in Adults (Adult Treatment Panel III) final report. Circulation 2002;106:3143–421.

23. Austin MA, McKnight B, Edwards KL, et al. Cardiovascular disease mortality in familial forms of hypertriglyceridemia: a 20-year prospective study. Circulation 2000;101:2777–82.

24. Voyiaziakis E, Goldberg IJ, Plump AS, et al. ApoA-I deficiency causes both hypertriglyceridemia and increased atherosclerosis in human apoB transgenic mice. J Lipid Res 1998;39:313–21.

25. Jacobson TA, Miller M, Schaefer EJ, et al. Hypertriglyceridemia and cardiovascular risk reduction. Clin Ther 2007;29:763–77.

26. Nordestgaard BG, Benn M, Schnohr P, et al. Nonfasting triglycerides and risk of myocardial infarction, ischemic heart disease, and death in men and women. J Am Med Assoc 2007;298:299–308.

27. Bansal S, Buring JE, Rifai N, et al. Fasting compared with nonfasting triglycerides and risk of cardiovascular events in women. J Am Med Assoc 2007;298:309–16.

28. Benlian P, De Gennes JL, Foubert L, et al. Premature atherosclerosis in patients with familial chylomicronemia caused by mutations in the lipoprotein lipase gene. N Engl J Med 1996;335:848–54.

29. Zhang X, Qi R, Xian X, et al. Spontaneous atherosclerosis in aged lipoprotein lipase deficient mice with severe hypertriglyceridemia on a normal chow diet. Circ Res 2008;102:250–6.

30. Nordestgaard BG, Zilversmit DB. Large lipoproteins are excluded from the arterial wall in diabetic cholesterol-fed rabbits. J Lipid Res 1988;29:1491–500.

31. Detrano R, Guerci AD, Carr JJ, et al. Coronary calcium as a predictor of coronary events in four racial or ethnic groups. N Engl J Med 2008;358:1336–45.

32. Lieber CS. Alcoholic fatty liver: its pathogenesis and mechanism of progression to inflammation and fibrosis. Alcohol 2004;34:9–19.

33. Le KA, Tappy L. Metabolic effects of fructose. Curr Opin Clin Nutr Metab Care 2006;9:469–75.

34. Lee CH, Olson P, Evans RM, et al. Minireview: lipid metabolism, metabolic diseases, and peroxisome proliferator-activated receptors. Endocrinology 2003; 144:2201–7.
35. Andersson Y, Majd Z, Lefebvre AM, et al. Developmental and pharmacological regulation of apolipoprotein C-II gene expression. Comparison with apo C-I and apo C-III gene regulation. Arterioscler Thromb Vasc Biol 1999;19:115–21.
36. Brown WV. Potential use of fenofibrate and other fibric acid derivatives in the clinic. Am J Med 1987;83:85–9.
37. Gotto AM Jr. Triglyceride as a risk factor for coronary artery disease. Am J Cardiol 1998;82:22Q–5Q.
38. Rubins HB, Robins SJ, Collins D, et al. Gemfibrozil for the secondary prevention of coronary heart disease in men with low levels of high-density lipoprotein cholesterol. Veterans Affairs High-Density Lipoprotein Cholesterol Intervention Trial Study Group. N Engl J Med 1999;341:410–8.
39. Robins SJ, Collins D, Wittes JT, et al. Relation of gemfibrozil treatment and lipid levels with major coronary events: VA-HIT: a randomized controlled trial. J Am Med Assoc 2001;285:1585–91.
40. Bellosta S, Paoletti R, Corsini A, et al. Safety of statins: focus on clinical pharmacokinetics and drug interactions. Circulation 2004;109(Suppl 1):III50–7.
41. Keech A, Simes RJ, Barter P, et al. Effects of long-term fenofibrate therapy on cardiovascular events in 9795 people with type 2 diabetes mellitus (the FIELD study): randomised controlled trial. Lancet 2005;366:1849–61.
42. McKenney JM, Sica D. Role of prescription omega-3 fatty acids in the treatment of hypertriglyceridemia. Pharmacotherapy 2007;27:715–28.
43. Pan M, Cederbaum AI, Zhang YL, et al. Lipid peroxidation and oxidant stress regulate hepatic apolipoprotein B degradation and VLDL production. J Clin Invest 2004;113:1277–87.
44. Qi K, Seo T, Al-Haideri M, et al. Omega-3 triglycerides modify blood clearance and tissue targeting pathways of lipid emulsions. Biochemistry 2002;41:3119–27.
45. Gruppo Italiano per lo Studio della Sopravvivenza nell'Infarto Miocardico. Dietary supplementation with n-3 polyunsaturated fatty acids and vitamin E after myocardial infarction: results of the GISSI-Prevenzione trial. Lancet 1999;354:447–55.
46. Arad Y, Ramakrishnan R, Ginsberg HN, et al. Effects of lovastatin therapy on very-low-density lipoprotein triglyceride metabolism in subjects with combined hyperlipidemia: evidence for reduced assembly and secretion of triglyceride-rich lipoproteins. Meta 1992;41:487–93.
47. Kusunoki M, Hara T, Tsutsumi K, et al. The lipoprotein lipase activator, NO-1886, suppresses fat accumulation and insulin resistance in rats fed a high-fat diet [in process citation]. Diabetologia 2000;43(7):875–80.
48. Goldberg RB, Kendall DM, Deeg MA, et al. A comparison of lipid and glycemic effects of pioglitazone and rosiglitazone in patients with type 2 diabetes and dyslipidemia. Diabetes Care 2005;28:1547–54.

Novel Therapies for Increasing Serum Levels of HDL

Peter P. Toth, MD, PhD[a,b,*]

KEYWORDS

- Cholesterol ester transfer protein inhibitors • Liver X-receptor
- High-density lipoprotein cholesterol (HDL-C)
- Reverse cholesterol transport • Infusible HDL mimetics
- PPAR-alpha agonists

The management of dyslipidemia in both the primary and secondary prevention settings has focused on low-density lipoprotein cholesterol (LDL-C) reduction as the primary target for decreasing risk for cardiovascular events. In recent years an enormous amount of both basic scientific and clinical research is suggesting that therapies that raise high-density lipoprotein cholesterol (HDL-C) may augment risk reduction in patients with coronary heart disease (CHD). Data from the Framingham Heart Study have shown that subjects with the highest HDL cholesterol levels exhibit the lowest risk of developing CHD.[1] Prospective, observational studies conducted throughout the world have consistently demonstrated that high serum levels of HDL-C are associated with reduced risk for CHD development and related complications such as myocardial infarction (MI), stroke, and death, whereas low serum levels of this lipoprotein are correlated with increased risk for cardiovascular morbidity and mortality in both men and women (**Table 1**).[2,3] Low serum levels of HDL-C also portend increased risk for cardiovascular morbidity and mortality in patients treated with drug-eluting stents.[4]

Multivariate analyses from a number of studies, including the Veterans Affairs High-Density Lipoprotein Cholesterol Intervention Trial Study Group (VA-HIT),[5] the Bezafibrate Infarction Prevention (BIP) trial,[6] and The Nurse's Health Study,[7] have shown that raising HDL-C is associated with reduced risk for cardiovascular events. Although some in the field of lipidology have suggested that the excess risk attributable to a low HDL-C can be obviated by dropping LDL-C to low levels, recent results from the Treating to New Targets trial do not support this approach. In this trial, even when LDL-C was reduced to less than 70 mg/dL in patients with stable CHD, as HDL-C decreased progressively below 42 mg/dL, there was a sharp increase in risk for cardiovascular events during the follow-up period.[8] It is also important to point out at the outset of

[a] Sterling Rock Falls Clinic, Ltd., 101 East Miller Road, Sterling, IL 61081, USA
[b] Department of Family and Community Medicine, University of Illinois College of Medicine, Peoria, IL 61656, USA
* Sterling Rock Falls Clinic, Ltd., 101 East Miller Road, Sterling, IL 61081.
E-mail address: peter.toth@srfc.com

Endocrinol Metab Clin N Am 38 (2009) 151–170
doi:10.1016/j.ecl.2008.11.012
0889-8529/08/$ – see front matter © 2009 Elsevier Inc. All rights reserved.

endo.theclinics.com

Table 1
Epidemiologic Evidence of Relationship Between HDL and CHD

Trial	Study Design	Sample	Results
Alsheikh-Ali et al[99]	Retrospective review of patient medical records of a large primary care practice	1512 patients with CHD or CHD risk equivalents, mean age 63 ± 12 years	66% of patients had low HDL (≤ 40 mg/dL in men; ≤ 50 mg/dL in women)
Apolipoprotein-related MOrtality RISk trial[100]	66.8 months for men; 64.4 months for women; prospective cohort	175,553; 43.8% women, 20–72 years	In both men and women, as apoAI and HDL-C levels decreased risk for nonfatal MI and sudden death increased
Atherosclerosis Risk in Communities Study[101]	10-year prospective cohort	12,339 African American and white men and women, 45–64 years	HDL was a strong, independent predictor of CHD, especially for women
Bezafibrate Infarction Preventions Study Group[6,102]	Cross-sectional	8257 patients with CHD, 18% women, 40–72 years	27% decreased in risk of CVD mortality for each 5 mg/dL increase in HDL
Cardiovascular Health Study[103,104]	7.5-year prospective, cohort study	5888 subjects, 60.2% women, ≥ 65 years	15% reduction in risk of MI per 15.7 mg/dL (0.4 mmol/L) increase in HDL
Cooperative Lipoprotein Phenotyping Study[105]	Case-control	8054 subjects, 22.2% women, 40–70+	Mean HDL was 3.4 mg/dL less in patients without CHD compared with those with CHD
Framingham Heart Study[106]	~50-year prospective cohort	5127 men and women, white, no CVD	1% HDL increase associated with 2% decreased CAD risk
Framingham Offspring Study[107]	~20 years prospective cohort	1446 men	1 mg/dL increase in HDL associated with 2% decreased CAD risk
Helsinki Heart Study[108]	5-year randomized, double-blind, placebo-controlled	4000 men w/dyslipidemia	Significant reduction in CAD independently associated with 11% increase in HDL
Honolulu Heart Program[109,110]	17-year prospective cohort	8006, Japanese-American men, 45–68 years	RR = 0.60 for CAD in men with HDL ≥ 60 mg/dL versus ≤ 40 mg/dL

Study	Design	Population	Finding
Lipid Research Clinics Coronary Primary Prevention Trial[111]	7.4-year randomized, double-blind, placebo-controlled	3806 men w/primary hypercholesterolemia, 35–59 years	2% and 3% decrease in CHD risk in men and women, respectively for each 1 mg/dL increase in HDL
Lipid Research Clinics Prevalence Mortality Follow-up Study[112]	8.5-year prospective cohort	6234 w/elevated lipid levels, 36.8% women, 30–69 years	CHD incidence rates significantly higher in subjects with low HDL (<40 mg/dL, 1.04 mmol/L) versus high HDL (≥50 mg/dL, 1.3 mmol/L)
Multiple Risk Factor Intervention Trial[113]	~30-year prospective cohort	10,950 men at high risk of CVD, 35–57	1 mg/dL increase in HDL resulted in 1% reduced incidence of CHD
Northern Manhattan Stroke Study[114]	Case-control	539 patients with first ischemic stroke, racially and ethnically diverse, 67% ≥ 65 years	OR = 0.52 for CAD in patients with HDL >35 mg/dL
Nurses Health Study[7]	~30-year prospective cohort	121,700 women, 30–55 years (initial cohort), 116,000 women, 25–42 years	17 mg/dL increase in HDL associated with 40% reduction in risk of CAD
Prospective Cardiovascular Munster Study[115]	6-year prospective cohort	4559 males, 40–65 years	HDL levels >45 mg/dL associated with reduced risk of CAD versus HDL <35 mg/dL
Tromso Heart Study[116]	2-year case-control	6595 men, 20–49 years	Low HDL associated with 3-fold increase in risk of CHD
Zutphen Elderly Study[117]	5-year prospective cohort	885 men, 64–84 years	20% reduction in incidence of first CHD event for each 0.26 mmol/L increase in HDL

Abbreviations: apoAI, apoprotein A-I; CAD, coronary artery disease; CHD, coronary heart disease; CVD, cardiovascular disease; HDL, high-density lipoprotein; HDL-C, high-density lipoprotein cholesterol; MI, myocardial infarction; OR, odds ratio; RR, relative risk.

this discussion that results from clinical trials with torcetrapib did not negate the hypothesis that raising HDL-C is of benefit in reducing risk for cardiovascular events. These trials were confounded by a number of off-target effects, such as increased serum aldosterone, changes in serum potassium and bicarbonate levels, and increases in blood pressure, all of which may have attenuated the benefit expected from changes in lipoprotein concentrations.[9,10]

The protectiveness of elevated HDL-C against CHD and its long-term sequelae is a subject of intense investigation throughout the world. HDL species have the capacity to modulate a large number of atherogenic mechanisms, such as inflammation, oxidation, thrombosis, and cell proliferation. Among lipoproteins, HDL is also unique, in that unlike atherogenic lipoproteins, which infiltrate arterial walls and deposit cholesterol and lipid within resident macrophages in the subendothelial space, HDL promotes the mobilization and clearance of excess lipid via the series of reactions collectively termed "reverse cholesterol transport." Numerous therapeutic agents are being developed in an attempt to modulate serum levels of HDL-C as well as its functionality. This article discusses the development of newer treatments targeted at raising HDL-C and HDL particle numbers to reduce residual risk in patients at risk for CHD.

HIGH-DENSITY LIPOPROTEIN FUNCTION

The HDLs are a multifunctional and heterogeneous class of lipoproteins that are involved in the transport of sterols and lipids.[11] HDL particles contain varying levels of antioxidants or pro-oxidants, which results in variation in HDL function.[12] This complex dual capacity of HDL-C to be both antiatherogenic and proatherogenic under certain conditions underscores the complexity of HDL functionality and requires considerable additional investigation. In the absence of systemic inflammation, a variety of antioxidant enzymes (paraoxonase, glutathione peroxidase, platelet activating factor acetylhydrolase) and apoproteins (AI and AII) bound to HDL aid in reducing the mass of oxidized lipid that peripheral tissues are exposed to. In contrast, in the presence of systemic inflammation, these antioxidant enzymes can dissociate or become inactivated, resulting in the generation of oxidized and peroxidized lipids that are atherogenic. The enzyme, apoprotein, complement pathway protein, and acute phase reactant cargo of HDLs can change rapidly in response to systemic inflammatory tone and these alterations can lead to sudden changes in the functionality of these lipoproteins.[13] HDL functionality can also be adversely impacted by such enzymes as myeloperoxidase, an enzyme produced in atherosclerotic plaque. Myeloperoxidase chemically modifies apoprotein A-I (apoA-I) and reduces its ability to interact with cell surface receptors.[14]

REVERSE CHOLESTEROL TRANSPORT

One of the major functions of HDL is to transport cholesterol from peripheral tissues to the liver for excretion in the bile.[11,15] The concept of reverse cholesterol transport (RCT), first introduced in 1968 by Glomset,[16] has been identified as the major function of HDL and is thought to lend biological plausibility to the inverse relationship between plasma HDL levels and risk for CHD. During RCT, a series of reactions serve to extract excess cholesterol from monocyte-derived macrophages in the subendothelial space and transport this cholesterol back to the liver for disposal as either biliary cholesterol or as bile acids via the activity of 7α-hydroxylase (**Fig. 1**).[17–19] Peripheral tissues transfer excess free cholesterol to lipid-poor apolipoprotein A-I (apoA-I) via the adenosine triphosphate binding membrane cassette transport protein A1 (ABCA1), resulting in the formation of nascent discoidal or pre-β HDL (ndHDL).[11] Free cholesterol on the surface of ndHDL is esterified by lecithin:cholesteryl acyltransferase and internalized into the hydrophobic core of the particle. As the ndHDL becomes progressively more lipidated and its core enlarges with more cholesteryl ester, it becomes increasingly larger and more spherical, forming HDL_3 and then HDL_2. Free cholesterol can also be effluxed from peripheral cells directly to more mature, spherical HDL particles (HDL_2 and HDL_3) via the scavenger receptor-B1 (SR-B1) receptor[20] or ABCG1 and ABCG4.[21,22]

Cholesterol in HDL may be transported back to the liver via two different receptors. In direct RCT, HDL binds via apoAI to SR-B1 receptors on the hepatocyte surface. SR-BI selectively delipidates HDL and then releases the depleted particle back into the circulation.[23,24] In indirect RCT, cholesteryl ester transfer protein (CETP) facilitates the transfer of cholesteryl ester from HDL in exchange for triglycerides in apoB100 containing lipoproteins such as very low-density lipoproteins (VLDL) and interme-diate-density lipoproteins (IDL). VLDL and IDL are then converted to LDL by the action of lipoprotein lipase (LPL). The LDL can then either return the cholesteryl ester to the liver via the LDL receptor or the LDL-related receptor protein, or it may travel to the periphery where it can be chemically modified via oxidation and be rendered athero-genic. The indirect RCT pathway is blocked by CETP inhibition. By blocking CETP activity, HDL particles become less enriched with triglyceride. When HDL is enriched with triglyceride it becomes a better target for lipolysis by hepatic lipase (HL). As HL lipolyzes HDL, the HDL particles become progressively smaller and can become ther-modynamically unstable, leading to the dissociation of apoAI. Free apoAI can be bound to cubulin or megalin and eliminated in urine. The relative physiologic and clin-ical significance of direct and indirect RCT is difficult to define at the present time.

OTHER ANTIATHEROGENIC EFFECTS OF HIGH-DENSITY LIPOPROTEIN

There are several well-established actions of HDL beyond RCT and reducing the formation of oxidized LDL that further delineate how HDLs may antagonize atherogen-esis (see **Table 1**). Endothelial cell dysfunction is associated with atherogenesis.[25] Endothelial dysfunction is characterized by reduced capacity for nitric oxide produc-tion, increased adhesion molecule expression, and reduced production of tissue plas-minogen activator (tPA) and increased synthesis of plasminogen activator inhibitor-1 (PAI-1). These changes are associated with increased vasoconstriction and a more thrombogenic surface. HDL stimulates endothelial nitric oxide production by stabi-lizing mRNA transcripts for nitric oxide synthase. Vasodilatation and myocardial perfu-sion both increase as a function of serum HDL levels.[26,27] The HDLs stimulate tPA and inhibit PAI-1 expression.[28] HDL inhibits sphingosine kinase, an enzyme that catalyzes the formation of sphingosine-1-phosphate. As sphingosine-1-phosphate levels decrease within the cell, activation of nuclear factor kappa-B (NK-κB) decreases, leading to a reduction in the expression of vascular cell adhesion molecule-1 (VCAM-1) and intercellular adhesion molecule-1 (ICAM-1).[29] Adhesion molecules potentiate the binding of inflammatory white blood cells, such as monocytes, to the endothelial cell surface. Once bound, monocytes follow a gradient of monocyte che-moattract protein-1 (MCP-1) down into the subendothelial space by either moving between endothelial cells at sites of weakened gap junctions or by transcytosis across the endothelial cell. HDL can inhibit the production of MCP-1.[30] HDL also stimulates the production of prostacyclin by functioning as an arachidonic acid to endothelial cell cyclooxygenase.[31] Prostacyclin is a potent vasodilator and augments the vasodi-latory effects of nitric oxide. HDL inhibits endothelial cell apoptosis by inhibiting acti-vation of caspases 3 and 9, and stimulates endothelial cell proliferation and migration, helping to restore the continuity of denuded areas of endothelium along the vascula-ture.[32] The effects of HDL on the endothelium are conceptually summarized in **Fig. 2**.

HDLs also appear to have intrinsic capacity to modulate risk for thrombosis. By increasing endothelial production of nitric oxide, prostacyclin, and tPA, platelet reac-tivity and coagulation are inhibited.[33] HDL inhibits platelet thromboxane A2 produc-tion, inhibits thrombin activation and thrombin-induced platelet aggregation, potentiates the activities of proteins C and S, and reduces production of the procoa-gulant tissue factor.[28,34–36] HDL is an important apoprotein carrier and is able to trans-fer a variety of apoproteins to other lipoproteins, thereby playing an important role in the dynamics of lipoprotein physiology (lipid transfer, lipolysis, cellular lipoprotein binding and uptake, and so forth).

In this context of HDL function, HDL is best viewed as a polymolecular supersystem that is in constant, dynamic flux. HDL responds to its environment by associating with, and dissociating from, a large number of proteins and lipids found in serum. HDL is a highly evolved and multifunctional lipoprotein. HDL is able to activate a broad variety of complex intracellular signaling systems that modulate whole families of genes. HDL interacts with a variety of cell types and is responsible for the mobilization and trans-port of cholesterol from peripheral tissues back to the liver. Importantly, HDL is the primary carrier of cholesterol to steroidogenic organs. HDL can significantly influence the function of endothelial cells and platelets, and can help to modulate the effects of

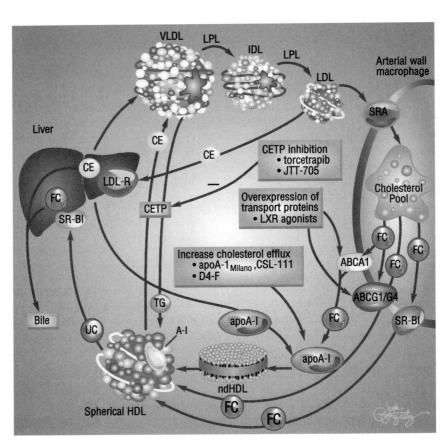

vascular inflammatory and oxidative tone. HDL also significantly impacts the capacity of inflammatory white blood cells to enter and take up residence in the subendothelial space of arteries.

NOVEL THERAPIES FOR INCREASING HIGH-DENSITY LIPOPROTEIN

The NCEP ATP III guidelines[37] recognize a low HDL-C as a categorical risk factor for CHD. A low serum HDL-C is a defining feature of the metabolic syndrome and there are many polymorphisms in a large number of genes (apoproteins, enzymes, cell surface receptors) that can predispose patients to isolated low HDL-C or combined forms of dyslipidemia with hypoalphalipoproteinemia.[3] It is estimated that approximately 35% of men and 39% of women residing in the United States have low serum levels of HDL-C.[38] This is an important and widely prevalent risk factor to address in the clinical contexts of primordial, primary, and secondary prevention. Whereas statin, niacin, and fibrate therapy have been demonstrated to increase HDL-C to varying extents, a number of newer treatments hold promise for reducing cardiovascular risk by raising HDL-C (**Box 1**). These include infusible HDL mimetics, novel peroxisome proliferator-activated receptor-α (PPAR-α) agonists, liver X receptor-α (LXR-α) agonists, CETP inhibitors, D-4F and other apoA mimetics, combination therapy with

◀──────

Fig. 1. Influence of high-density lipoprotein elevating therapies on pathways of reverse cholesterol transport (RCT). Peripheral tissues do not have the capacity to catabolize cholesterol. RCT is a complex pathway with built-in redundancy to ensure that whole-body cholesterol homeostasis is maintained. During RCT, cholesterol is mobilized from peripheral tissues and returned to the liver for disposal. In atherosclerotic disease, the capacity for recovering cholesterol from arterial walls does not keep pace with the rate at which atherogenic lipoproteins deliver cholesterol to subendothelial macrophages. VLDL secreted from the liver is sequentially converted to IDL and LDL via the lipolytic activity of lipoprotein lipase. Lipolyzed chylomicrons and VLDL particles can release surface coat mass that can be used to assimilate HDL in serum. LDL particles traverse the endothelial layer of arteries and interact with activated macrophages that express families of scavenging receptors, including scavenging receptor A (SRA). SRA promotes cholesterol uptake from LDL particles culminating in the formation of macrophage foam cells. Apoprotein AI (apoAI) is secreted from the small intestine and liver. Lipid-poor apoAI interacts with the ATP binding membrane cassette transporter A1 (ABCA1) and promotes the mobilization and externalization of cholesterol from intracellular lipid pools. The cholesterol bound to apoAI undergoes esterification by lecithin:cholesteryl acyltransferase. As the apoAI becomes more lipidated and cholesteryl esters move into the hydrophobic core of particles, it forms nascent discoidal HDL (ndHDL or "pre-β" HDL). ndHDL matures into the spherical particles HDL$_3$ (smaller) and then HDL$_2$ (larger). The macrophage expresses a variety of other transporters to ensure cholesterol homeostasis. Three other transport proteins (ABCG1, ABCG4, and scavenging receptor B-I) translocate intracellular cholesterol into HDL$_3$ and HDL$_2$. HDL$_2$ can transport cholesterol back to the liver via pathways described as "direct" and "indirect" RCT. In direct RCT, HDL$_2$ delivers cholesterol to the liver by binding to, and being delipidated by, SR-BI. In indirect RCT, cholesterol ester is exchanged 1:1 for triglyceride from apoB100-containing lipoproteins (VLDL, IDL). This enriches HDL with triglyceride, making it a better substrate for lipolysis and catabolism by hepatic lipase. The cholesterol exchanged into apoB100-containing lipoproteins can be returned to the liver via the LDL or LDL receptor–related protein or be transported into arterial walls. CETP inhibition decreases the cholesterol throughput of indirect RCT and inhibits the enrichment of HDL with triglyceride. Infusible apoAIs (apoAIMilano, CSL111) and HDL mimetics (D-4F) facilitate cholesterol mobilization and efflux from macrophages. Liver X receptor (LXR) agonists increase cellular cholesterol transport capacity by inducing increased expression of ABCA1 and ABCG1.

sustained-release niacin and a prostaglandin D1 (PGD1) receptor antagonist (Cordaptive), and farnesoid X receptor (FXR) antagonists. Each of these novel therapies will be briefly reviewed in the following sections.

Infusible High-Density Lipoprotein Mimetics

A number of studies have demonstrated that apoA-I correlates with HDL levels and, like HDL, correlates inversely with the development of atherosclerosis (see **Table 1**).[39–42] ApoAI is a major protein constituent of HDL and is secreted from both the liver and small intestine.[43] In addition to its role in promoting cellular cholesterol efflux, apoA-I is the major activator of lecithin:cholesteryl acyltransferase (LCAT).[44]

ApoA-I overexpression in transgenic mice and rabbits has been demonstrated to increase the number of circulating HDL particles and confers protection from the development of diet- or gene-induced atherosclerosis.[39,45–47] In contrast, carriers of the apoA-I$_{Milano}$ have severe hypoalphalipoproteinemia but are not at increased risk for premature CHD.[48] The cysteine substitution for arginine at position 173 in the apoA-I$_{Milano}$ variant allows dimerization via formation of a disulfide bond, resulting in the genesis of large HDL particles that have an increased serum half-life. The HDLs

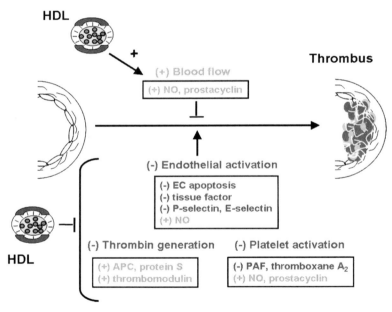

Fig. 2. Beneficial effects of HDL on endothelial function and thrombosis tendency. Stimulatory and inhibitory effects are indicated in green and red, respectively. HDLs interact with endothelial cells (EC) to promote secretion of the vasodilators, nitric oxide (NO), and prostacyclin. Both of these molecules also inhibit platelet aggregability. HDL inhibits endothelial activation, which reduces surface adhesion molecule expression (eg, selectins) and endothelial cell apoptosis. HDLs negatively modulate platelet activation and thrombin generation by inhibiting the production of tissue factor, plasminogen activator inhibitor-1, thromboxane A$_2$, and platelet activating factor (PAF), and stimulating the production of tissue plasminogen activator, thrombomodulin, and activated protein C (APC). (*Reproduced from* Mineo C, Deguchi H, Griffin JH, et al. Endothelial and antithrombotic actions of HDL. Circ Res 2006;98(11):1352–64; with permission.)

Box 1
Novel therapies for increasing HDL
Infusible HDL mimetics
PPAR-α agonists
LXR-α agonists
CETP inhibitors
D-4F and other apoA mimetics
Cordaptive (combination of extended-release niacin and PGD2 receptor antagonist)
Farnesoid X receptor antagonists

derived from patients with the apoA-I$_{Milano}$ phenotype have increased affinity for ABCA1, increased capacity for RCT, and augmented ability to antagonize oxidation and thrombosis.[49–52] Other proposed actions of apoA-I$_{Milano}$ are its increased affinity for ABCA1 as well as increased capacity to oppose lipid oxidation and antagonize thrombosis compared with native apoAI.[53] Given the antiatherogenic efficacy of both native ApoAI and apoA-I$_{Milano}$, it is both reasonable and scientifically valid to assess their therapeutic utility in the setting of established CHD.

Studies in mice and rabbits have used several approaches to increase HDL-C levels, including intravenous administration of synthetic HDL, apoA-I, and apoA-I$_{Milano}$ and have demonstrated significant capacity to induce atheromatous plaque regression.[51,54–58] Nissen and colleagues[59] examined the effect of once-weekly intravenous infusions of recombinant apoAI$_{Milano}$/phospholipid complexes (recombinant apoAI$_{Milano}$/1-palmitoyl-2-oleoyl phosphatidylcholine complex or ETC 216) on atheroma burden in 123 patients with established coronary artery disease (CAD), as measured by intravascular ultrasonography (IVUS). These workers demonstrated a significant regression of coronary atherosclerosis after 5 weeks of treatment compared with controls (change in percent atheroma volume -4.2% versus -0.8% [$P < .001$] in patients treated ETC 216 and placebo, respectively; mean change in total atheroma volume -14.1 versus -2.9 mm^3 [$P < .001$] in patients treated with ETC 216 and placebo, respectively).

Use of an infusion of HDL reconstituted with native apoAI HDL (CSL 111) was examined in the Atherosclerosis Safety and Efficacy (ERASE) Study. In this study, 183 patients were randomized to placebo or 40 mg/kg or 80 mg/kg of CSL-111, a reconstituted HDL consisting of apolipoprotein A-1 from human plasma combined with soybean phosphatidylcholine, which chemically and biologically resembles native HDL.[60] Short-term (4-week) infusion of CSL-111 at a dose of 40 mg/kg resulted in statistically significant improvements in plaque characterization indices on IVUS and quantitative coronary angiography. However, no significant differences were found in change in atheroma volume or nominal change in plaque volume compared with placebo. In addition, the higher dosage of CSL-III treatment group (80 mg/kg) was discontinued early because of liver function abnormalities.

Although infusible HDL mimetics have short-term capacity to induce coronary plaque regression based on IVUS studies, much more work must be done to better characterize the potential efficacy of these therapies in both the near and long term. Remaining questions include the impact of longer periods of treatment with apoA-I/ phospholipid infusions, optimal doses, dose sequencing, the amount of plaque regression that can ultimately be attained, and what effect plaque regression has on risk for cardiovascular morbidity and mortality.[61] In addition, safety concerns, such as anaphylactic reactions, and cost implications will quite likely impact further testing and use. This approach to therapeutic HDL modulation may offer clinicians a unique means by which to delipidate and stabilize atheromatous plaques vulnerable to rupture.

Novel Peroxisome Proliferator-Activated Receptor-α-Agonists

Agonizing the PPAR-α is another mechanism by which to influence HDL production and activity. PPARs are nuclear transcription factors. PPAR-α increases serum HDL levels by (1) stimulating hepatic apoAI expression and (2) promoting triglyceride catabolism by activating lipoprotein lipase, thereby decreasing the enrichment of HDL with triglyceride and reducing the lipolysis and catabolism of HDL by hepatic lipase. The fibric acid derivatives (gemfibrozil, fenofibrate, and bezafibrate) are PPAR-α agonists and modulate the expression of numerous genes within the nucleus.[62,63]

PPAR isoforms include PPAR-α, PPAR-β/σ, and PPAR-γ, and each manifest different physiologic and pharmacologic functions depending on their target genes and tissue distribution.[64,65] PPAR-α regulates genes involved in fatty acid uptake and storage, inflammation, and lipoprotein metabolism, whereas PPAR-γ regulates genes involved in glucose and fatty acid metabolism, inflammation, and macrophage lipid homeostasis.[66] PPAR-α activation increases hepatic apoA-I and apoA-II expression, increases HDL-C, promotes cholesterol efflux, and induces RCT.[67,68] PPAR-α agonists act to impact atherosclerosis in several ways including improving vascular wall reactivity, reducing expression of endothelial adhesion molecules, and decreasing levels of inflammatory cytokines such as tumor necrosis factor-α, interleukin (IL)-I, and IL-6.[65]

PPAR-α activators such as fibrates act to lower plasma triglycerides and VLDL particles and increase HDL-C and are therefore recognized as first-line agents in the treatment of primary hypertriglyceridemia, combined hyperlipidemia, and secondary lipid abnormalities. While fibrates were identified as ligands for the PPAR-α receptor, they demonstrated only weak agonist activity and require a high dosing (145 to 1200 mg/day) to achieve lipid-lowering effects. More potent and subtype-selective human PPAR-α agonists are in development including GFT505, a selective PPAR-α modulator that is 100-fold more potent than fenofibrate.[65] Newer selective PPAR-α agonists may prove beneficial in improved regulation of lipid metabolism as well as augmenting HDL functionality and concentrations in serum.

Liver X Receptor-α-Agonists

Liver X receptors (LXRs) are nuclear transcription factors involved in the regulation of lipid metabolism and inflammation. LXR agonists inhibit the progression of atherosclerosis in mice; however, the specific mechanisms are incompletely understood.[69] LXR agonists up-regulate the ABCA1 and ABCG1 in macrophages and may inhibit atherosclerosis by promoting RCT. The thiazolidinediones have also been shown activate LXR-α and increase expression of ABCA1 and ABCG1.[70] Synthetic LXR agonists induce atherosclerosis regression and promote macrophage cholesterol efflux and RCT in vivo and inhibit the progression of atherosclerosis in LDL receptor knockout and apoE knockout mice.[69,71–74] LXR agonists also inhibit lipopolysaccharide-induced expression of proinflammatory genes and decrease inflammation in mouse models.[42] The therapeutic benefit of LXR agonists is potentially dampened because of LXR-mediated increases in plasma and hepatic triglycerides resulting from LXR induction of lipogenic genes, including sterol response element binding protein-1c (SREBP-1c) and fatty acid synthase (FAS).[42,75] This can lead to increased risk for hepatic steatosis. Recently, the administration of a synthetic LXR agonist, GW3965, was found to increase the rate of RCT in vivo without inducing hepatic steatosis.[69] Continued interest in LXR agonism as a potential therapeutic approach and the use of more selective LXR modulators with less proclivity for inducing hypertriglyceridemia and hepatic steatosis will increase the likelihood that these agents will find a role in the prevention and management of CAD.

Cholesteryl Ester Transfer Protein Inhibitors

Another approach to elevating HDL-C is through the inhibition of CETP. CETP mediates the stoichiometric 1:1 exchange of triglycerides for cholesteryl ester between apolipoprotein B100–containing lipoproteins and HDL. Increased CETP activity may be proatherogenic as it lowers HDL-C and may reduce the amount of cholesterol delivered back to the liver via direct RCT. Therefore, inhibiting CETP activity has been proposed as a therapeutic benefit for patients with CHD.[76] Several approaches to inhibit CETP activity and increase HDL-C have been examined including anti-CETP antibodies, antisense oligonucleotides, and a vaccine that induces antibodies for the inhibition of CETP activity.[42]

Research on Japanese populations with CETP deficiency identified concurrent high serum levels of HDL-C and led to the development of CETP inhibitors to elevate HDL-C levels and potentially decrease cardiovascular risk.[77] CETP inhibitors have been demonstrated to induce considerable elevations in serum levels of HDL (up to 150%), with concomitant reductions in LDL-C. Yet results from recent clinical trials question the therapeutic efficacy of at least one CETP inhibitor—torcetrapib—which was demonstrated to increase blood pressure and serum levels of aldosterone and have no effect in decreasing the progression of coronary[78] and carotid atherosclerosis.[79] Although CETP inhibition with torcetrapib did not prove to be clinically beneficial, the concept of CETP inhibition continues to represent a potential approach to HDL therapeutics, and other CETP inhibitors are currently in development (anacetrapib, JTT-705).[10] In one recent study, anacetrapib increased serum HDL-C up to 129% and decreased LDL-C up to 38% in a dose-dependent manner and had no effect on blood pressure in human volunteers.[80] Given the adverse experience with torcetrapib, it is anticipated that the further development of CETP inhibitors will be cautious and slow, with intensive attention focused on patient safety in short-term dosing studies as well as surrogate and cardiovascular end point trials. Although torcetrapib exerted multiple forms of unanticipated off-target toxicities, additional investigation is under way to assess the functionality and the spectrum of HDL species generated by CETP inhibition.

D-4F and Other ApoA Mimetics

Apoproteins contain n amphipathic α-helices that stabilize the structure and size of lipoproteins.[81] These helical regions in apoAI also allow HDL to dock with such cell surface receptors as ABCA1 and SR-BI. Apoprotein mimetics are amphipathic α-helices that do not increase serum levels of HDL. Rather, these molecules augment the functionality of HDL. The apo A-I mimetic, D-4F, is an edible molecule that is resistant to hydrolysis by gastric peptidases because it is composed of D-amino acids (4F denotes the four phenylalanine residues in its amino acid sequence). D4-F has been shown to enhance HDL-C's antioxidant and anti-inflammatory properties, as well as increase rates of RCT. Given orally, D-4F functions as small amphipathic helices that mimic the effects and functions of apo AI. The antiatherogenic effect of D-4F has been demonstrated in hyperlipidemic mice[82] and in apolipoprotein E-null mice.[83] When given orally to mice and monkeys, D-4F results in the formation of pre-β HDL, improved HDL-mediated cholesterol efflux from macrophages, reduced lipoprotein lipid hydroperoxide formation, and increased paraoxonase activity. Importantly, D-4F stimulates the conversion of proinflammatory HDL to anti-inflammatory HDL.[84] Oral D-4F administered to LDL receptor–null mice on a Western diet and apoE-null mice on a chow diet results in reductions of atherosclerotic lesions by 79% and 75%, respectively, without significantly altering plasma lipid levels.[85] Taken together, the studies on D-4F suggest that it may have therapeutic potential; however, additional research on its optimal use and further characterization of its systemic effects and safety profile in humans are needed. If ultimately successful, D-4F offers an appealing and more cost-effective way of delivering an apo AI mimetic to patients with low HDL-C and/or compromised capacity for RCT. A number of other apoA-I mimetic peptides are also in development.[86]

Cordaptive

Niacin, or nicotinic acid, is a soluble B vitamin that has favorable effects on all major lipid subfractions, including HDL. Niacin binds to a receptor labeled HM74 (or alternative nomenclature gp109A) on the surface of adipocytes.[87] This leads to the inhibition of hormone-sensitive lipase, which in turn reduces the mobilization of fatty acids into the portal circulation. Niacin also reduces the esterification of mono- and diglycerides to reform triglycerides by inhibiting acyl-coenzyme A: diglycerol acyltransferase 2 (DGAT2) and increase apoB100 catabolism. This leads to reduced VLDL and triglyceride secretion by the liver. Niacin increases serum HDL levels by down-regulating the expression of the F1 moiety of the F1F0 ATP synthetase, a holoparticle HDL receptor.[88] This leads to reduced hepatic HDL catabolism. HDL levels are likely also increased secondary to reduced enrichment of HDL with triglyceride and its subsequent catabolism by hepatic lipase. Despite the ability of niacin to raise HDL (by 15% to 30%), the use of niacin therapy has been limited because of its side-effect profile, notably cutaneous vasodilation leading to skin flushing, warmth, and pruritis. Niacin mediates vasodilatation by activating production of prostaglandin D2, which binds to the prostaglandin D2 receptor 1 (PGD1).

Cordaptive is a combination of sustained-release niacin and a PGD1 receptor blocker (laropiprant), which functions to prevent activation of vasodilatation by prostaglandin D2. Formerly known as MK-0524A, Cordaptive has been shown in limited clinical studies to reduce symptoms of flushing.[89] Current ongoing studies will further assess the effects of Cordaptive on cardiovascular outcomes in both the ACHIEVE trial and in the Treatment of HDL to Reduce the Incidence of Vascular Events (HPS2-THRIVE) trial (http://www.ctsu.ox.ac.uk/projects/hps2-thrive). This agent may increase use of niacin augmentation, especially if flushing is inhibited significantly. A downstream metabolite of PGD2 (15-deoxy-D12,14-prostaglandin J2) is a potent endogenous PPAR-γ agonist that promotes expression of ABCA1 and increases transfer of cholesterol from macrophages to HDL.[90] One potential unforeseen toxicity of Cordaptive may be a reduction in the capacity of 15-deoxy-D12,14-prostaglandin J2 to stimulate expression of ABCA1 on the surface of macrophages. Although approved for use in the European Union, the US Food and Drug Administration issued a "not approvable" letter for Cordaptive. This stance may change as clinical trial data with the drug become available and the benefit/risk ratio may be more adequately assessed.

Farnesoid X Receptor Antagonists

The Farnesoid X receptor (FXR), a member of the nuclear receptor family, is a modulator of lipid, bile acid, and glucose homeostasis.[91] FXR regulates bile acid synthesis, conjugation, and transport; induces the expression of phospholipid transfer protein, an enzyme involved in HDL remodeling; and decreases triglyceride levels by increasing their clearance by modulating LPL activity and inducing PPARα.[91] One of the most important functions of FXR activation is to inhibit cholesterol 7-alpha-hydroxylase, the rate-limiting enzyme in bile acid biosynthesis. FXR is expressed in a wide variety of tissues, including the heart, kidney, thymus, and spleen.[92] Studies have identified FXR in the vasculature in vivo and in cultured vascular smooth muscle cells, which indicate that FXR is functional in vascular smooth muscle.[93] Chenodeoxycholate is a natural ligand for FXR. The role of FXR in HDL metabolism is not well understood, but apoA-I and hepatic lipase expression are both inhibited by activated FXR.[94,95] The implications for antagonizing FXR function to favorably influence HDL metabolism and RCT are unknown.[74] FXR agonists may be potentially beneficial for triglyceride lowering while FXR antagonists may have a role in LDL lowering.[74] Studies on the use of guggolipid as an antagonist of FXR have not demonstrated consistent results in lowering LDL-C and raising HDL-C.[96,97] Considerable additional study is needed to determine how FXR functions in HDL metabolism and what if any role FXR agonists, antagonists, or modulators have in CHD prevention.[98]

SAFETY AND EFFICACY CONSIDERATIONS

HDL metabolism is clearly extremely complex. As research on novel therapies targeting HDL-C continues to evolve, the regulatory circuitry of HDL metabolism will clarify. Many new genetic polymorphisms affecting the rate of production and the functionality of HDL are being identified. It is possible that in many of these patients, interventions will have to be matched with specific alterations in HDL metabolism. This will require considerable additional insight into the genomics, lipidomics, and metabolomics of dyslipidemia and HDL speciation and function. Many patients with impairments in HDL metabolism may ultimately require combinations of drugs to achieve optimal regulation of HDL synthesis, function, and capacity for RCT. Infusible apoproteins and HDLs, apoAI mimetics, the agonism of nuclear transcription factors, modulation of macrophage ABC transporters, stimulating hepatic and intestinal expression of apoAI, and the therapeutic adjustment of enzymes that remodel HDLs and facilitate transfer reactions among lipoproteins (CETP, phospholipid transfer protein, endothelial lipase, lipoprotein lipase, hepatic lipase) may assume therapeutic roles in lipid management. Sorting these issues out will require well-designed clinical studies and large clinical trials, which will require much time and incur considerable expense. Given the difficulties and lessons learned from the torcetrapib trials, it is likely that these novel HDL therapies will be required to demonstrate both safety as well as capacity for reducing cardiovascular morbidity and mortality before regulatory approval. It is unclear how much credence will be placed on surrogate end point studies using IVUS and carotid intima media thickness measurements when evaluating the clinical efficacy of these newer forms of intervention in patients with low HDL or poorly functional HDL.

SUMMARY

Low serum levels of HDL-C are an important risk factor for all forms of atherosclerotic disease. Comprehensive risk factor management is crucial to ensuring that risk for developing atherosclerotic disease and sustaining acute cardiovascular events is optimally reduced. Some studies do show that HDL elevation contributes to risk reduction in patients with CHD. HDL is among the most fascinating and complex molecular assemblies yet to evolve in mammalian systems. The continued exploration of HDL biogenesis and the nature of its interactions with the histologic components of arterial walls will reveal a far more rich and challenging landscape against which the war against atherogenesis will be waged. It is likely that the modulation of HDL function and its concentrations in serum will significantly impact future approaches to the management of cardiovascular disease in both the primary and secondary prevention settings. There will be considerable challenges intrinsic to the process of elucidating which specific therapies best meet the needs of patients with particular forms of hypoalphalipoproteinemia and/or compromised HDL functionality.

REFERENCES

1. Castelli WP. Cholesterol and lipids in the risk of coronary artery disease–the Framingham Heart Study. Can J Cardiol 1988;4(Suppl A):5A–10A.
2. Gotto AM Jr, Brinton EA. Assessing low levels of high-density lipoprotein cholesterol as a risk factor in coronary heart disease: a working group report and update. J Am Coll Cardiol 2004;43(5):717–24.
3. Toth PP. High-density lipoprotein: epidemiology, metabolism, and antiatherogenic effects. Dis Mon 2001;47(8):369–416.
4. Wolfram RM, Brewer HB, Xue Z, et al. Impact of low high-density lipoproteins on in-hospital events and one-year clinical outcomes in patients with non-ST-elevation myocardial infarction acute coronary syndrome treated with drug-eluting stent implantation. Am J Cardiol 2006;98(6):711–7.
5. Rubins HB, Robins SJ, Collins D, et al. Gemfibrozil for the secondary prevention of coronary heart disease in men with low levels of high-density lipoprotein cholesterol. Veterans Affairs High-Density Lipoprotein Cholesterol Intervention Trial Study Group. N Engl J Med 1999;341(6):410–8.
6. Secondary prevention by raising HDL cholesterol and reducing triglycerides in patients with coronary artery disease. The Bezafibrate Infarction Prevention (BIP) study. Circulation 2000;102(1):21–7.
7. Shai I, Rimm EB, Hankinson SE, et al. Multivariate assessment of lipid parameters as predictors of coronary heart disease among postmenopausal women: potential implications for clinical guidelines. Circulation 2004;110(18):2824–30.
8. Barter P, Gotto AM, LaRosa JC, et al. HDL cholesterol, very low levels of LDL cholesterol, and cardiovascular events. N Engl J Med 2007;357(13):1301–10.
9. Tall AR, Yvan-Charvet L, Wang N. The failure of torcetrapib: was it the molecule or the mechanism? Arterioscler Thromb Vasc Biol 2007;27(2):257–60.
10. Toth P. Torcetrapib and atherosclerosis: what happened and where do we go from here? Future Lipidol 2007;2:277–84.
11. Oram JF, Heinecke JW. ATP-binding cassette transporter A1: a cell cholesterol exporter that protects against cardiovascular disease. Physiol Rev 2005;85(4): 1343–72.
12. Navab M, Anantharamaiah GM, Reddy ST, et al. Mechanisms of disease: proatherogenic HDL—an evolving field. Nat Clin Pract Endocrinol Metab 2006;2(9): 504–11.
13. Vaisar T, Pennathur S, Green PS, et al. Shotgun proteomics implicates protease inhibition and complement activation in the antiinflammatory properties of HDL. J Clin Invest 2007;117(3):746–56.
14. Shao B, Oda MN, Oram JF, et al. Myeloperoxidase: an inflammatory enzyme for generating dysfunctional high density lipoprotein. Curr Opin Cardiol 2006;21(4): 322–8.
15. Fielding CJ, Fielding PE. Molecular physiology of reverse cholesterol transport. J Lipid Res 1995;36(2):211–28.

16. Glomset JA. The plasma lecithins:cholesterol acyltransferase reaction. J Lipid Res 1968;9(2):155–67.
17. Brewer HB Jr, Remaley AT, Neufeld EB, et al. Regulation of plasma high-density lipoprotein levels by the ABCA1 transporter and the emerging role of high-density lipoprotein in the treatment of cardiovascular disease. Arterioscler Thromb Vasc Biol 2004;24(10):1755–60.
18. Rader DJ. Molecular regulation of HDL metabolism and function: implications for novel therapies. J Clin Invest 2006;116(12):3090–100.
19. Toth PP. Reverse cholesterol transport: high-density lipoprotein's magnificent mile. Curr Atheroscler Rep 2003;5(5):386–93.
20. Yancey PG, Bortnick AE, Kellner-Weibel G, et al. Importance of different pathways of cellular cholesterol efflux. Arterioscler Thromb Vasc Biol 2003;23(5):712–9.
21. Wang N, Lan D, Chen W, et al. ATP-binding cassette transporters G1 and G4 mediate cellular cholesterol efflux to high-density lipoproteins. Proc Natl Acad Sci U S A 2004;101(26):9774–9.
22. Wang N, Yvan-Charvet L, Lutjohann D, et al. ATP-binding cassette transporters G1 and G4 mediate cholesterol and desmosterol efflux to HDL and regulate sterol accumulation in the brain. FASEB J 2008;22:1073–82.
23. Krieger M. Charting the fate of the "good cholesterol": identification and characterization of the high-density lipoprotein receptor SR-BI. Annu Rev Biochem 1999;68:523–58.
24. Krieger M. Scavenger receptor class B type I is a multiligand HDL receptor that influences diverse physiologic systems. J Clin Invest 2001;108(6):793–7.
25. Anderson TJ, Gerhard MD, Meredith IT, et al. Systemic nature of endothelial dysfunction in atherosclerosis. Am J Cardiol 1995;75(6):71B–4B.
26. Li XP, Zhao SP, Zhang XY, et al. Protective effect of high density lipoprotein on endothelium-dependent vasodilatation. Int J Cardiol 2000;73(3):231–6.
27. Levkau B, Hermann S, Theilmeier G, et al. High-density lipoprotein stimulates myocardial perfusion in vivo. Circulation 2004;110(21):3355–9.
28. O'Connell BJ, Genest J Jr. High-density lipoproteins and endothelial function. Circulation 2001;104(16):1978–83.
29. Baker PW, Rye KA, Gamble JR, et al. Ability of reconstituted high density lipoproteins to inhibit cytokine-induced expression of vascular cell adhesion molecule-1 in human umbilical vein endothelial cells. J Lipid Res 1999;40(2):345–53.
30. Navab M, Imes SS, Hama SY, et al. Monocyte transmigration induced by modification of low density lipoprotein in cocultures of human aortic wall cells is due to induction of monocyte chemotactic protein 1 synthesis and is abolished by high density lipoprotein. J Clin Invest 1991;88(6):2039–46.
31. Fleisher LN, Tall AR, Witte LD, et al. Stimulation of arterial endothelial cell prostacyclin synthesis by high density lipoproteins. J Biol Chem 1982;257(12):6653–5.
32. Nofer JR, Levkau B, Wolinska I, et al. Suppression of endothelial cell apoptosis by high density lipoproteins (HDL) and HDL-associated lysosphingolipids. J Biol Chem 2001;276(37):34480–5.
33. Mineo C, Deguchi H, Griffin JH, et al. Endothelial and antithrombotic actions of HDL. Circ Res 2006;98(11):1352–64.
34. Nofer JR, Walter M, Kehrel B, et al. HDL3-mediated inhibition of thrombin-induced platelet aggregation and fibrinogen binding occurs via decreased production of phosphoinositide-derived second messengers 1,2-diacylglycerol and inositol 1,4,5-tris-phosphate. Arterioscler Thromb Vasc Biol 1998;18(6):861–9.

35. Aviram M, Brook JG. Characterization of the effect of plasma lipoproteins on platelet function in vitro. Haemostasis 1983;13(6):344–50.
36. Griffin JH, Kojima K, Banka CL, et al. High-density lipoprotein enhancement of anticoagulant activities of plasma protein S and activated protein C. J Clin Invest 1999;103(2):219–27.
37. National Cholesterol Education Panel. Third Report of the National Cholesterol Education Program (NCEP) Expert Panel on Detection, Evaluation, and Treatment of High Blood Cholesterol in Adults (Adult Treatment Panel III) Final Report. Circulation 2002;106:3143–421.
38. Ford ES, Giles WH, Dietz WH. Prevalence of the metabolic syndrome among US adults: findings from the third National Health and Nutrition Examination Survey. JAMA 2002;287(3):356–9.
39. Rubin EM, Krauss RM, Spangler EA, et al. Inhibition of early atherogenesis in transgenic mice by human apolipoprotein AI. Nature 1991;353(6341):265–7.
40. Plump AS, Scott CJ, Breslow JL. Human apolipoprotein A-I gene expression increases high density lipoprotein and suppresses atherosclerosis in the apolipoprotein E-deficient mouse. Proc Natl Acad Sci U S A 1994;91(20):9607–11.
41. Tangirala RK, Tsukamoto K, Chun SH, et al. Regression of atherosclerosis induced by liver-directed gene transfer of apolipoprotein A-I in mice. Circulation 1999;100(17):1816–22.
42. Pal M, Pillarisetti S. HDL elevators and mimetics—emerging therapies for atherosclerosis. Cardiovasc Hematol Agents Med Chem 2007;5(1):55–66.
43. Sirtori CR, Calabresi L, Franceschini G. Recombinant apolipoproteins for the treatment of vascular diseases. Atherosclerosis 1999;142(1):29–40.
44. Rothblat GH, Mahlberg FH, Johnson WJ, et al. Apolipoproteins, membrane cholesterol domains, and the regulation of cholesterol efflux. J Lipid Res 1992; 33:1091–7.
45. Duverger N, Kruth H, Emmanuel F, et al. Inhibition of atherosclerosis development in cholesterol-fed human apolipoprotein A-I-transgenic rabbits. Circulation 1996;94(4):713–7.
46. Paszty C, Maeda N, Verstuyft J, et al. Apolipoprotein AI transgene corrects apolipoprotein E deficiency-induced atherosclerosis in mice. J Clin Invest 1994;94(2):899–903.
47. Calabresi L, Tedeschi G, Treu C, et al. Limited proteolysis of a disulfide-linked apoA-I dimer in reconstituted HDL. J Lipid Res 2001;42(6):935–42.
48. Franceschini G, Calabresi L, Chiesa G, et al. Increased cholesterol efflux potential of sera from ApoA-IMilano carriers and transgenic mice. Arterioscler Thromb Vasc Biol 1999;19(5):1257–62.
49. Sirtori CR, Calabresi L, Franceschini G, et al. Cardiovascular status of carriers of the apolipoprotein A-I(Milano) mutant: the Limone sul Garda study. Circulation 2001;103(15):1949–54.
50. Shah PK, Yano J, Reyes O, et al. High-dose recombinant apolipoprotein A-I(milano) mobilizes tissue cholesterol and rapidly reduces plaque lipid and macrophage content in apolipoprotein e-deficient mice. Potential implications for acute plaque stabilization. Circulation 2001;103(25):3047–50.
51. Chiesa G, Monteggia E, Marchesi M, et al. Recombinant apolipoprotein A-I(Milano) infusion into rabbit carotid artery rapidly removes lipid from fatty streaks. Circ Res 2002;90(9):974–80.
52. Bielicki JK, Oda MN. Apolipoprotein A-I(Milano) and apolipoprotein A-I(Paris) exhibit an antioxidant activity distinct from that of wild-type apolipoprotein A-I. Biochemistry 2002;41(6):2089–96.

53. Toth PP, Davidson MH. Therapeutic interventions targeted at the augmentation of reverse cholesterol transport. Curr Opin Cardiol 2004;19(4):374–9.
54. Ameli S, Hultgardh-Nilsson A, Cercek B, et al. Recombinant apolipoprotein A-I Milano reduces intimal thickening after balloon injury in hypercholesterolemic rabbits. Circulation 1994;90(4):1935–41.
55. Badimon JJ, Badimon L, Fuster V. Regression of atherosclerotic lesions by high density lipoprotein plasma fraction in the cholesterol-fed rabbit. J Clin Invest 1990;85(4):1234–41.
56. Ibanez BB, Cimmino G, Vilahur G, et al. Rapid change in plaque size, composition, and molecular footprint after recombinant apolipoprotein A-I Milano (ETC 216) administration. J Am Coll Cardiol 2008;51:1104–9.
57. Li D, Weng S, Yang B, et al. Inhibition of arterial thrombus formation by ApoA1 Milano. Arterioscler Thromb Vasc Biol 1999;19(2):378–83.
58. Parolini C, Marchesi M, Lorenzon P, et al. Dose-related effects of repeated ETC-216 (recombinant apolipoprotein A-I MIlano/1-palmitoyl-2-oleoyl phosphatidylcholine complex) administrations on rabbit lipid-rich soft plaques: in vivo assessment by intravascular ultrasound and magnetic resonance imaging. J Am Coll Cardiol 2008;51:1098–103.
59. Nissen SE, Tsunoda T, Tuzcu EM, et al. Effect of recombinant ApoA-I Milano on coronary atherosclerosis in patients with acute coronary syndromes: a randomized controlled trial. JAMA 2003;290(17):2292–300.
60. Tardif JC, Gregoire J, L'Allier PL, et al. Effects of reconstituted high-density lipoprotein infusions on coronary atherosclerosis: a randomized controlled trial. JAMA 2007;297(15):1675–82.
61. Zhao XB, Brown BG. ApoA-I milano/phospholipids complex. J Am Coll Cardiol 2008;51:1110–1.
62. Blanquart C, Barbier O, Fruchart JC, et al. Peroxisome proliferator-activated receptors: regulation of transcriptional activities and roles in inflammation. J Steroid Biochem Mol Biol 2003;85(2–5):267–73.
63. Zambon A, Gervois P, Pauletto P, et al. Modulation of hepatic inflammatory risk markers of cardiovascular diseases by PPAR-alpha activators: clinical and experimental evidence. Arterioscler Thromb Vasc Biol 2006;26(5):977–86.
64. Bordet R, Gele P, Duriez P, et al. PPARs: a new target for neuroprotection. J Neurol Neurosurg Psychiatr 2006;77(3):285–7.
65. Fruchart JC. Novel peroxisome proliferator activated receptor-alpha agonists. Am J Cardiol 2007;100(11A):n41–6.
66. Staels B, Fruchart JC. Therapeutic roles of peroxisome proliferator-activated receptor agonists. Diabetes 2005;54(8):2460–70.
67. Chinetti G, Lestavel S, Bocher V, et al. PPAR-alpha and PPAR-gamma activators induce cholesterol removal from human macrophage foam cells through stimulation of the ABCA1 pathway. Nat Med 2001;7(1):53–8.
68. Chinetti-Gbaguidi G, Rigamonti E, Helin L, et al. Peroxisome proliferator-activated receptor alpha controls cellular cholesterol trafficking in macrophages. J Lipid Res 2005;46(12):2717–25.
69. Naik SU, Wang X, Da Silva JS, et al. Pharmacological activation of liver X receptors promotes reverse cholesterol transport in vivo. Circulation 2006;113(1):90–7.
70. Zelcer N, Tontonoz P. Liver X receptors as integrators of metabolic and inflammatory signaling. J Clin Invest 2006;116(3):607–14.
71. Joseph SB, McKilligin E, Pei L, et al. Synthetic LXR ligand inhibits the development of atherosclerosis in mice. Proc Natl Acad Sci U S A 2002;99(11):7604–9.

72. Terasaka N, Hiroshima A, Koieyama T, et al. T-0901317, a synthetic liver X receptor ligand, inhibits development of atherosclerosis in LDL receptor-deficient mice. FEBS Lett 2003;536(1–3):6–11.

73. Levin N, Bischoff ED, Daige CL, et al. Macrophage liver X receptor is required for antiatherogenic activity of LXR agonists. Arterioscler Thromb Vasc Biol 2005;25(1):135–42.

74. Rader DJ. Liver X receptor and farnesoid X receptor as therapeutic targets. Am J Cardiol 2007;100(11A):n15–9.

75. Li AC, Glass CK. PPAR- and LXR-dependent pathways controlling lipid metabolism and the development of atherosclerosis. J Lipid Res 2004;45(12):2161–73.

76. Barter PJ, Brewer HB Jr, Chapman MJ, et al. Cholesteryl ester transfer protein: a novel target for raising HDL and inhibiting atherosclerosis. Arterioscler Thromb Vasc Biol 2003;23(2):160–7.

77. Barter PJ, Kastelein JJ. Targeting cholesteryl ester transfer protein for the prevention and management of cardiovascular disease. J Am Coll Cardiol 2006;47(3):492–9.

78. Nissen SE, Tardif JC, Nicholls SJ, et al. Effect of torcetrapib on the progression of coronary atherosclerosis. N Engl J Med 2007;356(13):1304–16.

79. Kastelein JJ, van Leuven SI, Burgess L, et al. Effect of torcetrapib on carotid atherosclerosis in familial hypercholesterolemia. N Engl J Med 2007;356(16):1620–30.

80. Krishna R, Anderson MS, Bergman AJ, et al. Effect of the cholesteryl ester transfer protein inhibitor, anacetrapib, on lipoproteins in patients with dyslipidaemia and on 24-h ambulatory blood pressure in healthy individuals: two double-blind, randomised placebo-controlled phase I studies. Lancet 2007;370(9603):1907–14.

81. Segrest JP, Li L, Anantharamaiah GM, et al. Structure and function of apolipoprotein A-I and high-density lipoprotein. Curr Opin Lipidol 2000;11(2):105–15.

82. Navab M, Anantharamaiah GM, Reddy ST, et al. Oral D-4F causes formation of pre-beta high-density lipoprotein and improves high-density lipoprotein-mediated cholesterol efflux and reverse cholesterol transport from macrophages in apolipoprotein E-null mice. Circulation 2004;109(25):3215–20.

83. Li X, Chyu KY, Faria Neto JR, et al. Differential effects of apolipoprotein A-I-mimetic peptide on evolving and established atherosclerosis in apolipoprotein E-null mice. Circulation 2004;110(12):1701–5.

84. Navab M, Anantharamaiah GM, Reddy ST, et al. Apolipoprotein A-I mimetic peptides. Arterioscler Thromb Vasc Biol 2005;25(7):1325–31.

85. Navab M, Anantharamaiah GM, Hama S, et al. Oral administration of an Apo A-I mimetic Peptide synthesized from D-amino acids dramatically reduces atherosclerosis in mice independent of plasma cholesterol. Circulation 2002;105(3):290–2.

86. Anantharamaiah GM, Mishra VK, Garber DW, et al. Structural requirements for antioxidative and anti-inflammatory properties of apolipoprotein A-I mimetic peptides. J Lipid Res 2007;48(9):1915–23.

87. Tunaru S, Kero J, Schaub A, et al. PUMA-G and HM74 are receptors for nicotinic acid and mediate its anti-lipolytic effect. Nat Med 2003;9(3):352–5.

88. Kamanna VS, Kashyap ML. Nicotinic acid (niacin) receptor agonists: will they be useful therapeutic agents? Am J Cardiol 2007;100(11 A):S53–61.

89. Cheng K, Wu TJ, Wu KK, et al. Antagonism of the prostaglandin D2 receptor 1 suppresses nicotinic acid-induced vasodilation in mice and humans. Proc Natl Acad Sci U S A 2006;103(17):6682–7.

90. Rubic T, Trottmann M, Lorenz RL. Stimulation of CD36 and the key effector of reverse cholesterol transport ATP-binding cassette A1 in monocytoid cells by niacin. Biochem Pharmacol 2004;67(3):411–9.
91. Claudel T, Staels B, Kuipers F. The farnesoid X receptor: a molecular link between bile acid and lipid and glucose metabolism. Arterioscler Thromb Vasc Biol 2005;25(10):2020–30.
92. Otte K, Kranz H, Kober I, et al. Identification of farnesoid X receptor beta as a novel mammalian nuclear receptor sensing lanosterol. Mol Cell Biol 2003; 23(3):864–72.
93. Bishop-Bailey D, Walsh DT, Warner TD. Expression and activation of the farnesoid X receptor in the vasculature. Proc Natl Acad Sci U S A 2004;101(10): 3668–73.
94. Claudel T, Sturm E, Duez H, et al. Bile acid-activated nuclear receptor FXR suppresses apolipoprotein A-I transcription via a negative FXR response element. J Clin Invest 2002;109(7):961–71.
95. Sirvent A, Verhoeven AJ, Jansen H, et al. Farnesoid X receptor represses hepatic lipase gene expression. J Lipid Res 2004;45(11):2110–5.
96. Szapary PO, Wolfe ML, Bloedon LT, et al. Guggulipid for the treatment of hypercholesterolemia: a randomized controlled trial. JAMA 2003;290(6):765–72.
97. Ulbricht C, Basch E, Szapary P, et al. Guggul for hyperlipidemia: a review by the Natural Standard Research Collaboration. Complement Ther Med 2005;13(4): 279–90.
98. Ory DS. Nuclear receptor signaling in the control of cholesterol homeostasis: have the orphans found a home? Circ Res 2004;95(7):660–70.
99. Alsheikh-Ali AA, Lin JL, Abourjaily P, et al. Prevalence of low high-density lipoprotein cholesterol in patients with documented coronary heart disease or risk equivalent and controlled low-density lipoprotein cholesterol. Am J Cardiol 2007;100(10):1499–501.
100. Walldius G, Jungner I, Holme I, et al. High apolipoprotein B, low apolipoprotein A-1, and improvement in the prediction of fatal myocardial infarction (AMORIS study): a prospective study. Lancet 2001;358(9298):2026–33.
101. Sharrett AR, Ballantyne CM, Coady SA, et al. Coronary heart disease prediction from lipoprotein cholesterol levels, triglycerides, lipoprotein(a), apolipoproteins A-I and B, and HDL density subfractions: the Atherosclerosis Risk in Communities (ARIC) study. Circulation 2001;104(10):1108–13.
102. The Bezafibrate Infarction Prevention (BIP) Study Group, Israel. Lipids and lipoproteins in symptomatic coronary heart disease. Distribution, intercorrelations, and significance for risk classification in 6,700 men and 1,500 women. Circulation 1992;86(3):839–48.
103. Psaty BM, Furberg CD, Kuller LH, et al. Traditional risk factors and subclinical disease measures as predictors of first myocardial infarction in older adults. The Cardiovascular Health Study. Arch Intern Med 1999;159: 1339–47.
104. Psaty BM, Anderson M, Kronmal RA, et al. The association between lipid levels and the risks of incident myocardial infarction, stroke, and total mortality: the Cardiovascular Health Study. J Am Geriatr Soc 2004;52(10):1639–47.
105. Castelli WP, Doyle TG, Hames CG, et al. HDL cholesterol and other lipids in coronary heart disease. The cooperative lipoprotein phenotyping study. Circulation 1977;55(5):767–72.
106. Kannel WB. High-density lipoproteins: epidemiologic profile and risks of coronary artery disease. Am J Cardiol 1983;52(4):9B–12B.

107. Asztalos BF, Cupples LA, Demissie S, et al. High-density lipoprotein subpopulation profile and coronary heart disease prevalence in male participants of the Framingham Offspring Study. Arterioscler Thromb Vasc Biol 2004;24(11): 2181–7.

108. Manninen V, Elo MO, Frick MH, et al. Lipid alterations and decline in the incidence of coronary heart disease in the Helsinki Heart Study. JAMA 1988; 260(5):641–5.

109. Kitamura A, Iso H, Naito Y, et al. High-density lipoprotein cholesterol and premature coronary heart disease in urban Japanese men. Circulation 1994;89(6): 2533–9.

110. Reed D, Benfante R. Lipid and lipoprotein predictors of coronary heart disease in elderly men in the Honolulu Heart Program. Ann Epidemiol 1992;2(1–2): 29–34.

111. Gordon DJ, Knoke J, Probstfield JL, et al. High-density lipoprotein cholesterol and coronary heart disease in hypercholesterolemic men: the lipid research clinics coronary primary prevention trial. Circulation 1986;74(6):1217–25.

112. Gordon DJ, Probstfield JL, Garrison RJ, et al. High-density lipoprotein cholesterol and cardiovascular disease. Four prospective American studies. Circulation 1989;79:8–15.

113. Shaten BJ, Kuller LH, Neaton JD. Association between baseline risk factors, cigarette smoking, and CHD mortality after 10.5 years. MRFIT Research Group. Prev Med 1991;20(5):655–9.

114. Sacco RL, Benson RT, Kargman DE, et al. High-density lipoprotein cholesterol and ischemic stroke in the elderly: the Northern Manhattan Stroke Study. JAMA 2001;285(21):2729–35.

115. Assmann G, Cullen P, Schulte H. The Muenster Heart Study (PROCAM), results of follow-up at 8 years. Eur Heart J 1998;19(Suppl A):A2–11.

116. Miller NE, Thelle DS, Forde OH, et al. The Tromsø heart-study. High-density lipoprotein and coronary heart-disease: a prospective case-control study. Lancet 1977;1(8019):965–8.

117. Weijenberg MP, Feskens EJ, Kromhout D. Total and high density lipoprotein cholesterol as risk factors for coronary heart disease in elderly men during 5 years of follow-up. The Zutphen Elderly Study. Am J Epidemiol 1996;143(2): 151–8.

Lipid Management in Children

Frances R. Zappalla, DO, Samuel S. Gidding, MD*

KEYWORDS

- Cholesterol • Risk factors • Atherosclerosis
- Nutrition metabolic syndrome • Obesity

Atherosclerosis begins in youth, and the initiation of atherosclerosis is related to traditional cardiovascular risk factors, including dyslipidemia.[1] Rapid progression of atherosclerosis is related to the presence of multiple risk factors or one severe risk factor such as familial hypercholesterolemia (present in about 1 in 500 children), or diabetes mellitus (type 1 and 2 (present in about 1 in 500 children).[1–4] Using measures of subclinical atherosclerosis (carotid intima media thickness [IMT] and coronary artery calcium on CT scan), four longitudinal studies in diverse populations have shown that risk factors measured in youth are better predictors of subclinical atherosclerosis than risk factors measured at the time of the noninvasive assessment.[5–8]

Although the prevention of risk factor development through behavioral means remains the mainstay of pediatric management, a significant subgroup of children may require lipid management before reaching adulthood.[9–11] This article reviews evidence that atherosclerosis begins in childhood, briefly discusses the impact of the obesity epidemic on lipids in childhood, and identifies children at high risk for accelerated atherosclerosis who might require more than behavioral management of lipid abnormalities. Medical conditions that place children and adolescents at higher risk for premature cardiovascular disease are categorized and summarized in **Box 1**.

EARLY ATHEROSCLEROSIS

Although the advanced lesions of atherosclerosis are seen in adult life, it has been well established that fatty streaks are present in the aorta by age 10 years and in the coronary arteries by age 20 years. The presence of atherosclerotic lesions in young adults was documented first during the Korean War when autopsy studies showed evidence of coronary atherosclerosis in 45% of soldiers with a mean age of 22 years.[12] The Pathobiological Determinants of Atherosclerosis in Youth study is a multicenter study looking at the relationship of cardiovascular risk factors measured post mortem and the presence of atherosclerosis in adolescents and young adults, age 15 through

---

Nemours Cardiac Center, A. I. DuPont Hospital for Children, 1600 Rockland Road, Wilmington, DE 19803, USA
* Corresponding author.
E-mail address: sgidding@nemours.org (S.S. Gidding).

Endocrinol Metab Clin N Am 38 (2009) 171–183
doi:10.1016/j.ecl.2008.11.006
0889-8529/08/$ – see front matter © 2009 Elsevier Inc. All rights reserved.

Box 1
Conditions associated with accelerated atherosclerosis in children and adolescents

Conditions in which coronary artery disease is well documented

Familial hypercholesterolemia

Diabetes mellitus, types 1 and 2

End-stage renal disease

Kawasaki disease with aneurysms

Heart transplantation

Conditions in which premature coronary artery disease may be present

Kawasaki disease without aneurysms

HIV

After cancer treatment

Chronic inflammatory diseases (eg, rheumatoid arthritis, systemic lupus)

Certain congenital heart diseases (eg, coarctation of the aorta, single coronary anomalies, transposition corrected by arterial switch procedure)

---

34 years, who died accidentally.[13] Risk factors for atherosclerosis included blood lipids, height, weight, tobacco smoke exposure, diabetes mellitus, and renal artery thickness as a measure of hypertension. The non–high-density lipoprotein (HDL) cholesterol concentration had a positive association with more extensive fatty streaks and raised lesions, and every 30-mg/dL increase in non-HDL cholesterol concentration was associated with increased atherosclerosis. HDL cholesterol was associated negatively with these lesions. Smoking, obesity, hyperglycemia, and hypertension also were associated positively with the presence of lesions even when lipid profiles were normal. For each 5-year increase in age, the lesion location was similar, but the grade of atherosclerosis increased from grades I and II to grades IV and V. In the Bogalusa Heart Study autopsies were performed on participants who died accidentally or by suicide. The risk factors measured in childhood correlated with atherosclerosis assessed at autopsy. Fatty streaks were present in 50% of the children, increased with age, and were seen in 85% of adults. The presence of fibrous streaks also increased with age, being found in 8% of children and 69% of adults. The extent of these lesions correlated with elevated total cholesterol level, low-density lipoprotein (LDL) cholesterol level, triglyceride level, blood pressure, and body mass index (BMI).[14] It has been proposed that passive in utero exposure to a hyperlipidemic environment may program individuals for accelerated atherosclerosis. Napoli and colleagues[15] demonstrated early atherosclerotic lesions on autopsies of fetuses, young infants, and children of mothers known to have hyperlipidemia.

In contrast, low levels of cardiovascular risk factors are associated with minimal early development of atherosclerosis.[1] Just as genetic defects contribute to elevated cholesterol increase risk, genetic mutations associated with low cholesterol confer cardiovascular protection. Cohen and colleagues[16] found that patients who had the proprotein convertase subtilisin/kexin type 9 serine protease (*PCSK9*) gene had reduced plasma levels of LDL cholesterol and a 47% to 88% reduction in the risk of coronary heart disease at age 40 to 55 years.

An important recent advance in understanding the natural history of atherosclerosis has been the use of noninvasive imaging techniques, including assessment of endothelial dysfunction by brachial artery ultrasound, the carotid IMT by ultrasound, and of coronary calcification by CT scanning. In children who have familial hypercholesterol-emia, carotid IMT is increased, endothelial dysfunction has been demonstrated, and the prevalence of coronary calcium in adolescents is 28%.[17–19] The rate of change in carotid IMT was much greater in young adults who have familial hypercholesterol-emia than in a control population.[20] Cholesterol levels at very young ages may impact endothelial function later in life.[21] With regard to cardiovascular risk factors in general, a consistent observation across several studies has been that risk factors measured in youth or young adulthood, including LDL cholesterol, are better predictors of carotid IMT or the presence of coronary artery calcium than risk factors measured at the time of the noninvasive study.[7,8,22]

THE OBESITY EPIDEMIC AND THE METABOLIC SYNDROME

Childhood obesity now is an epidemic in the United States and worldwide. In 2007 the World Health Organization estimated that throughout the world 22 million children under the age of 5 years were overweight. Since the 1980s the obesity rate has tripled in many countries, including the United States and in Europe.[23] Overweight children and adolescents are more likely to become obese adults.[24] Recent population surveil-lance has suggested that cardiovascular disease rates are increasing in young adults.[25] As a consequence of the childhood obesity epidemic, certain risks factors such as hypertension, hyperinsulinemia, high triglyceride level, low HDL cholesterol level, and type 2 diabetes are being seen in with increased frequency in childhood. Investigators have applied variations of the Adult Treatment Panel III definition of the metabolic syndrome to the childhood and adolescent population. In the National Health and Nutrition Examination Survey III cohort, for example, one adaptation shows a prevalence of the metabolic syndrome of 28.7% in overweight children, with 89% having least one of the abnormalities of the metabolic syndrome and 56% having two abnormalities. Weiss and colleagues[26] reported that the prevalence of the meta-bolic syndrome was as high as 50% in severely obese youngsters. In a longitudinal study from Princeton High School outside Cincinnati, Ohio, children who had meta-bolic syndrome in adolescence were more likely to have premature cardiovascular disease in young adulthood.[27]

DIAGNOSING DYSLIPIDEMIA

Lipid panels are recommended in several contexts. They should be drawn in all children who are considered at high risk for cardiovascular disease as defined in **Box 1**. In addition, screening lipid profiles have been recommended in a wide range of clinical settings, as summarized in **Box 2**, because of the increased likelihood of finding a lipid abnormality (obesity, positive family history) or in the presence of other established risk factors. Lipid profiles can be obtained after the age of 2 years. Useful ages to consider lipid measurement for screening purposes are between 5 and 8 years, because of the opportunity to teach health behaviors, and after puberty, because of the strong tracking relationships between values at this age and in adulthood.

Table 1 presents a classification of lipid levels in youth. Protective, optimal, border-line, elevated, and extreme levels are shown for LDL cholesterol, HDL cholesterol, and triglycerides.[28] The table is based on the most recent comprehensive guideline published in 1992[29,30] with additional modifications from recent guidelines published by various groups and current research. As a general rule, LDL cholesterol levels above 130 mg/dL are considered high, and values above 100 mg/dL are considered borderline. Triglyceride levels over 200 mg/dL are unambiguously high, and values

Box 2
Clinical characteristics of children requiring lipid screening
BMI $\geq$ 85% of age-/gender-specific value
A parent with a total cholesterol level > 240 mg/dL
A parent, grandparent, or sibling of a parent with cardiovascular disease < age 55 years (included are those undergoing coronary angiography with evidence of atherosclerosis, stent placement, balloon angioplasty, and/or coronary by-pass)
Hypertension
Cigarette smoking
Unknown family history

between 500 and 1000 mg/dL are of clinical concern. HDL cholesterol levels are stratified as in adults.

There are several hereditary dyslipidemias. A family history and measurement of parental lipid panels are helpful in establishing a genetic diagnosis.

Familial hypercholesterolemia is present in 1 in 500 individuals. It is characterized by elevated LDL (generally > 160 mg/dL) and normal triglyceride level. A family history of elevated cholesterol and/or premature cardiovascular disease helps establish the diagnosis. The elevated serum cholesterol and LDL levels are caused by a deficiency of functional LDL receptors on the liver cell membrane. A rare disorder with similar presentation involves an abnormality of apolipoprotein B preventing uptake of LDL particles by LDL receptors.[31]

The homozygous form can present in the first year of life with serum cholesterol levels higher than 500 mg/dL. The LDL level in the homozygous form is about twice as high as the level in a heterozygous family member. In this form of familial hypercholesterolemia, both parents have elevated serum cholesterol levels. Xanthomas can appear before age 10 years, and vascular disease can present before age the age of 20 years. The disorder is rare, occurring in 1 in 1 million persons. These children need LDL apheresis as part of their treatment. Other disorders causing secondary hyperlipidemia must be excluded to make the diagnosis. The heterozygote condition usually has no xanthomas, and the serum cholesterol level usually is less than 500 mg/dL.

Familial combined hyperlipidemia, a general term for other hereditary dyslipidemias, presents with elevated triglyceride and/or serum cholesterol levels (increased LDL and very-low-density lipoprotein) often in association with low HDL cholesterol. It is the

Table 1					
Classification of dyslipidemia in childhood					
Lipid Type	Protective Level (mg/dL)	Optimal Level (mg/dL)	Borderline Level (mg/dL)	Elevated Level (mg/dL)	Extreme, Gene-Related Abnormality (mg/dL)
LDL-C	40–60	< 100	100–129	$\geq$ 130	$\geq$ 160
HDL-C	> 80	$\geq$ 60	40–59	< 40	< 30 (?)
TG	< 100	< 100	100–200	> 200	> 400

Abbreviations: HDL-C, high-density lipoprotein cholesterol; LDL-C, low-density lipoprotein cholesterol; TG, triglycerides.

dyslipidemia most frequently seen in childhood. Parents may have varying types of dyslipidemia resulting triglyceride or serum cholesterol elevations of varying severity. A unifying feature is the presence of elevated levels of apolipoprotein B. This type of dyslipidemia is associated with the metabolic syndrome and may be a consequence of the obesity epidemic.[32] In familial lipoprotein lipase deficiency, triglyceride levels are elevated dramatically. It is a relatively rare disorder in children and is associated with pancreatitis and abdominal pain. The activity of lipoprotein lipase is diminished or absent, causing the hydrolysis and removal of chylomicrons from the blood to be impaired. The condition also may occur acutely and secondarily in systemic lupus, pancreatitis, diabetic ketoacidosis, or immunologic disorders. The risk for atherosclerotic heart disease is debated.

TREATMENT OF HYPERLIPIDEMIA IN YOUTH

For the general population, the American Heart Association/American Academy of Pediatrics guidelines stress a low-fat, low-cholesterol diet rich in fruit, vegetables, whole grains, and lean protein for all children over the age of 2 years.[33] The diet should be low in saturated fat (< 10%) and cholesterol (< 300 mg/d). Trans fats or partially hydrogenated oils ideally should be eliminated from the diet or should comprise less than 1% of total calories. Because trans fats occur naturally in meat and dairy products, there is not much room in the suggested diet for the additional trans fats found in many processed and fast foods. Sugar and salt intakes should be minimized also. Children over the age of 2 years should be encouraged to consume low-fat (1%) or nonfat milk and low-fat diary products. Calorie intake should match physical activity, and physical activity should be emphasized.

Physical activity in youth should include at least 60 minutes of moderate to strenuous activity daily. Screen time, including television, video games, and hand-held games, should be restricted to 2 hours or less a day.

Dietary fat should not be restricted in children younger than 2 years. The emphasis in this age group, as with the older children, should be on food that is nutrient dense and in appropriate portions for age and physical activity. Breastfeeding is recommended for infants.

Therapeutic Lifestyle Recommendations

Diet is the initial management for all children and adolescents who have dyslipidemia (**Box 3**), including all those who have LDL cholesterol levels of 100 mg/dL or higher. There are no specific recommendations for diet counseling for elevated triglyceride levels, but special attention should be given to lean children who have triglyceride levels higher than 200 mg/dL and to overweight children who have levels higher than 150 mg/dL.

If there is little improvement in elevated LDL cholesterol after using the general population diet for 3 months, a more aggressive dietary approach is necessary. In these children the saturated fat should be limited to less than 7% of the total daily calories, and the dietary cholesterol intake should be less than 200 mg/d. Families should consult a nutritionist or dietitian for help in planning a balanced diet with adequate calories and nutrition. The American Heart Association recommends an adequate trial of diet for at least 6 to 12 months along with lifestyle changes.[9,29] These guidelines should be followed by the entire family.

Several studies have demonstrated the safety and effectiveness of a low-fat diet in children.

Box 3
Dietary recommendations to improve dyslipidemia in children

For LDL cholesterol

Use nonfat (skim) and low-fat milk products daily.

Use vegetable oils and soft margarines that are low in saturated fat and transfatty acids instead of butter or most other animal fats.

Choose a range of main meal entrees including fish and legumes to limit saturated fat consumption from meats and poultry.

Avoid prepared meats and lunch products with high saturated fat content (eg, bacon, sausage) and organ meats (eg, liver).

Limit egg yolk consumption to 2–3/week.

For high triglycerides/low HDL

Balance dietary calories to maintain normal growth.

Eat vegetables and fruits daily, limit juice intake.

Use vegetable oils and soft margarines.

Eat whole grain breads and cereals; limit refined carbohydrates.

Reduce the intake of sugar sweetened beverages and foods.

Data from American Heart Association/American Academy of Pediatrics diet recommendations for children (AHA nutrition). Pediatrics 2006;117(2):544–59.

The Dietary Intervention Study in Children involved 8- to 10-year-old children who had hyperlipidemia.[34] These children were placed on a low-fat diet that limited dietary cholesterol to less than 200 mg/d. This 3-year study demonstrated that a low-fat diet is safe in children and results in normal growth and development. Total fat intake was reduced to 28% to 29% as a consequence of a reduction in cholesterol and saturated fat intake. The LDL cholesterol level was 5 to 7 mg/dL lower in the intervention group than in the control group at the conclusion of follow-up. The Special Turku Atherosclerosis Risk Factor Intervention Project for Children is an ongoing study aimed at decreasing a child's exposure to known risk factors for atherosclerosis. Children and their families were assigned randomly to a control or an intervention group when the child was 7 months old. The families in the intervention group received individualized nutritional and lifestyle counseling and reduced the intake of saturated fat intake. The families in the control group received the routine information given at the well baby and childcare clinics. Through early adolescence total cholesterol and LDL cholesterol levels have been about 3–5 mg/dL lower in the boys in the intervention group than the control group.[34] There has been no difference in the growth and development of the children as they enter adolescence, but those in the intervention group, particularly the girls, are less overweight.[35] The children in the intervention group demonstrated greater nutrition knowledge than those in the control group and were able to explain the reasons for their choices on a nutrition test.[36] In this study, cholesterol levels before 3 years of age affected endothelial function later in life.[21]

The treatment of hyperlipidemia caused by obesity (high triglyceride/low HDL phenotype) is weight loss and exercise (see **Box 3**). Weight loss of about 10% of current BMI, particularly when accomplished in association with regular exercise, can improve lipid profiles substantially.[37] In these children, dietary change can have dramatic results. Because high intake of processed foods, including simple carbohydrates (sugar and white flour), worsens the high triglyceride/low HDL phenotype, these foods should be restricted or eliminated. Healthy fats (mono- and polyunsaturated fats) lower triglyceride levels and raise HDL cholesterol levels; therefore only saturated fats and cholesterol should be limited in the diet. Dietary and behavioral counseling should include advice on controlling portion size, restricting snacks, eliminating sugar-sweetened beverages, increasing dietary fiber, limiting meals away from the home, and ordering wisely in restaurants.

Additional diet components may be beneficial. Intake of dietary fiber, particularly soluble fiber, has been shown to have an inverse association with insulin levels, weight gain, lipid levels, and other risk factors for cardiovascular disease in young adults.[38] There is increasing evidence that omega-3 fatty acids reduce risk of cardiovascular disease.[39] Omega-3 fatty acids are found in seafood and specific seeds, nuts, and plant oils. The omega-3 fatty acids found in fish and fish oils contain the 20-carbon eicosapentaenoic acid (EPA) and the 22-carbon docosahexaenoic acid (DHA). The plant sources of omega-3 fatty acids (canola, walnut, soybean, and flaxseed oils) contain the 18-carbon α-linolenic acid (ALA). ALA is considered an essential fatty acid because it cannot be produced by humans. EPA and DHA can be obtained directly through foods or by the enzymatic conversion of ALA. Thus, consumption of high-fiber foods and two to three servings of fatty fish per week has been recommended for children over the age of 2 years. There is some concern about environmental contamination of fish, particularly for children and pregnant women. The highest levels of these contaminants are in older and larger fatty fish, and intake of these fish should be limited. In particular, the Food and Drug Administration (FDA) recommends that pregnant women and children should avoid tilefish, shark, swordfish, and king mackerel. The Environmental Protection Agency Web site lists the local fish advisories for each state. The Environmental Defense Fund Web site also has a printable pocket guide of fish that are safe and those to be avoided.

PHARMACOLOGIC TREATMENT

The National Heart, Lung, and Blood Institute has new evidence-based and integrated cardiovascular risk guidelines in preparation for children; this work was not completed in time for this article. These guidelines should be consulted for specific recommendations when published in 2009. The following discussion is based on the guidelines in effect at the time of this writing.

The evidence base for pharmacologic intervention for dyslipidemia in childhood is limited, and recommendations are based largely on expert consensus and short- to medium-term randomized trials conducted for the statins. There are limited trial data for medications other than the statins, although there is substantial clinical experience with bile acid–binding resins. The role of pharmacologic treatment of dyslipidemia has been reviewed recently.[9] In general, pharmacologic treatment is reserved for those at highest risk, that is children at least 10 years of age who have LDL levels of 190 mg/dL or higher or of 160 mg/dL or higher and other risk factors such as diabetes mellitus, end-stage renal disease, or multiple other major risk factors such as hypertension, tobacco use, or severe obesity after a trial of diet management. The medications preferably should be started after menses, and a Tanner stage of II or higher is preferred. Treatment at younger ages is considered for homozygosity for LDL receptor deficiency. There is no evidence base for the proper age at which to start medication. Because advanced grades of atherosclerosis can be demonstrated by the early part of the third decade in individuals who have multiple risk factors or who are at the extremes of the lipid distribution, it seems reasonable to start at some point in adolescence based on risk stratification.[1] A recent American Academy of Pediatrics statement, however, has suggested that statins can be started at 8 years of age.[30] **Box 4** summarizes pharmacologic treatment recommendations for children.

There are no consensus recommendations for pharmacologic management of elevated triglycerides at this time; pharmacologic management usually is reserved for those at risk for pancreatitis, such as homozygotes for lipoprotein lipase deficiency, or for children who have multiple cardiovascular risk factors.

Historically, the bile acid–binding resins were the recommended therapy for hyperlipidemia in children. Bile acids bind to the resin in the intestinal lumen, preventing enterohepatic uptake, up-regulating the formation of bile acids from hepatocyte cholesterol, and thus reducing the intracellular cholesterol concentration. This action results in an up-regulation of the LDL receptors on the hepatocyte surface, increasing clearance of LDL cholesterol. The bile acid–binding resins are not absorbed systemically, making them safe for use in children. Dosing of the bile acids begin at 4 to 5 g/d (which lowers LDL cholesterol about 30 mg/dL) and can be titrated up to 20 g/d. The resins may increase triglyceride levels and interfere with absorption of the fat-soluble vitamins, particularly vitamins A, D, and K, although no clinical toxicity has been reported. An increase in homocysteine levels also has been noted. Gastrointestinal side effects including constipation, bloating, and flatulence result in poor compliance. A study using two forms of cholestyramine (powder and tablet form) showed patients preferred the tablet form. Gastrointestinal complaints were common, however, and compliance remained low in both groups.[40]

Statins have been shown to reduce the risk of cardiovascular disease and cardiovascular mortality significantly in the adult population. The statins work by inhibiting the enzyme hydroxymethylglutaryl coenzyme A reductase (HMG CoA reductase) needed for the endogenous production of cholesterol. The depletion of intracellular cholesterol pool triggers an up-regulation of the LDL surface receptors. This

---

Box 4
American Heart Association recommendations for pharmacologic treatment of dyslipidemias in children

Treatment is recommended in children age 10 years or older who have

LDL cholesterol ≥ 190 mg/dL or

LDL cholesterol ≥ 160 mg/dL plus

Diabetes mellitus or

Two additional risk factors for cardiovascular disease (hypertension, tobacco use, insulin resistance, HDL cholesterol < 40 mg/dL)

Mitigating factors to consider in delaying initiation of treatment

Elevated HDL cholesterol (≥ 60 mg/dL)

Absence of family history of cardiovascular disease

Female gender

Modified from McCrindle BW, Urbina EM, Dennison BA, et al. Drug therapy of high-risk lipid abnormalities in children and adolescents: a scientific statement from the American Heart Association Atherosclerosis, Hypertension, and Obesity in Youth Committee, Council of Cardiovascular Disease in the Young, with the Council on Cardiovascular Nursing. Circulation 2007;115(14):1962.

up-regulation of the receptors leads to increased clearance of LDL cholesterol. Statins now are the agents of choice in children and adolescents who have hyperlipidemia.[9] The statins approved for adolescents by the FDA as a result of studies showing up to 2-year efficacy and safety include lovastatin, simvastatin, pravastatin, and atorvastatin.

Adverse effects are infrequent in childhood and include gastrointestinal upset, an increase in liver transaminase (alanine aminotransferase and aspartate aminotransferase) levels, muscle cramps, and rhabdomyolysis. Rhabdomyolysis is rare, but fear of the side effect is a frequent reason for discontinuation of the medication. The risk of rhabomyolisis increases with concomitant use of cyclosporine, erythromycin, and gemfibrozil.[41] Creatine kinase and liver transaminase levels should be monitored periodically in patients taking the medication. Warning signs include an increase in creatine kinase 10 times the upper limit of normal or alanine aminotransferase or aspartate aminotransferase levels three times above the normal limit. If the increases are noted, or there are any symptoms of muscle cramps or pain, the medications should be withheld until the symptoms resolve. The laboratory tests should be repeated in 2 weeks; the medication can be restarted with careful monitoring when the test results return to normal. Mild to severe sporadic increases in creatinine kinase can be observed after vigorous exercise, weight lifting, and contact sports. These increases may not be caused by statins.

Statins are contraindicated in pregnancy, and adolescent females need to be counseled about pregnancy prevention while taking the medication, although the evidence for significant teratogenic effects is limited.[42] Central nervous system and limb defects have been reported in newborns exposed to statins in utero. Animal toxicity studies also suggest that statins are teratogenic.[4] The data are not conclusive, but they suggest that statins should be avoided during pregnancy and that pregnant women exposed to cholesterol-lowering drugs should be monitored very closely.

Before initiating treatment with statins, a baseline lipid panel, creatine kinase, and liver transaminases should be obtained.[9] The medication should be started with the lowest dose given once a day in the evening. The child and family should be advised to report any adverse effects such as muscle cramps, weakness, or asthenia. The lipid panel, creatinine kinase, alanine aminotransferase, and aspartate aminotransferase levels should be rechecked in 4 weeks. If the LDL cholesterol level is less than 130 mg/dL, medications are continued, and the laboratory results are rechecked in 8 weeks and again in 3 months. If the LDL cholesterol level is above 130 mg/dL, the medication dose can be doubled and laboratory tests rechecked in 4 weeks. Growth (height, weight, and BMI), development, and laboratory tests should be rechecked at 3 and 6 months.

Two studies have assessed the impact of statin treatment on change in carotid IMT progression in adolescents and young adults who have familial hypercholesterolemia and average cholesterol levels in excess of 225 mg/dL.[41,43,44] Pravastatin treatment, achieving an average LDL cholesterol reduction of 24%, was associated with a slight reduction in carotid IMT compared with an untreated control group in which IMT increased. After 2 years of treatment, both simvastatin (cholesterol reduction in the 40% range) and a combination of simvastatin with ezetimibe (cholesterol reduction of just over 50%) showed no progression of carotid IMT. Thus, statin treatment slows the progression of carotid IMT thickening; the amount of cholesterol lowering needed to achieve this result has not been established but may not be nearly as great as recommended for secondary prevention in adults who have diabetes mellitus or prior disease events.

Niacin is used rarely in pediatric patients. It lowers LDL cholesterol and triglyceride levels and increases the HDL cholesterol level by decreasing hepatic production and the release of very-low-density lipoprotein. It also can lower lipoprotein (a) levels. There has been one study in the pediatric population using a dose ranging from 500 to 2200 mg over an 8.1-month period. Adverse effects, which were reversible and included flushing, glucose intolerance, hyperuricemia, myopathy, and hepatic failure, were seen in 76% of the children.[45] The most common side effect with niacin is flushing, which can be minimized by taking an aspirin with niacin at meal time; however, the use of aspirin on a regular basis in children has been discouraged because of an association with Reye's syndrome.

Fibrates increase HDL cholesterol and decrease triglyceride levels. Gastrointestinal upset and cholelithiasis can occur. The risk of myopathy also is increased with the use of other drugs, particularly statins or in patients who have renal insufficiency. There is little pediatric experience with these drugs. They are used in patients who have severely elevated triglyceride levels when there is a risk of pancreatitis.

Ezetimibe lowers cholesterol by preventing intestinal absorption. The drug works at the brush border of the small intestine and prevents the absorption of dietary cholesterol as well as the reabsorption of excreted endogenous cholesterol. It has been shown to lower LDL cholesterol by 20%. There are no specific studies in children; however, a study by Gaigne[44] of 50 patients who had severe LDL cholesterol elevation included children age 12 years and older. Ezetimibe may be a useful adjunct in patients intolerant of statins, with an additional LDL reduction of approximately 15%.

Omega-3 fatty acids have been shown to be beneficial in the prevention of cardiovascular disease.[39] Omega-3 fatty acids decrease the risk for arrhythmias leading to sudden death, decrease the risk of thrombosis, decrease triglyceride levels, decrease the rate of growth of the atherosclerotic plaque, improve endothelial function, and reduce inflammatory responses. Omega-3 fatty acid supplements have been shown to improve the cholesterol profile of children who have hyperlipidemia.[41–46] They may be useful as primary agents in the treatment of elevated triglyceride levels, but no clinical trial data in children exist.

Plant stanols and sterols also have been found to be effective in lowering cholesterol by inhibiting cholesterol absorption. Studies in children using dietary stanols have show a reduction in LDL cholesterol of 11% with a dose of 1.2 g/d.[47,48]

SUMMARY

Cardiovascular disease is the leading cause of death in the United States and has origins in childhood. Familial hyperlipidemia, childhood obesity, and certain systemic diseases increase the risk of atherosclerosis in childhood. Hyperlipidemia in childhood and adolescence should be identified and treated with medication in the setting of genetic hyperlipidemia or the presence of multiple cardiovascular risk factors. Healthy lifestyle choices should be stressed to all families, especially those who are a high risk for cardiovascular disease.

REFERENCES

1. McGill HC Jr, McMahan CA, Gidding SS. Preventing heart disease in the 21st century: implications of the pathobiological determinants of atherosclerosis in youth (PDAY) study. Circulation 2008;117(9):1216–27.
2. Gidding S. Noninvasive cardiac imaging: implications for risk assessment in adolescents and young adults. Ann Med 2008;40:506–13.
3. National Institute of Diabetes and Digestive Diseases. National diabetes statistics fact sheet: general information and national estimates on diabetes in the United

States. Bethesda (MD): U.S. Department of Health and Human Services, National Institutes of Health; 2005.

4. Kaufman FR. Type 2 diabetes mellitus in children and youth: a new epidemic. J Pediatr Endocrinol Metab 2002;15(Suppl 2):737–44.

5. McMahan CA, Gidding SS, Fayad ZA, et al. Risk scores predict atherosclerotic lesions in young people. Arch Intern Med 2005;165(8):883–90.

6. Mahoney LT, Burns TL, Stanford W, et al. Coronary risk factors measured in childhood and young adult life are associated with coronary artery calcification in young adults: the Muscatine study. J Am Coll Cardiol 1996;27(2):277–84.

7. Raitakari OT, Juonala M, Kahonen M, et al. Cardiovascular risk factors in childhood and carotid artery intima-media thickness in adulthood: the cardiovascular risk in young Finns study. JAMA 2003;290(17):2277–83.

8. Li S, Chen W, Srinivasan SR, et al. Childhood cardiovascular risk factors and carotid vascular changes in adulthood: the Bogalusa heart study. JAMA 2003; 290(17):2271–6.

9. McCrindle BW, Urbina EM, Dennison BA, et al. Drug therapy of high-risk lipid abnormalities in children and adolescents: a scientific statement from the American Heart Association Atherosclerosis, Hypertension, and Obesity in Youth Committee, Council of Cardiovascular Disease in the Young, with the Council on Cardiovascular Nursing. Circulation 2007;115(14):1948–67.

10. Kavey RE, Allada V, Daniels SR, et al. Cardiovascular risk reduction in high-risk pediatric patients: a scientific statement from the American Heart Association Expert Panel on Population and Prevention Science; the Councils on Cardiovascular Disease in the Young, Epidemiology and Prevention, Nutrition, Physical Activity and Metabolism, High Blood Pressure Research, Cardiovascular Nursing, and the Kidney in Heart Disease; and the Interdisciplinary Working Group on Quality of Care and Outcomes Research: endorsed by the American Academy of Pediatrics. Circulation 2006;114(24):2710–38.

11. Management of dyslipidemias in children and adolescents with diabetes: consensus statement American Diabetes Association. Diabetes Care 2003;26(7):2194–7.

12. McNamara JJ, Molot MA, Stremple JF, et al. Coronary artery disease in combat casualties in Vietnam. JAMA 1971;216(7):1185–7.

13. Relationship of atherosclerosis in young men to serum lipoprotein cholesterol concentrations and smoking. A preliminary report from the Pathobiological Determinants of Atherosclerosis in Youth (PDAY) Research Group. JAMA 1990; 264(23):3018–24.

14. Berenson GS, Srinivasan SR, Bao W, et al. The Bogalusa heart study. Association between multiple cardiovascular risk factors and atherosclerosis in children and young adults. N Engl J Med 1998;338(23):1650–6.

15. Napoli C, Glass CK, Witztum JL, et al. Influence of maternal hypercholesterolaemia during pregnancy on progression of early atherosclerotic lesions in childhood: fate of early lesions in children (FELIC) study. Lancet 1999;354(9186): 1234–41.

16. Cohen JC, Boerwinkle E, Mosley TH Jr, et al. Sequence variations in PCSK9, low LDL, and protection against coronary heart disease. N Engl J Med 2006;354(12):1264–72.

17. Gidding S, Chomka E, Bookstein L. Usefulness of electron beam tomography in adolescents and young adults with heterozygous familial hypercholesterolemia. Circulation 1998;98:2580–3.

18. Mietus-Snyder M, Malloy MJ. Endothelial dysfunction occurs in children with two genetic hyperlipidemias: improvement with antioxidant vitamin therapy. J Pediatr 1998;133(1):35–40.

19. Tonstad S, Joakimsen O, Stensland-Bugge E, et al. Risk factors related to carotid intima-media thickness and plaque in children with familial hypercholesterolemia and control subjects. Arterioscler Thromb Vasc Biol 1996;16(8):984–91.
20. De Groot E, Hovingh GK, Zwinderman AH, et al. Data density curves of B-mode ultrasound arterial wall thickness measurements in unaffected control and at-risk populations. Int Angiol 2005;24(4):359–65.
21. Raitakari OT, Ronnemaa T, Jarvisalo MJ, et al. Endothelial function in healthy 11-year-old children after dietary intervention with onset in infancy: the Special Turku Coronary Risk Factor Intervention Project for children (STRIP). Circulation 2005;112(24):3786–94.
22. Loria CM, Liu K, Lewis CE, et al. Early adult risk factor levels and subsequent coronary artery calcification: the CARDIA Study. J Am Coll Cardiol 2007;49(20):2013–20.
23. Obesity: preventing and managing the global epidemic. Report of a WHO consultation 1997.
24. Whitaker RC, Wright JA, Pepe MS, et al. Predicting obesity in young adulthood from childhood and parental obesity. N Engl J Med 1997;337(13):869–73.
25. Ford ES, Capewell S. Coronary heart disease mortality among young adults in the U.S. from 1980 through 2002: concealed leveling of mortality rates. J Am Coll Cardiol 2007;50(22):2128–32.
26. Weiss R, Dziura J, Burgert TS, et al. Obesity and the metabolic syndrome in children and adolescents. N Engl J Med 2004;350(23):2362–74.
27. Morrison JA, Friedman LA, Gray-McGuire C. Metabolic syndrome in childhood predicts adult cardiovascular disease 25 years later: the Princeton Lipid Research Clinics Follow-Up Study. Pediatrics 2007;120(2):340–5.
28. Jolliffe CJ, Janssen I. Distribution of lipoproteins by age and gender in adolescents. Circulation 2006;114(10):1056–62.
29. National Cholesterol Education Program (NCEP). Highlights of the report of the Expert Panel on Blood Cholesterol Levels in Children and Adolescents. Pediatrics 1992;89(3):495–501.
30. Daniels SR, Greer FR. Lipid screening and cardiovascular health in childhood. Pediatrics 2008;122(1):198–208.
31. Scriver C, Beaudet A, Sly W, et al. In: Stanbury JB, Wyngaarden JB, Fredrickson DS, editors. The metabolic basis of inherited disease. 6th edition. New York: McGraw-Hill Information Services Co.; 1989.
32. Shamir R, Tershakovec AM, Gallagher PR, et al. The influence of age and relative weight on the presentation of familial combined hyperlipidemia in childhood. Atherosclerosis 1996;121(1):85–91.
33. Gidding SS, Dennison BA, Birch LL, et al. Dietary recommendations for children and adolescents: a guide for practitioners. Pediatrics 2006;117(2):544–59.
34. Obarzanek E, Kimm SY, Barton BA, et al. Long-term safety and efficacy of a cholesterol-lowering diet in children with elevated low-density lipoprotein cholesterol: seven-year results of the Dietary Intervention Study in Children (DISC). Pediatrics 2001;107(2):256–64.
35. Hakanen M, Lagstrom H, Kaitosaari T, et al. Development of overweight in an atherosclerosis prevention trial starting in early childhood. The STRIP study. Int J Obes (Lond) 2006;30(4):618–26.
36. Rasanen M, Niinikoski H, Keskinen S, et al. Nutrition knowledge and food intake of seven-year-old children in an atherosclerosis prevention project with onset in infancy: the impact of child-targeted nutrition counselling given to the parents. Eur J Clin Nutr 2001;55(4):260–7.

37. Becque MD, Katch VL, Rocchini AP, et al. Coronary risk incidence of obese adolescents: reduction by exercise plus diet intervention. Pediatrics 1988; 81(5):605–12.
38. Ludwig DS, Pereira MA, Kroenke CH, et al. Dietary fiber, weight gain, and cardiovascular disease risk factors in young adults. JAMA 1999;282(16):1539–46.
39. Kris-Etherton P, Harris W, Appel L. Omega-3 fatty acids and cardiovascular disease. New recommendations from the American Heart Association. Arterioscler Thromb Vasc Biol 2003;23:151–2.
40. McCrindle BW, O'Neill MB, Cullen-Dean G, et al. Acceptability and compliance with two forms of cholestyramine in the treatment of hypercholesterolemia in children: a randomized, crossover trial. J Pediatr 1997;130(2):266–73.
41. Davidson MH, Robins on JG. Safety of aggressive lipid management. J Am Coll Cardiol 2007;49(17):1753–62.
42. Kazmin A, Garcia-Bournissen F, Koren G. Risks of statin use during pregnancy: a systematic review. J Obstet Gynaecol Can 2007;29(11):906–8.
43. Wiegman A, Hutten BA, de Groot E, et al. Efficacy and safety of statin therapy in children with familial hypercholesterolemia: a randomized controlled trial. JAMA 2004;292(3):331–7.
44. Kastelein JJ, Akdim F, Stroes ES, et al. Simvastatin with or without ezetimibe in familial hypercholesterolemia. N Engl J Med 2008;358(14):1431–43.
45. Coletti RB, Neufeld EJ, Roff NK, et al. Niacin treatment of hypercholesterolemia in children. Pediatrics 1993;92:78–82.
46. Gagne C, Gaudet D, Bruckert E. Efficacy and safety of ezetimibe coadministered with atorvastatin or simvastatin in patients with homozygous familial hypercholesterolemia. Circulation 2002;105(21):2469–75.
47. Engler MM, Engler MB, Malloy MJ, et al. Effect of docosahexaenoic acid on lipoprotein subclasses in hyperlipidemic children (the early study). Am J Cardiol 2005;95(7):869–71.
48. Amundsen AL, Ntanios F, Put N, et al. Long-term compliance and changes in plasma lipids, plant sterols and carotenoids in children and parents with FH consuming plant sterol ester-enriched spread. Eur J Clin Nutr 2004;58(12): 1612–20.

Lipid Management in the Geriatric Patient

Ajith P. Nair, MD, Bruce Darrow, MD, PhD*

KEYWORDS

- Geriatric • Elderly • Cholesterol • Lipids
- Statins • Fibrates • Niacin • Ezetimibe

In the United States, the proportion of the population older than 65 years will increase from 12.4% in 2000 to 19.6% in 2030, and the number of persons older than 80 years will increase from approximately 9.3 million in 2000 to an estimated 19.5 million in 2030.[1] As the population ages, the number of persons at risk for adverse cardiovascular events will increase. Although octogenarians represent only 5% of the United States population, they account for 20% of all hospitalizations for myocardial infarctions (MI) and 30% of all MI-related hospital deaths.[2] Prevention of cardiovascular disease and modification of risk factors in the elderly population thus demands significant attention. Paradoxically, despite their increased risk of cardiac events, elderly patients are less likely to receive appropriate therapy.[3] Reluctance in treating geriatric patients classically stems from concerns regarding the ultimate benefits of therapy when weighed against the side effects. In a Canadian study of 396,077 patients older than 66 years who had a history of cardiovascular disease or diabetes, only 19.1% were treated with statins. Furthermore, the adjusted probabilities of statin prescription declined with increasing cardiovascular risk; rates were 37.7%, 26.7%, and 23.4%, respectively, in low-, intermediate-, and high- risk patients between the ages of 66 and 74 years.[4] Although the relative risk reduction (RRR) of cholesterol-lowering therapy may be equivalent among the young and old, the absolute magnitude of risk reduction (ARR), or number of cardiovascular events prevented, is greater in elderly patients.[5] Treatment for dyslipidemia therefore is indicated in elderly patients and should include consideration of high-dose therapy as well as combination therapy for maximum risk reduction.[6,7]

CHOLESTEROL PROFILES AND CARDIOVASCULAR RISK IN ELDERLY PATIENTS

Although some studies failed to detect an association between high serum cholesterol levels and cardiovascular risk in elderly patients,[8,9] other prospective studies reported a significant correlation between coronary heart disease (CHD) mortality and both total cholesterol and low-density lipoprotein (LDL) cholesterol levels.[10,11] In the studies that

Cardiovascular Institute, Mount Sinai Medical Center, One Gustave L. Levy Place, NY 10029, USA
* Corresponding author.
E-mail address: bruce.darrow@mountsinai.org (B. Darrow).

Endocrinol Metab Clin N Am 38 (2009) 185–206
doi:10.1016/j.ecl.2008.11.003
0889-8529/08/$ – see front matter © 2009 Elsevier Inc. All rights reserved.

endo.theclinics.com

found an association between lower cholesterol levels and increased cardiovascular mortality,[12,13] there may be an element of reverse epidemiology.[14] Chronic illnesses, including end-stage renal and liver diseases and cancer, often are associated with poor nutritional status, low cholesterol profiles, and higher overall mortality rates. Congestive heart failure, often caused by CHD, can lead to debilitation and lower cholesterol levels. Death results from cardiovascular causes, thus eliminating the beneficial association between low cholesterol levels and cardiovascular mortality. After adjusting for overall nutritional status by using other measures including albumin and ferritin, total cholesterol and LDL cholesterol have, in fact, been demonstrated to have the same correlation to cardiovascular risk as seen in younger patients.

Cholesterol profiles vary with increasing age, and declines in total cholesterol and LDL cholesterol have been noted after reaching a plateau between the ages of 50 and 60 years in men and 60 and 70 years in women.[15,16] In cross-sectional studies this decline may be caused by depletion of individuals who have higher cholesterol levels because of earlier cardiovascular-related mortality. In prospective studies in the elderly, this decline in cholesterol may be secondary to decreasing weight.[17] LDL cholesterol increases more rapidly in men than in women after the age of 20. By age 55 to 60 years, however women may have concentrations that exceed those in men because of an accelerated increase after menopause. High-density lipoprotein (HDL) cholesterol decreases in men after puberty and remains lower than in women at all age groups.[18] In the Systolic Hypertension in the Elderly Program (4763 persons; mean age, 72 years), the mean baseline total cholesterol level was 236 mg/dL, the mean HDL cholesterol level was 54 mg/dL; and the LDL cholesterol level averaged 154 mg/dL.[11] Over a follow-up of 4.5 years, higher baseline total, non-HDL, and LDL cholesterol levels and the ratios of total cholesterol, non-HDL cholesterol, and LDL cholesterol to HDL cholesterol were associated with a 30% to 35% higher rate of CHD events. Likewise, Framingham data established that a 1% increase in total cholesterol produced a 2% increase in the incidence of CHD, and this relation has been demonstrated to apply to persons age 60 to 70 years.[19]

Other studies have demonstrated that there is a U-shaped relationship between cholesterol and total mortality in the elderly. In a study of 4066 elderly patients, persons with the lowest total cholesterol levels ($\leq$ 160 mg/dL) had the highest rate of death from coronary artery disease (CAD), whereas those who had elevated total cholesterol levels seemed to have a lower risk for death from CHD.[10] After adjustment for markers of poor health (eg, low serum iron and albumin levels), elevated total cholesterol remained predictive of increased CHD death. It is unclear whether chronic illness has a direct pathophysiologic effect (eg, through procoagulant and proinflammatory mediators) on CHD or if a lifelong burden of atherosclerotic disease and its consequences, such as congestive heart failure, results in frailty and subsequent low cholesterol levels at the terminal stages of life. Other markers, such as apolipoprotein A1, have been shown to be prognostic markers for ischemic heart disease but may not improve prediction significantly over HDL cholesterol.[20]

TREATMENT OF ELDERLY PATIENTS WHO HAVE DYSLIPIDEMIA

Data supporting the use of statins for the prevention of cardiovascular events in the elderly stem from the results of several subgroup analyses of large, randomized trials. Despite the potential for error in subgroup analysis,[21,22] data provided by these studies have been consistent in demonstrating the benefit of lipid-lowering therapy in the elderly.

Multiple trials have demonstrated that the benefits of statin therapy for secondary prevention of cardiac events in elderly patients are equivalent to or greater than the benefits in younger patients.[23] Based on this finding, the National Cholesterol Education Program (NCEP) issued an update to the Adult Treatment Panel III (ATP III) guidelines recommending that elderly patients (> 65 years) at higher risk receive lipid-lowering therapy.[24] Although other lipid-lowering therapies also have proven beneficial in elderly patients, treatment with 3-hydroxy-3-methyl-glutaryl coenzyme A (HMG CoA) reductase inhibitors (statins) have demonstrated efficacy in both the secondary and primary prevention of cardiovascular events in elderly patients.

Secondary Prevention of Coronary Heart Disease in Elderly Patients

Subgroup analyses of the Scandinavian Simvastatin Survival Study (4S), the Cholesterol and Recurrent Events (CARE) trial, the Long-Term Intervention with Pravastatin in Ischemic Disease (LIPID) trial, and the Heart Protection Study (HPS) have demonstrated that the benefits of statins in elderly patients are equivalent to or greater than the benefits seen in the overall study cohorts (**Table 1**).

Scandinavian simvastatin survival study

The 4S trial randomly assigned 4444 patients between the ages of 35 and 70 years who had moderate hypercholesterolemia and a history of MI or angina pectoris to simvastatin or placebo. Treatment with simvastatin resulted in a 30% reduction in the risk of death from all causes ($P < .0003$) and a 42% reduction in CHD death ($P < .0001$) over a median follow-up period of 5.4 years.[25] Patients enrolled in this trial had total serum cholesterol levels between 213 and 309 mg/dL and initially were assigned randomly to simvastatin, 20 mg/d, or placebo. The simvastatin dose was increased to 40 mg/d in patients whose total cholesterol remained above 201 mg/dL.

The trial included 1021 patients older than 65 years at study enrollment. In post hoc analysis, patients were divided into two groups, 65 years of age or older (mean age, 67 years) and younger than 65 years (mean age, 56 years).[26] The changes observed in each of the subpopulations were similar at 6 weeks and remained stable over the entire study period. All-cause mortality was significantly reduced in the patients in the simvastatin group aged 65 years or older, with a relative risk (RR) of 0.66 (95% confidence interval [CI], 0.48–0.90; $P < .009$). This 34% RRR was greater than the 28% RRR in patients younger than 65 years (RR, 0.72; 95% CI, 0.57–0.91; $P < .007$). The RR for CHD mortality in the simvastatin group was reduced equivalently by 43% in patients aged 65 years and older and by 42% in patients younger than 65 years. Despite similarities in RRR, the ARR in the group aged 65 years and older was more than twice that in group under 65 years of age for both all-cause and CHD mortality because of the substantial increase in the all-cause mortality rates among patients more than 65 years old (number needed to treat [NNT], 16 for patients age 65 years or older, versus 40 for patients younger than 65 years).

Heart protection study

The HPS randomly allocated 20,536 United Kingdom adults (age 65–79 years) who had a history of coronary disease, other occlusive arterial disease, diabetes, or high-risk hypertension to simvastatin, 40 mg/d, or placebo over an average 5-year treatment period.[27] The study's primary outcomes were overall mortality and fatal or nonfatal vascular events. The average compliance with simvastatin was 85%, and the average non-study statin use in the placebo arm was 17%. Approximately 28% of patients studied were age 70 years and older. Monotherapy with simvastatin, 40 mg/d, reduced LDL cholesterol by approximately 58 mg/dL from a mean of 131 mg/dL at baseline. All-cause mortality was significantly reduced by 1.8% in the 10,269 patients in the simvastatin group versus the 10,267 patients in the placebo

Table 1
Secondary prevention trials using statins in the elderly

Study	Patients	Statin	End Point	Duration	Description	Results[a]
4S[26]	4444 total; 1021 were age ≥ 65 years at the start of study; post hoc assessment of trial	Simvastatin, 20 mg or 40 mg, versus placebo	All-cause mortality, cardiovascular mortality	5.4 years	Patients had total cholesterol levels between 213 and 309 mg/dL and triglyceride levels ≤ 2.5 mmol/L	Simvastatin produced a 34% RRR in all-cause mortality ($P = .009$) and 43% RRR in CHD mortality ($P = .003$). There was a greater ARR in elderly patients (NNT, 15 versus 67)
Heart Protection Study[27]	20,536 adults in the United Kingdom; 28% age > 70 years	Simvastatin, 40 mg, versus placebo	Overall mortality and fatal/nonfatal vascular events	5 years	Subgroup analysis; mean LDL 131.4 mg/dL at baseline	There was an ARR of 9.2% and a RRR of 28% for major vascular events (NNT, 11)
CARE trial[31]	4159 US and Canadian patients who had average cholesterol levels (≤ 240 mg/dL); 1283 age 65–75 years	Pravastatin, 40 mg, versus placebo	Coronary death, recurrent MI, need for revascularization, stroke	5 years	Subset analysis of the CARE trial: patients who had baseline cholesterol levels of 155–271 mg/dL	Pravachol treatment led to a 32% RRR (NNT, 11) in major coronary events
LIPID trial[33]	9014 patients post-MI or who had unstable angina from 87 centers in New Zealand and Australia; 3514 age 65–75 years	Pravastatin, 40 mg, versus placebo	All-cause mortality, CHD death and non-fatal MI, stroke	6 years	Subgroup analysis; baseline cholesterol levels 155–271 mg/dL	RRR in mortality by 21%, death from CHD by 24%, CHD death or nonfatal MI by 22%, and MI by 26%; stroke reduction NS
Prospective Pravastatin Pooling Project[34]	Pooled analysis of 19,768 patients from the WOSCOPS, CARE, and LIPID trials; 4843 age 65–75 years	Pravastatin versus placebo	Coronary death or nonfatal MI	5–6 years	Baseline cholesterol levels between 177–297 mg/dL, LDL-C between 125–212 mg/dL	RRR in primary end point of 26%

Abbreviations: 4S, Scandinavian simvastatin survival study; ARR, absolute risk reduction; CARE, cholesterol and recurrent events trial; CHD, coronary heart disease; LDL-C, low-density lipoprotein cholesterol; LIPID, long-term intervention with pravastatin in ischemic disease study group; MI, myocardial infarction; NNT, number needed to treat; RRR, relative risk reduction; WOSCOPS, west of Scotland coronary prevention study.

[a] All reductions are statistically significant ($P < .05$).

group because of a significant reduction in the coronary death rate. Overall, therapy with simvastatin, 40 mg/d, led to a 25% reduction in the rates of MI, stoke, and revascularization. After adjusting for the rate of non-adherence in the treatment group and for statin use in the placebo group, statin use was estimated to reduce the rates of these events by about a third.

Among all patients, major vascular events occurred in 19.8% in the simvastatin group versus 25.2% in the placebo group (P = .002).[28] In older patients, the respective rates for major vascular events in the simvastatin versus placebo groups were 20.9% versus 27.2% in patients between the ages of 65 and 70 years and 23.6% versus 28.7% in patients older than 70 years (NNT, 16 and 20, respectively). The stroke rate also was reduced in elderly patients.[29] Over 5 years, in the patients between the ages of 65 and 70 years, stokes occurred in 4.5% of the patients allocated to simvastatin and in 6.3% of those allocated to placebo (NNT, 56). In patients older than 70 years, the rate of stroke was 5.8% in the simvastatin group versus 8.2% in the placebo group (NNT, 42).

Side effects from simvastatin were minimal. The rates of new primary cancer were similar in the simvastatin and placebo groups (7.9% versus 7.8%; RR, 1.0; 95% CI, 0.91–1.11). There was no significant difference in cancer deaths. Furthermore, there was no significant difference between the groups in treatment cessation because of elevated liver enzymes. Unexplained muscle pain or weakness was reported by similar percentages in each group (32.9% of the simvastatin-allocated versus 33.2% of the placebo-allocated participants).

Cholesterol and recurrent events trial

The CARE trial randomly assigned 4159 patients recruited from 80 United States and Canadian medical centers who had a history of MI and plasma total cholesterol levels less than 240 mg/dL to pravastatin, 40 mg/d, or placebo.[30] Over a mean follow-up of 5 years, pravastatin led to a 24% (P = .003) reduction in the risk for coronary death or recurrent MI, a 26% (P = .005) reduction in the need for coronary bypass surgery, a 23% (P = .01) reduction in the need for coronary angioplasty, and a 31% reduction (P = .01) in the frequency of strokes. A subset analysis of 1283 patients age 65 to 75 years demonstrated greater RRR and ARR in major coronary events and stroke.[31] Major coronary events occurred in 28.1% of patients in the placebo arm and in 19.7% of patients in the pravastatin arm, leading to an RRR of 32% and a NNT of 11 to prevent a major coronary event. In older patients in the pravastatin group, coronary death decreased from 7.3% to 4.5% (NNT, 33), and the incidence of stroke decreased from 7.3% to 4.4% (absolute reduction, 2.9%; 95% CI, 0.3–4.5%; NNT, 33).

Long-term intervention with pravastatin in ischemic disease trial

A similar subgroup analysis from the LIPID trial, which randomly assigned 9014 patients age 31 to 75 years who had previous MI or unstable angina and baseline plasma cholesterol levels of 155 to 271 mg/dL to pravastatin, 40 mg/d, or placebo, was consistent with the results previously described.[32] In this trial, patients were followed for a 6-year period, and the prespecified primary outcome was death from CHD. Secondary outcomes included death from any cause, death from CHD or nonfatal MI, nonhemorrhagic stroke, coronary revascularization, and duration of hospital stay. Of the total number of enrolled patients, 3514 patients between the ages of 65 and 75 years were selected. Compared to younger patients in the placebo arm, older patients had significant differences (all P < .001) in the rates of death (20.6% versus 9.8%), MI (11.4% versus 9.5%), unstable angina (26.7% versus 23.2%), and stroke (6.7% versus 3.1%).[33] Older patients randomly assigned to pravastatin had lower rates of overall morality (16.5% versus 20.6%; P = .003; NNT, 22) and CHD or nonfatal MI (15.5% versus 19.7%; P = .002; NNT, 21). The authors concluded that for every 1000 elderly patients treated over 6 years, pravastatin prevented 45 deaths, 33 MIs, 32 unstable angina events, 34 coronary revascularization procedures, and 133 major cardiovascular events, compared with 22 deaths and 107 major cardiovascular events per 1000 younger patients.

Pooled pravastatin trials

In pooled analysis of three trials using pravastatin, 40 mg/d, a total of 19,768 patients were evaluated via a prospectively defined protocol initiated after the start of each of the three individual trials.[34] These trials were the West of Scotland Coronary Prevention Study (WOSCOPS)[35] and the CARE[30] and LIPID[32] studies reviewed previously. The primary end points of coronary death or nonfatal MI were reduced significantly in younger (age < 65 years) and older (age ≥ 65 years) patients. Among the 4843 patients age 65 to 75 years, the RRR in the primary end point was 26% (95% CI, 14%–35%; P < .001). The RRR in older patients did not differ from that seen in younger patients (21% RRR in patients aged 55–64 years and 32% RRR in patients aged < 55 years).

The CARE and LIPID studies excluded patients over 75 years of age, the 4S trial included only those less than 70 years old, and the HPS included persons younger than 80 years. Subgroup analysis of the aforementioned trials included only patients age 65 to 75 years. In the Intermountain Heart Collaborative Study, 7220 consecutive patients who had angiographically defined CAD (stenosis ≥ 70%) were followed after hospital discharge, and therapy with statins was associated with significant mortality reduction across all age groups.[36] Overall morality over a mean follow-up period of 3.3 ± 1.8 years was 16%. Mortality rates in patients age 80 years and older was 29.5% among patients not taking statins versus 8.5% among those taking statins (hazard ratio [HR] 0.50; P = .036; NNT, 5). In patients age 65 to 79 years, the rates were 18.7% without statins versus 6.0% with statins (HR 0.56; P < .001; NNT = 8); in those younger than 65 years the rates were 8.9% versus 3.1% (HR 0.70; P = .097; NNT, 18). Elderly patients were less likely than younger patients to receive statins (19.8% of patients age 80 years and older, 21.1% of patients age 65–79 years, 28% among patients < 65 years; P < .0001). Despite the limitations of a single-center, observational study with potential confounders, this study nonetheless demonstrated similar RRRs in elderly patients, especially those age 80 years or older.

In a meta-analysis of nine secondary interventional prevention trials with statins that included a total of 19,569 patients ranging in age from 65 to 82 years, all-cause mortality was 15.6% with statins compared with 18.7% with placebo (NNT, 30). The 5-year relative risk reduction was 22% (RR, 0.78; 95% CI, 0.65–0.89). CHD mortality was reduced by 30% (RR, 0.70; 95% CI, 0.53–0.83), nonfatal MI by 26% (RR, 0.74; 95% CI, 0.60–0.89), and stroke by 25% (RR, 0.75; CI 0.56–0.94).[37]

Primary Prevention of Coronary Heart Disease in Elderly Patients

In patients who do not have a previous history of cardiovascular events, modification of risk factors for cardiovascular disease is essential, especially in patients at higher risk. The primary prevention of cardiovascular events in elderly patients also has been demonstrated through subgroup analysis of several large-scale statin trials and prospective cohort studies (**Table 2**).

Air force/Texas coronary atherosclerosis prevention study

The Air Force/Texas Coronary Atherosclerosis Prevention Study (AFCAPS/TexCAPS) was the first large-scale study to evaluate the effects of a statin on the primary

Table 2
Primary prevention trials using statins in the elderly

Study	Patients	Statin	End Point	Duration	Description	Results[a]
AFCAPS/ TexCAPS[38]	6605 patients; 1416 age > 65 years	Lovastatin, 40 mg, versus placebo	Fatal/nonfatal MI, unstable angina, sudden cardiac death	5.2 years	Subgroup analysis; baseline triglyceride level was 221 mg/dL; mean LDL-C level was 150 mg/dL	37% RRR in primary end point apparent in men > 57 years and women > 62 years
CARDS[40]	2838 type 2 diabetic patients with LDL < 160 mg/dL and the presence of one other CVD risk factor; 1129 age 65–75 years	Atorvastatin, 10 mg, versus placebo	Acute CHD events, revascularization and stokes	3.9 years	Post hoc analysis comparing 1129 patients age 65–75 years with 1079 patients age < 65 years	ARR of 3.9% in older patients versus 2.7% in younger patients
Cardiovascular Health Study[41]	5201 patients age > 65 years at study entry	General statin use	MI, stroke, CAD-related death	7.3 years	Cohort study	Statin use associated with decrease in CV events (HR, 0.44) and all-cause mortality (HR, 0.56)
PROSPER[b,42]	5804 men and women age 70–82 years with a history of or at risk for vascular disease; cholesterol levels 154–351 mg/dL	Pravachol, 40 mg, versus placebo	Primary outcome was combined end point of definite or suspected death from CHD, nonfatal MI, or fatal or nonfatal stroke	3.2 years	Randomized, placebo-controlled trial in elderly patients	Pravastatin reduced the risk of the primary end point by 15%; risk of CHD death was 24% lower; no difference in all-cause mortality; increase in new cancer diagnosis by 25%

Abbreviations: AFCAPS/TexCAPS, air force/Texas coronary atherosclerosis prevention study; ARR, absolute risk reduction; CAD, coronary artery disease; CARDS, collaborative atorvastatin diabetes study; CHD, coronary heart disease; CV, cardiovascular; CVD, cardiovascular disease; HR, hazards ratio; LDL-C, low-density lipoprotein cholesterol; MI, myocardial infarction; PROSPER, pravastatin in elderly individuals at risk of vascular disease; RRR, relative risk reduction.
[a] All reductions are statistically significant ($P < .05$).
[b] The PROSPER trial evaluated secondary prevention in patients who had vascular disease and primary prevention of events in those at risk for vascular disease.

prevention of cardiovascular events.[38] When compared with placebo, treatment with lovastatin (20 mg–40 mg) produced a 37% reduction (P = .001) in the risk for a first acute major coronary event (defined as fatal or nonfatal MI, unstable angina, or sudden cardiac death) over an average follow-up of 5.2 years. The event rate in the lovastatin group was 7 per 1000 patient years versus 11 per 1000 patient years in the placebo group. Of the 6605 patients studied, 1416 patients were older than 65 years. The event rate in the older cohort of patients was higher, and the RRR with lovastatin was similar in both men and women older than the median age.

Collaborative atorvastatin diabetes study

The Collaborative Atorvastatin Diabetes Study evaluated the use of atorvastatin, 10 mg/d, for the primary prevention of acute CHD events, coronary revascularization, and strokes in patients age 40 to 75 years who had type 2 diabetes, LDL cholesterol concentrations of less than 160 mg/dL, and one other risk factor for CVD (hypertension, retinopathy, microalbuminuria, macroalbuminuria, or active smoking).[39] A total of 2838 patients were enrolled in the randomized trial. A separate post hoc analysis coompared 1129 patients age 65 to 75 years with 1709 younger patients.[40] The ARR in a first major cardiovascular event in older patients was 3.9% (38% RRR; P = .001; NNT, 21) versus 2.7% in younger patients (37% RRR; P = .017; NNT 33). There was no significant difference in ARR between the two groups (P = .546). There was no significant decrease in all-cause mortality in either group.

Cardiovascular health study

The Cardiovascular Health Study (CHS) was a prospective cohort study of risk factors for cardiovascular disease in men and women age 65 years and older at entry. Data from the CHS demonstrated the benefits of statins in the primary prevention of cardiovascular events. The CHS cohort consisted of 5201 patients. After the exclusion of patients who had a previous history of cardiovascular events and patients who did not receive cholesterol-lowering medications, 1914 subjects were evaluated.[41] During a follow-up period of 7.3 years, there were 382 cardiovascular events that included MIs, strokes, and CAD-related death, and there were 362 total deaths.[41] When compared with patients who did not use cholesterol-lowering agents, statin use was associated with decreased risk of cardiovascular events (multivariate HR, 0.44; 95% CI, 0.27–0.71) and all-cause mortality (HR, 0.56; 95% CI, 0.36–0.88). A subgroup of patients older than 74 years also demonstrated a benefit from statin use.

Pravastatin in elderly individuals at risk of vascular disease trial

The largest trial designed to evaluate the benefit of statin therapy in exclusively elderly patients was the Pravastatin in Elderly Individuals at Risk of Vascular Disease (PROSPER) trial. Unlike the aforementioned studies, the PROSPER trial evaluated the benefit of pravastatin in the primary prevention of CHD events and cerebrovascular events in elderly patients at risk for developing vascular disease and the secondary prevention of these events in elderly patients who had existing vascular disease.[42] The trial randomly assigned 5804 men (n = 2804) and women (n = 3000) age 70 to 82 years with cholesterol levels ranging from 154 mg/dL to 351 mg/dL to pravastatin, 40 mg/d (n = 2891) or placebo (n = 2913). All patients had risk factors for or a history of vascular disease. The primary end point was a composite of coronary death, nonfatal MI, and fatal or nonfatal stroke. Treatment with pravastatin lowered LDL cholesterol levels by 34%. Over an average follow-up period of 3.2 years, the incidence of the primary end point in the pravastatin group was 14.1%, versus 16.2% in the placebo group (NNT, 48; HR, 0.85; 95% CI, 0.74–0.97; P = .014). The incidence of CHD death and nonfatal MI also was reduced from 12.2% to 10.1% (HR, 0.81; CI, 0.69–0.94; P = .006). The risk of stroke was unaffected, although the 4.5% overall rate in the group was half the expected rate, thus decreasing the power to detect a difference. Despite a tendency toward greater benefit in patients who had a history of vascular disease, the RRR was similar in the primary and secondary arms of the trial.

Of note, there was a significant increase in the risk of new cancers in the treatment group (HR, 1.25; CI, 1.04–1.51; $P = .020$), which the authors concluded may have been a chance finding, given the results of meta-analysis that have failed to draw similar conclusions.[43] A meta-analysis including the 4S, CARE, LIPID, WOSCOPS, and AFCAPS trials evaluated the risk for cancer and determined that there was no difference in absolute risk for cancer between patients randomly assigned to statins and those taking the placebo. The estimated differences were 0.0% for all nonfatal cancers (95% CI, −0.8% to −0.8%) and −0.1% for all fatal cancers (95% CI, −0.7% to 0.4%).[43] Likewise, the PROSPER trial investigators conducted a meta-analysis of trials lasting more than 3 years and using pravastatin (WOSCOPS, CARE, LIPID, and PROSPER).[42] The investigators found that the risk for cancer with pravastatin was not significantly higher than with placebo (HR, 1.06; 95% CI, 0.96–1.17).

Intensive Lipid Therapy in the Elderly

The benefit of intensive statin therapy in patients at high risk for vascular events has been proved in several trials.[44–46] The apprehension about treating elderly patients with intensive statin therapy stems from concern regarding side effects and a question whether the benefit is similar to that in younger patients. Despite these concerns, analysis of several trials has supported the use of intensive statin therapy in high-risk elderly patients (**Table 3**).[6]

Myocardial ischemia reduction with acute cholesterol lowering trial

The Myocardial Ischemia Reduction with Acute Cholesterol Lowering trial randomly assigned 3086 patients to atorvastatin, 80 mg, or placebo between 24 and 96 hours after hospital admission for an acute coronary syndrome (ACS).[44] The primary end point was a combination of death, nonfatal acute MI, cardiac arrest with resuscitation, or recurrent symptomatic myocardial ischemia requiring hospitalization. Atorvastatin was continued for 16 weeks, and treatment led to a reduction in LDL cholesterol from 124 mg/dL to 72 mg/dL. There was 15% RRR in the primary end point with atorvastatin and a greater than 50% reduction in the incidence of stroke.[47] In post hoc analysis, there was a 14% decrease in the primary end point among older patients, which was less than the 22% seen in younger patients ($P = .11$).[48] Both primary and secondary end points occurred more often in the elderly patients, however. The primary end point occurred in 12.4% and 21.7% of the younger and older placebo populations, respectively. Therefore, the ARR was similar in younger (2.9%) and older patients (2 2.5%). Older patients discontinued statin therapy more often than younger patients (5.3% versus 3.5%, respectively), and serious adverse events occurred in 1.2% of elderly patients.

Pravastatin or atorvastatin evaluation and infection therapy—thrombolysis in myocardial infarction 22 trial

The efficacy of pravastatin, 40 mg/d, versus atorvastatin, 80 mg/d, in preventing adverse CHD outcomes in patients presenting with ACS was evaluated in the Pravastatin or Atorvastatin Evaluation and Infection Therapy—Thrombolysis in Myocardial Infarction 22 (PROVE-IT TIMI 22) trial.[45] Patients were assigned randomly to therapy within 10 days of presentation, and the primary end point was a composite of death from any cause, MI, unstable angina requiring hospitalization, revascularization at least 30 days after randomization, and stroke. Treatment with pravastatin reduced the mean LDL cholesterol level from 106 mg/dL to 95 mg/dL, whereas atorvastatin

Table 3
Intensive statin therapy and secondary prevention in the elderly

Study	Patients	Statins	Endo Point	Duration	Description	Results[a]
MIRACL trial[48]	3086 patients who had ACS	Atorvastatin, 80 mg, versus placebo	Combined death, nonfatal acute MI, cardiac arrest with resuscitation, recurrent myocardial ischemia	16 weeks	Patients randomly assigned within 24–96 hours of ACS admission	ARR similar in old and young patients; 14% reduction in primary end point in older patients versus 22% in younger patients
PROVE-IT TIMI 22 trial[49]	4162 patients who had ACS; 624 age > 70 years	Atorvastatin, 80 mg, versus pravastatin 40 mg	Death, MI, and unstable angina	6 months	Substudy analysis; patients randomly assigned to therapy within 10 days of ACS presentation	Older patients with LDL < 70 mg/dL had an ARR of 8% and RRR of 40% compared with 2.3% and 26%, respectively, in younger patients
TNT trial[50]	10,001 patients who had stable CHD; 3809 age > 65 years	Atorvastatin, 80 mg, versus atorvastatin, 10 mg	CHD death, nonfatal MI, resuscitated cardiac arrest, stroke	4.9 years	Subgroup analysis	ARR of 2.3% and RRR of 19% in the high-intensity arm; NNT 34 in older patients versus 26 in younger patients
SAGE trial[51]	893 patients age 65–85 years who had a history of CAD	Atorvastatin, 80 mg, versus pravastatin 40 mg	Primary end point was absolute change in duration of ischemia as assessed by 48-hour ambulatory ECG; secondary MACE end points	12 months	Prospective, randomized, double-blind trial in older patients	Pravastatin and atorvastatin reduced the total duration of myocardial ischemia equally; 77% reduction in all-cause mortality with high-dose atorvastatin versus pravastatin

Abbreviations: ACS, acute coronary syndrome; ARR, absolute risk reduction; CAD, coronary artery disease; CHD, Coronary heart disease; MACE, major adverse cardiovascular events; MI, myocardial infarction; MIRACL, myocardial ischemia reduction with acute cholesterol lowering trial; NNT, number needed to treat; PROVE-IT, pravastatin or atorvastatin evaluation and infection therapy; RRR, relative risk reduction; SAGE, study assessing goals in the elderly; TNT, treating to new targets.
[a] All reductions are statistically significant (*P* < .05).

reduced the mean LDL cholesterol level from 106 mg/dL to 62 mg/dL. The RRR in the primary end point was 15% with atorvastatin; this benefit was noted at 30 days and persisted through 6 months. Among the 4162 patients enrolled, 624 patients older than 70 years were identified in a subsequent substudy and were compared with younger patients using a composite end point of death, MI and unstable angina.[49] Older patients who reached the LDL cholesterol goal of less than 70 mg/dL had an 8% ARR (NNT, 12) and a 40% RRR (P = .008) for major CHD events; younger patients had an ARR of 2.3% (NNT, 40) and a RRR of 26% (P = .013).

Treating to new targets study

Secondary analysis of the Treating to New Targets (TNT) study demonstrated that more aggressive reduction in LDL cholesterol in older patients led to a reduction in major cardiovascular events without significant adverse side effects.[46,50] Of the 10,001 patients enrolled in the trial who had stable CHD and LDL cholesterol levels below 130 mg/dL, 3809 were older than 65 years. Patients were assigned randomly to atorvastatin, 10 mg/d or 80 mg/d, and were evaluated over a median 4.9 years. The primary outcome was the time to first occurrence of a major cardiovascular event (death caused by CHD, nonfatal MI, resuscitated cardiac arrest, or stroke).

The mean age of the older cohort was 69.9 years. After 12 weeks of therapy, the LDL cholesterol level was 72 mg/dL in patients assigned to atorvastatin, 80 mg/d, versus 97 mg/dL in those receiving 10 mg/d. There was a negligible increase in HDL cholesterol in both groups. Elderly patients assigned to the higher dose experienced a 2.3% ARR in the primary end point (12.6% versus 10.3%; P = .032) and a 19% RRR. This ARR in the primary end point was similar to that in patients less than 65 years old (2.3%; HR, 0.76; CI, 0.64–0.90; P = .001). Despite the increase in the rate of strokes in the elderly, there was no difference in stroke rates between high-dose and low-dose atorvastatin.

The study assessing goals in the elderly trial

The Study Assessing Goals in the Elderly (SAGE) trial was a 12-month, prospective, multicenter, randomized, double-blind trial that evaluated the effects of intensive versus moderate lipid-lowering therapy in older patients who had CHD.[51] Like the PROSPER trial, the SAGE trial was designed to evaluate high-intensity lipid therapy in an exclusively elderly population. A total of 893 patients age 65 to 85 years who had a history of CAD and more than one episode of myocardial ischemia that lasted longer than 3 minutes during ambulatory ECG were assigned randomly to atorvastatin, 80 mg/d, or pravastatin, 40 mg/d. The primary end point was absolute change from baseline in total duration of ischemia as assessed by 48-hour ambulatory ECG. Ischemia was defined as an ST-segment depression of 1 mm or more below the baseline in more than two leads and lasting for more than 1 minute. The ischemic burden was defined as the depression amplitude multiplied by the duration of ischemia. Major cardiovascular events were defined as cardiovascular death, nonfatal MI, resuscitated cardiac arrest, coronary revascularization procedures, fatal and nonfatal stroke, and hospitalization for unstable angina.

Baseline LDL cholesterol levels were between 100 mg/dL and 250 mg/dL. The average patient age was 72.4 ± 5.1 years in the atorvastatin group and 72.6 ± 5.2 years in the pravastatin group. At 12 months, atorvastatin produced greater decreases than pravastatin in mean LDL cholesterol level (55.4% versus 32.4%; P < .001), triglycerides (26.3% versus 7.0%; P < .001), and apolipoprotein B (44.8% versus 24.5%; P < .001). Pravastatin, however, did lead to a greater increase in HDL cholesterol than atorvastatin (7.6% versus 5.0%; P = .009).

Both pravastatin and atorvastatin reduced the total duration of myocardial ischemia at 12 months (both, $P < .001$). The mean ischemia time was reduced by 42.7 minutes, from 113.5 minutes to 70.8 minutes, in the atorvastatin group ($P < .001$) and by 45.6 minutes, from 124.3 to 78.7 minutes, in the pravastatin group ($P < .001$). There was a trend toward fewer major adverse cardiovascular events and a 77% reduction in all-cause mortality in the group taking atorvastatin 80-mg/d group relative to pravastatin, 40 mg/d, over 12 months (1.3% versus 4.0%; $P = .014$).

Rosuvastatin

There are limited studies on the use of rosuvastatin in the elderly. The Statin Therapies for Elevated Lipid Levels Compared Across Doses to Rosuvastatin study was a 6-week randomized, open-label trial comparing the effects of rosuvastatin, atorvastatin, simvastatin, and pravastatin on lipid profiles in patients who had hypercholesterolemia.[52] In a subgroup analysis of patients older than 65 years (mean age, 71 years), rosuvastatin, 10 mg, decreased LDL cholesterol levels by a mean of 52 mg/dL (27%) from a mean baseline of 190 mg/dL.

The Controlled Rosuvastatin Multinational Trial in Heart Failure (CORONA) trial evaluated the benefits of statin therapy in elderly patients who had heart failure. Of the trials discussed previously, only the PROSPER trial[42] and the HPS[29] included patients who had left ventricular dysfunction, and both these trials excluded patients who had severe systolic dysfunction. Previous retrospective analysis had demonstrated mortality benefit with statin use in elderly patients who had heart failure.[53,54] The CORONA trial sought to evaluate this potential benefit in a randomized, prospective fashion. A total of 5011 patients older than 60 years (mean age, 73 years) who had New York Heart Association class II, III, or IV heart failure who were receiving optimal medical therapy were assigned randomly to receive rosuvastatin, 10 mg/d, or placebo.[55] Patients were followed for a median duration of 32.8 months. The primary composite outcome was death from cardiovascular causes, nonfatal MI, or nonfatal stroke. Secondary outcomes included death from any cause, any coronary event, death from cardiovascular causes, and the number of hospitalizations. The average ejection fraction was $31 \pm 7\%$ in both groups. Despite significant reductions in LDL cholesterol levels from 137 mg/dL to 76 mg/dL (43.8%; $P < .001$) and C-reactive protein, there was no significant difference in the primary end point, death, coronary outcomes, or death from coronary causes. In prespecified secondary analysis, there was a 19% reduction in hospitalizations among patients receiving rosuvastatin (2193 in the rosuvastatin group versus 2694 in the placebo group; $P < .001$). There was no difference in creatinine kinase elevations, muscle-related symptoms, or elevated aminotransferases in the rosuvastatin group. The results of the CORONA trial bring into question the benefit of statins in elderly patients who have ischemic heart failure. The lack of benefit has been postulated to result from other coexisting conditions that may not be affected by statins or from a significant portion of deaths caused by scar-associated sudden cardiac death.[56]

Despite the lack of published data regarding reduction in clinic events, rosuvastatin has demonstrated benefit in delaying the progression of atherosclerosis, as measured by carotid intima media thickness, in patients who have subclinical atherosclerosis and low Framingham risk.[57] In higher-risk patients, many of whom had previous MIs, rosuvastatin promoted atherosclerotic plaque reduction as assessed by intravascular ultrasound and quantitative coronary angiography.[58,59] Data from the Justification for the Use of statins in Primary prevention: an Intervention Trial Evaluating Rosuvastatin trial,[60] which was halted early, probably will demonstrate the benefits of rosuvastatin in decreasing major adverse cardiovascular events, and the potential benefits in elderly patients remain to be seen.

Adverse Effects from Statins

Despite the relative safety of statins, the risks of side effects in the elderly may be increased because of polypharmacy.[6] In a study of elderly patients presenting to a Canadian emergency room, the average number of prescribed medications was 4.2 per patient, and 10.6% of 283 visits were attributed to adverse drug-related events.[61] In the United States, a survey of non-institutionalized adults demonstrated that 40% of persons older than 65 years of age used five or more medications, and 12% used 10 or more medications.[62] Despite the potential for adverse effects, stream-lining therapies to those with demonstrated clinical benefit may maximize outcomes and limit the potential for adverse side effects.

Data from the aforementioned trials note that side effects from statin use are equivalent, or at times higher, than in younger patients. Adverse effects from statins are more common with high doses and when combined with gemfibrozil. In the subgroup analysis of the PROVE-IT trial, the side-effect profiles were similar between elderly and younger patients receiving high-dose atorvastatin therapy. Liver function elevations occurred in 2.3% of older and 2.2% of younger patients, and creatinine phosphoki-nase elevations occurred in 1.1% versus 1.3%.[49] The TNT and SAGE trials noted an increased number of treatment-related adverse events, however. In the TNT subgroup study, an increased number of withdrawals and side effects were noted in older patients who were receiving atorvastatin, 80 mg/d, versus 10 mg/d, and this increased rate was similar to the rates observed in the 4S trial substudy.[50] Adverse events occurred in 8.3% of patients receiving higher doses versus 5.2% of those receiving lower doses, and the withdrawal rate was 4.4% in the high-dose group versus 2.2% in the low-dose group. There also was a slightly greater incidence of elevation in the liver function values (1.2% versus 0.2%) in the high-intensity group, but no difference in myalgias or muscle toxicity was observed. The SAGE trial also noted more frequent elevations in liver function tests (4.3% versus 0.2%; $P < .001$) in the atorvastatin, 80 mg, group versus the pravastatin, 40 mg, group. Myalgias were similar in both groups (3.1% with atorvastatin versus 2.7% with pravastatin; $P = .70$), and there were no cases of rhabdomyolysis.[51] In the "Z phase" (Zocor, chronic phase) of the A to Z trial, 2265 patients who experienced ACS and received simvastatin, 80 mg/d, after a 1-month period of receiving 40 mg/d were compared with 2232 ACS patients who received placebo for 4 months followed by simvastatin, 20 mg/d.[63] The primary end point, which was a composite of cardiovascular death, nonfatal MI, readmission for ACS, and stroke, was not achieved. Therapy with high-dose simvastatin increased myopathy, with nine patients (0.4%) experiencing creati-nine phosphokinase elevations more than 10 times the upper limit of normal and three patients developing overt rhabdomyolysis.

Awareness of the potential for adverse side effects with statins is important. Patients experiencing such effects can be switched to other statins that are metabolized differ-ently. Lipophilic statins include lovastatin, simvastatin, atorvastatin, and fluvastatin. The first three drugs are metabolized by the cytochrome p450 3A4 enzyme for conver-sion to water-soluble metabolites. Hydrophilic statins include pravastatin and rosu-vastatin, and like fluvastatin, are not metabolized by the cytochrome p450 3A4 system and thus are less likely to have interactions with substances that inhibit this pathway (including amiodarone, diltiazem, verapamil, high intake of grapefruit juice, azole fungals, cyclosporine, and macrolides).[6] Moreover, gemfibrozil has the potential to increase side effects from all statins except fluvastatin (Lescol), increasing serum levels to sixfold by blocking the glucuronidation pathway. Fortunately fenofibrate does not block this pathway and does not increase statin levels. Thus, substituting fenofibrate and using statins that are not metabolized by the cytochrome P450 3A4 isoenzyme system such as fluvastatin, pravastatin, and rosuvastatin may limit drug interactions.

Although there have been reports of an association between statin use and dementia in the elderly,[64] data on this risk are equivocal. Initial studies suggested decreased risk for dementia with the use of statins.[65,66] Subsequent contradictory reports suggested that statins provide no therapeutic benefit in preventing dementia.[67] Retrospective analysis and flaws in study design have been suggested as reasons for these discrepant conclusions.[68] Although clinical evidence is lacking, laboratory data suggest a decrease in beta-amyloid generation and cerebral deposition through cholesterol lowering.[69] Preliminary studies suggest that atorvastatin might be of clinical benefit in the treatment of Alzheimer's disease;[70] larger, prospective studies on this subject are warranted to offer more definitive conclusions. Likewise, conflicting data exist on an association between statin use and age-related macular degeneration.[71,72] Although the use of statins has been linked to advanced neurovascular age-related macular degeneration, confounding factors may play a role, and no definitive conclusions can be made regarding the role of statins in age-related macular degeneration.[73]

Other Lipid-Lowering Therapies and Combination Therapy

Although the benefits of statin use in geriatric patients are well established, little has been published describing the efficacy and safety of use of non-statin therapies (**Table 4**).

Ezetimibe: efficacy and safety

Ezetimibe is indicated for the reduction of LDL cholesterol, either as monotherapy or in combination with statins. The Effect of Combination Ezetimibe and High-Dose Simvastatin versus Simvastatin Alone on the Atherosclerotic Process in Patients with Heterozygous Familial Hypercholesterolemia trial focused attention on the absence of data regarding the efficacy of simvastatin, 80 mg, plus ezetimibe, 10 mg, in improving carotid intima media thickness versus simvastatin alone, although LDL cholesterol levels were significantly lower in the combination group (141 mg/dL versus 193 mg/dL).[74] Although this study had design flaws that may have precluded beneficial effects of the combination being observed, the most appropriate use of ezetimibe may be either in combination with statin therapy in patients who cannot reach LDL cholesterol goals on statin monotherapy or in patients who cannot tolerate statins.

A pooled analysis of 1861 patients showed that in patients over age 65 years the addition of ezetimibe made no significant difference in the incidence of serious side effects after 12 weeks of therapy, although discontinuation for possible side effects was greater in the small population of patients over age 75 years.[75] Substantially more patients taking ezetimibe-plus-statin therapy in this meta-analysis were at or below target LDL cholesterol levels, irrespective of age. The product-prescribing supplement for both ezetimibe and combination ezetimibe/simvastatin (Vytorin) noted no increase in adverse events in geriatric patients in the trials reviewed for Food and Drug Administration (FDA) approval.

Fibrates: efficacy and safety

Fibrates, including gemfibrozil and fenofibrate, are indicated for monotherapy or for adjunctive therapy for treatment of dyslipidemias, particularly in patients who have hypertriglyceridemia and/or low HDL cholesterol. Few data, however, support the

Table 4
Non-statin lipid-lowering therapies

Drug	Suggested Use	Side Effects
Ezetimibe	Combined use with high-dose statins for goal LDL reduction or with low statin doses to minimize side effects	No increase in side effects with use in elderly
Fibrates (gemfibrozil, fenofibrate)	Monotherapy or combination therapy in patients who have hypertriglyceridemia and/or low HDL; limited study of their benefits in geriatric patients	Increased risk for rhabdomyolysis with combined use of gemfibrozil and statins; gemfibrozil also decreases warfarin metabolism
Niacin	Monotherapy or combination therapy for elevated LDL, hypertriglyceridemia, and low HDL	Flushing (less common with sustained-release formulation), worsening glycemic control in diabetics; no increase in side effects among geriatric patients
Omega-3 fatty acids	Combined with statins; outcomes data limited in geriatric patients	No serious side effects

Abbreviations: HDL, high-density lipoprotein; LDL, low-density lipoprotein.

efficacy of these medications in patients over age 65 years. Many of the largest randomized trials of fibrate limited or disallowed the enrollment of geriatric patients: the maximum age was 72 years in the Veterans Affairs High-Density Lipoprotein Cholesterol Intervention Trial,[76] 74 years in the Bezafibrate Infarction Prevention Trial,[77,78] and 55 years in the Helsinki Heart Study.[79]

The Fenofibrate Intervention and Event Lowering in Diabetes study investigated the use of fenofibrate versus placebo in 9795 patients who had diabetes and reported a small decrease in the overall number of total cardiovascular events in the fenofibrate group. Patients between age 65 and 75 years composed about 40% of the study population,[80] but in subgroup analysis these patients did not have any significant benefit from fibrate treatment.[81] The Action to Control Cardiovascular Risk in Diabetes (ACCORD) trial, still in progress, has a maximum age of 79 years and may help clarify the benefit of fenofibrate in geriatric patients.[82]

Fibrate therapy is associated with a low incidence of several potential side effects, including increased rash, gastrointestinal complaints, increased serum creatinine level, muscle aches, rhabdomyolysis, liver function abnormalities, and deep vein thrombosis.[83–85] An increase in adverse events has been noted with gemfibrozil in patients who concurrently are using statins or who have renal insufficiency, and thus caution should be used in geriatric patients who fall into these categories.[85,86] A significant increase in serum creatinine during fibric acid therapy should prompt lowering the dose by one half to one third; and with a glomerular filtration rate less than 30 mL/min/1.73 m^2 body surface area, the fenofibrate dose should be 48 mg/d rather than 145 mg/d. It is not clear that incidence of adverse effects of fibrate monotherapy is otherwise increased in geriatric patients. There are isolated reports of increased prothrombin time in two geriatric patients[87,88] and one non-geriatric patient[89] taking stable doses of warfarin after starting fibrate therapy.

Niacin: efficacy and safety

Niacin, or nicotinic acid, also is indicated as either monotherapy or adjunctive therapy for treatment of elevated LDL cholesterol, hypertriglyceridemia, and/or low HDL cholesterol. The largest outcome trial, the Coronary Drug Project, showed reduced incidence of MI and a mortality benefit for niacin compared with placebo, but enrollment was restricted to patients age 35 to 64 years. The Arterial Biology for the Investigation of the Treatment Effects of Reducing Cholesterol 2 trial compared carotid intima media thickness in 167 patients (mean age, 67 years) receiving moderate-dose statin therapy and randomly assigned to 1 g niacin or placebo and found a significant benefit in the niacin group. Adverse cardiac events were fewer in the niacin group; the study was not powered to detect a significant effect on clinical events.[90]

Niacin has been associated with flushing, as well as gastrointestinal side effects and rare hepatotoxicity.[83] Flushing is less common with sustained-release niacin (eg, Slo-Niacin) than with immediate-release niacin, but hepatotoxicity at higher doses is greater. In addition to the side effects, concerns about worsening glycemic control in diabetics have limited use of this medication, but a recent review of the subject concluded that this risk may be limited.[91] The product-prescribing supplement for extended-release niacin (Niaspan) noted no increase in adverse events in geriatric patients in the trials reviewed for FDA approval.

Omega-3 fatty acids: efficacy and safety

Omega-3 fatty acids are dietary supplements and thus are not regulated by the FDA, with the exception of a proprietary formulation (Lovaza) indicated for treatment of patients who have hypertriglyceridemia. They have little effect on the serum levels of LDL cholesterol and HDL cholesterol[92] and thus may be most effective when combined with statins; this combination seems to be both safe and effective.[93,94] The Gruppo Italiano per lo Studio della Sporavvivenza nell'Infarto Miocardico-Prevenzione study demonstrated a decrease in sudden cardiac death after MI among patients receiving n-3 polyunsaturated fatty acid (850–882 mg eicosapentaenoic acid and docosahexaenoic acid).[95,96] Data on the benefits in of omega-3 fatty acid therapy in geriatric patients are lacking, however.

The safety of omega-3 fatty acid supplements has been demonstrated in geriatric patients, particularly in studies investigating their effects on the progression of dementia.[97] Despite the antiplatelet effects, there does not seem to be a significant clinical risk of bleeding, even when with omega-3 fatty acid therapy is added to other antithrombotic agents.[92,98]

SUMMARY

Despite the proven benefits of lipid-lowering therapy in elderly patients, the agents are underused in this population. A retrospective cohort study of 34,501 persons older than 65 years noted that the persistence of statin therapy in older patients declines over time, and nonwhite race, lower income, older age, depression, dementia, and occurrence of CHD events after starting treatment were independent risk factors for the discontinuation of therapy.[99] Nonetheless, increased awareness of the importance of risk-factor modification in the elderly has led to earlier treatment of dyslipidemia. After the publication of the NCEP ATP III guidelines, the use of statins in the elderly increased,[100] and it is hoped that this change will translate into clinical benefit. Multiple primary and secondary trials have demonstrated that the benefits of statins in geriatric patients are equivalent to or greater than the benefits in younger patients because there is the same RRR in older persons and a greater ARR. Although side effects may be slightly increased with high-dose statin therapy, careful vigilance in monitoring drug interactions and limiting polypharmacy can reduce these effects. In patients who do not meet LDL cholesterol targets or who have concomitant hypertriglyceridemia or low HDL cholesterol, combination therapy with non-statin agents can be considered. Considering the burden of atherosclerotic disease in the geriatric population, modification of risk factors is essential. Anti-lipid therapy plays a vital role in reducing cardiovascular events and should be considered in most geriatric patients when applicable.

REFERENCES

1. US Census Bureau. State and national population projections. Available at: http://www.census.gov/population/www/projections/popproj.html. Accessed June 2, 2008.
2. Williams MA, Fleg JL, Ades PA, et al. Secondary prevention of coronary heart disease in the elderly (with emphasis on patients > or =75 years of age): an American Heart Association scientific statement from The Council on Clinical Cardiology Subcommittee on Exercise, Cardiac Rehabilitation, And Prevention. Circulation 2002;105(14):1735–43.
3. Ko DT, Mamdani M, Alter DA. Lipid-lowering therapy with statins in high-risk elderly patients: the treatment-risk paradox. JAMA 2004;291(15):1864–70.
4. Malenka DJ, Baron JA. Cholesterol and coronary heart disease. The importance of patient-specific attributable risk. Arch Intern Med 1988;148(10):2247–52.
5. Grundy SM, Cleeman JI, Rifkind BM, et al. Cholesterol lowering in the elderly population. Coordinating Committee of the National Cholesterol Education Program. Arch Intern Med 1999;159(15):1670–8.
6. Maroo BP, Lavie CJ, Milani RV. Efficacy and safety of intensive statin therapy in the elderly. Am J Geriatr Cardiol 2008;17(2):92–100.
7. Shepherd J. Monotherapy vs combination therapy for dyslipidemia in the elderly. Am J Geriatr Cardiol 2008;17(2):108–13.
8. Kronmal RA, Cain KC, Ye Z, et al. Total serum cholesterol levels and mortality risk as a function of age. A report based on the Framingham data. Arch Intern Med 1993;153(9):1065–73.
9. Krumholz HM, Seeman TE, Merrill SS, et al. Lack of association between cholesterol and coronary heart disease mortality and morbidity and all-cause mortality in persons older than 70 years. JAMA 1994;272(17):1335–40.
10. Corti MC, Guralnik JM, Salive ME, et al. Clarifying the direct relation between total cholesterol levels and death from coronary heart disease in older persons. Ann Intern Med 1997;126(10):753–60.
11. Frost PH, Davis BR, Burlando AJ, et al. Serum lipids and incidence of coronary heart disease. Findings from the Systolic Hypertension in the Elderly Program (SHEP). Circulation 1996;94(10):2381–8.
12. Onder G, Landi F, Volpato S, et al. Serum cholesterol levels and in-hospital mortality in the elderly. Am J Med 2003;115(4):265–71.
13. Schatz IJ, Masaki K, Yano K, et al. Cholesterol and all-cause mortality in elderly people from the Honolulu Heart Program: a cohort study. Lancet 2001; 358(9279):351–5.
14. Kalantar-Zadeh K, Block G, Horwich T, et al. Reverse epidemiology of conventional cardiovascular risk factors in patients with chronic heart failure. J Am Coll Cardiol 2004;43(8):1439–44.

15. Tiyyagura SR, Smith DA. Standard lipid profile. Clin Lab Med 2006;26(4): 707–32.
16. Kreisberg RA, Kasim S. Cholesterol metabolism and aging. Am J Med 1987; 82(1B):54–60.
17. Ferrara A, Barrett-Connor E, Shan J. Total, LDL, and HDL cholesterol decrease with age in older men and women. The Rancho Bernardo Study 1984–1994. Circulation 1997;96(1):37–43.
18. Choi BG, Vilahur G, Viles-Gonzalez JF, et al. The role of high-density lipoprotein cholesterol in atherothrombosis. Mt Sinai J Med 2006;73(4):690–701.
19. Castelli WP, Wilson PW, Levy D, et al. Cardiovascular risk factors in the elderly. Am J Cardiol 1989;63(16):12H–9H.
20. Florvall G, Basu S, Larsson A. Apolipoprotein A1 is a stronger prognostic marker than are HDL and LDL cholesterol for cardiovascular disease and mortality in elderly men. J Gerontol A Biol Sci Med Sci 2006;61(12):1262–6.
21. Lagakos SW. The challenge of subgroup analyses—reporting without distorting. N Engl J Med 2006;354(16):1667–9.
22. Wang R, Lagakos SW, Ware JH, et al. Statistics in medicine—reporting of subgroup analyses in clinical trials. N Engl J Med 2007;357(21):2189–94.
23. Dornbrook-Lavender KA, Roth MT, Pieper JA. Secondary prevention of coronary heart disease in the elderly. Ann Pharmacother 2003;37(12):1867–76.
24. Third report of the National Cholesterol Education Program (NCEP) expert panel on detection, evaluation, and treatment of high blood cholesterol in adults (Adult Treatment Panel III) final report. Circulation 2002;106(25):3143–421.
25. Randomised trial of cholesterol lowering in 4444 patients with coronary heart disease: the Scandinavian Simvastatin Survival Study (4S). Lancet 1994; 344(8934):1383–9.
26. Miettinen TA, Pyorala K, Olsson AG, et al. Cholesterol-lowering therapy in women and elderly patients with myocardial infarction or angina pectoris: findings from the Scandinavian Simvastatin Survival Study (4S). Circulation 1997; 96(12):4211–8.
27. Heart Protection Study Collaborative Group. MRC/BHF Heart Protection Study of cholesterol lowering with simvastatin in 20,536 high-risk individuals: a randomised placebo-controlled trial. Lancet 2002;360(9326):7–22.
28. Farmer JA, Gotto AM Jr. The Heart protection study: expanding the boundaries for high-risk coronary disease prevention. Am J Cardiol 2003;92(1A):3i–9i.
29. Collins R, Armitage J, Parish S, et al. Effects of cholesterol-lowering with simvastatin on stroke and other major vascular events in 20536 people with cerebrovascular disease or other high-risk conditions. Lancet 2004;363(9411):757–67.
30. Sacks FM, Pfeffer MA, Moye LA, et al. The effect of pravastatin on coronary events after myocardial infarction in patients with average cholesterol levels. Cholesterol and Recurrent Events trial investigators. N Engl J Med 1996;335(14):1001–9.
31. Lewis SJ, Moye LA, Sacks FM, et al. Effect of pravastatin on cardiovascular events in older patients with myocardial infarction and cholesterol levels in the average range. Results of the Cholesterol and Recurrent Events (CARE) trial. Ann Intern Med 1998;129(9):681–9.
32. Prevention of cardiovascular events and death with pravastatin in patients with coronary heart disease and a broad range of initial cholesterol levels. The Long-Term Intervention with Pravastatin in Ischaemic Disease (LIPID) study group. N Engl J Med 1998;339(19):1349–57.
33. Hunt D, Young P, Simes J, et al. Benefits of pravastatin on cardiovascular events and mortality in older patients with coronary heart disease are equal to or

exceed those seen in younger patients: results from the LIPID trial. Ann Intern Med 2001;134(10):931–40.

34. Sacks FM, Tonkin AM, Shepherd J, et al. Effect of pravastatin on coronary disease events in subgroups defined by coronary risk factors: the Prospective Pravastatin Pooling Project. Circulation 2000;102(16):1893–900.

35. Shepherd J, Cobbe SM, Ford I, et al. Prevention of coronary heart disease with pravastatin in men with hypercholesterolemia. West of Scotland Coronary Prevention Study Group. N Engl J Med 1995;333(20):1301–7.

36. Allen Maycock CA, Muhlestein JB, Horne BD, et al. Statin therapy is associated with reduced mortality across all age groups of individuals with significant coronary disease, including very elderly patients. J Am Coll Cardiol 2002;40(10):1777–85.

37. Afilalo J, Duque G, Steele R, et al. Statins for secondary prevention in elderly patients: a hierarchical bayesian meta-analysis. J Am Coll Cardiol 2008;51(1):37–45.

38. Downs JR, Clearfield M, Weis S, et al. Primary prevention of acute coronary events with lovastatin in men and women with average cholesterol levels: results of AFCAPS/TexCAPS. Air Force/Texas Coronary Atherosclerosis Prevention Study. JAMA 1998;279(20):1615–22.

39. Colhoun HM, Betteridge DJ, Durrington PN, et al. Primary prevention of cardio-vascular disease with atorvastatin in type 2 diabetes in the Collaborative Ator-vastatin Diabetes Study (CARDS): multicentre randomised placebo-controlled trial. Lancet 2004;364(9435):685–96.

40. Neil HA, DeMicco DA, Luo D, et al. Analysis of efficacy and safety in patients aged 65–75 years at randomization: Collaborative Atorvastatin Diabetes Study (CARDS). Diabetes Care 2006;29(11):2378–84.

41. Lemaitre RN, Psaty BM, Heckbert SR, et al. Therapy with hydroxymethylglutaryl coenzyme a reductase inhibitors (statins) and associated risk of incident cardio-vascular events in older adults: evidence from the Cardiovascular Health Study. Arch Intern Med 2002;162(12):1395–400.

42. Shepherd J, Blauw GJ, Murphy MB, et al. Pravastatin in elderly individuals at risk of vascular disease (PROSPER): a randomised controlled trial. Lancet 2002; 360(9346):1623–30.

43. Bjerre LM, LeLorier J. Do statins cause cancer? A meta-analysis of large randomized clinical trials. Am J Med 2001;110(9):716–23.

44. Schwartz GG, Olsson AG, Ezekowitz MD, et al. Effects of atorvastatin on early recurrent ischemic events in acute coronary syndromes: the MIRACL study: a randomized controlled trial. JAMA 2001;285(13):1711–8.

45. Cannon CP, Braunwald E, McCabe CH, et al. Intensive versus moderate lipid lowering with statins after acute coronary syndromes. N Engl J Med 2004; 350(15):1495–504.

46. LaRosa JC, Grundy SM, Waters DD, et al. Intensive lipid lowering with atorvastatin in patients with stable coronary disease. N Engl J Med 2005;352(14):1425–35.

47. Waters DD, Schwartz GG, Olsson AG, et al. Effects of atorvastatin on stroke in patients with unstable angina or non-Q-wave myocardial infarction: a Myocardial Ischemia Reduction with Aggressive Cholesterol Lowering (MIRACL) substudy. Circulation 2002;106(13):1690–5.

48. Olsson AG, Schwartz GG, Szarek M, et al. Effects of high-dose atorvastatin in patients > or = 65 years of age with acute coronary syndrome (from the Myocar-dial Ischemia Reduction with Aggressive Cholesterol Lowering [MIRACL] study). Am J Cardiol 2007;99(5):632–5.

49. Ray KK, Bach RG, Cannon CP, et al. Benefits of achieving the NCEP optional LDL-C goal among elderly patients with ACS. Eur Heart J 2006;27(19):2310–6.

50. Wenger NK, Lewis SJ, Herrington DM, et al. Outcomes of using high- or low-dose atorvastatin in patients 65 years of age or older with stable coronary heart disease. Ann Intern Med 2007;147(1):1–9.

51. Deedwania P, Stone PH, Bairey Merz CN, et al. Effects of intensive versus moderate lipid-lowering therapy on myocardial ischemia in older patients with coronary heart disease: results of the Study Assessing Goals in the Elderly (SAGE). Circulation 2007;115(6):700–7.

52. Jones PH, Davidson MH, Stein EA, et al. Comparison of the efficacy and safety of rosuvastatin versus atorvastatin, simvastatin, and pravastatin across doses (STELLAR* Trial). Am J Cardiol 2003;92(2):152–60.

53. Foody JM, Shah R, Galusha D, et al. Statins and mortality among elderly patients hospitalized with heart failure. Circulation 2006;113(8):1086–92.

54. Ray JG, Gong Y, Sykora K, et al. Statin use and survival outcomes in elderly patients with heart failure. Arch Intern Med 2005;165(1):62–7.

55. Kjekshus J, Apetrei E, Barrios V, et al. Rosuvastatin in older patients with systolic heart failure. N Engl J Med 2007;357(22):2248–61.

56. Masoudi FA. Statins for ischemic systolic heart failure. N Engl J Med 2007; 357(22):2301–4.

57. Crouse JR 3rd, Raichlen JS, Riley WA, et al. Effect of rosuvastatin on progression of carotid intima-media thickness in low-risk individuals with subclinical athero-sclerosis: the METEOR trial. JAMA 2007;297(12):1344–53.

58. Ballantyne CM, Raichlen JS, Nicholls SJ, et al. Effect of rosuvastatin therapy on coronary artery stenoses assessed by quantitative coronary angiography. A study to evaluate the effect of rosuvastatin on intravascular ultrasound-derived coronary atheroma burden. Circulation 2008;117:2458–66.

59. Nissen SE, Nicholls SJ, Sipahi I, et al. Effect of very high-intensity statin therapy on regression of coronary atherosclerosis: the ASTEROID trial. JAMA 2006; 295(13):1556–65.

60. Ridker PM. Rosuvastatin in the primary prevention of cardiovascular disease among patients with low levels of low-density lipoprotein cholesterol and elevated high-sensitivity C-reactive protein: rationale and design of the JUPITER trial. Circulation 2003;108(19):2292–7.

61. Hohl CM, Dankoff J, Colacone A, et al. Polypharmacy, adverse drug-related events, and potential adverse drug interactions in elderly patients presenting to an emergency department. Ann Emerg Med 2001;38(6):666–71.

62. Kaufman DW, Kelly JP, Rosenberg L, et al. Recent patterns of medication use in the ambulatory adult population of the United States: the Slone survey. JAMA 2002;287(3):337–44.

63. de Lemos JA, Blazing MA, Wiviott SD, et al. Early intensive vs a delayed conser-vative simvastatin strategy in patients with acute coronary syndromes: phase Z of the A to Z trial. JAMA 2004;292(11):1307–16.

64. Bernick C, Katz R, Smith NL, et al. Statins and cognitive function in the elderly: the Cardiovascular Health Study. Neurology 2005;65(9):1388–94.

65. Jick H, Zornberg GL, Jick SS, et al. Statins and the risk of dementia. Lancet 2000;356(9242):1627–31.

66. Rockwood K, Kirkland S, Hogan DB, et al. Use of lipid-lowering agents, indica-tion bias, and the risk of dementia in community-dwelling elderly people. Arch Neurol 2002;59(2):223–7.

67. Zandi PP, Sparks DL, Khachaturian AS, et al. Do statins reduce risk of incident dementia and Alzheimer disease? The Cache County study. Arch Gen Psychi-atry 2005;62(2):217–24.

68. Li G, Higdon R, Kukull WA, et al. Statin therapy and risk of dementia in the elderly: a community-based prospective cohort study. Neurology 2004;63(9):1624–8.
69. Simons M, Keller P, De Strooper B, et al. Cholesterol depletion inhibits the generation of beta-amyloid in hippocampal neurons. Proc Natl Acad Sci U S A 1998; 95(11):6460–4.
70. Sparks DL, Sabbagh MN, Connor DJ, et al. Atorvastatin for the treatment of mild to moderate Alzheimer disease: preliminary results. Arch Neurol 2005;62(5):753–7.
71. Klein R, Knudtson MD, Klein BE. Statin use and the five-year incidence and progression of age-related macular degeneration. Am J Ophthalmol 2007; 144(1):1–6.
72. McGwin G Jr, Modjarrad K, Hall TA, et al. 3-hydroxy-3-methylglutaryl coenzyme a reductase inhibitors and the presence of age-related macular degeneration in the Cardiovascular Health Study. Arch Ophthalmol 2006;124(1):33–7.
73. Cukras CA, Agron E, SanGiovanni JP, et al. The use of statins and the development of AMD in AREDS [abstract 3772]. Association for Research in Vision and Ophthalmology 2008 Annual Meeting. Ft Lauderdale, FL; 2008.
74. Kastelein JJ, Akdim F, Stroes ES, et al. Simvastatin with or without ezetimibe in familial hypercholesterolemia. N Engl J Med 2008;358(14):1431–43.
75. Lipka L, Sager P, Strony J, et al. Efficacy and safety of coadministration of ezetimibe and statins in elderly patients with primary hypercholesterolaemia. Drugs Aging 2004;21(15):1025–32.
76. Rubins HB, Robins SJ, Iwane MK, et al. Rationale and design of the Department of Veterans Affairs High-Density Lipoprotein Cholesterol Intervention Trial (HIT) for secondary prevention of coronary artery disease in men with low high-density lipoprotein cholesterol and desirable low-density lipoprotein cholesterol. Am J Cardiol 1993;71(1):45–52.
77. Goldbourt U, Behar S, Reicher-Reiss H, et al. Rationale and design of a secondary prevention trial of increasing serum high-density lipoprotein cholesterol and reducing triglycerides in patients with clinically manifest atherosclerotic heart disease (the Bezafibrate Infarction Prevention Trial). Am J Cardiol 1993; 71(11):909–15.
78. The Coronary Primary Prevention trial: design and implementation: the Lipid Research Clinics Program. J Chronic Dis 1979;32(9–10):609–31.
79. Manttari M, Elo O, Frick MH, et al. The Helsinki Heart Study: basic design and randomization procedure. Eur Heart J 1987;8(Suppl I):1–29.
80. Scott R, Best J, Forder P, et al. Fenofibrate Intervention and Event Lowering in Diabetes (FIELD) study: baseline characteristics and short-term effects of fenofibrate [ISRCTN64783481]. Cardiovasc Diabetol 2005;4:13–22.
81. Keech A, Simes RJ, Barter P, et al. Effects of long-term fenofibrate therapy on cardiovascular events in 9795 people with type 2 diabetes mellitus (the FIELD study): randomised controlled trial. Lancet 2005;366(9500):1849–61.
82. Buse JB, Bigger JT, Byington RP, et al. Action to Control Cardiovascular Risk in Diabetes (ACCORD) trial: design and methods. Am J Cardiol 2007;99(12A):21i–33i.
83. Birjmohun RS, Hutten BA, Kastelein JJ, et al. Efficacy and safety of high-density lipoprotein cholesterol-increasing compounds: a meta-analysis of randomized controlled trials. J Am Coll Cardiol 2005;45(2):185–97.
84. Davidson MH, Armani A, McKenney JM, et al. Safety considerations with fibrate therapy. Am J Cardiol 2007;99(6A):3C–18C.
85. Holoshitz N, Alsheikh-Ali AA, Karas RH. Relative safety of gemfibrozil and fenofibrate in the absence of concomitant cerivastatin use. Am J Cardiol 2008; 101(1):95–7.

86. Guay DR. Micronized fenofibrate: a new fibric acid hypolipidemic agent. Ann Pharmacother 1999;33(10):1083–103.
87. Rindone JP, Keng HC. Gemfibrozil-warfarin drug interaction resulting in profound hypoprothrombinemia. Chest 1998;114(2):641–2.
88. Aldridge MA, Ito MK. Fenofibrate and warfarin interaction. Pharmacotherapy 2001;21(7):886–9.
89. Ahmad S. Gemfibrozil interaction with warfarin sodium (Coumadin). Chest 1990; 98(4):1041–2.
90. Taylor AJ, Sullenberger LE, Lee HJ, et al. Arterial Biology for the Investigation of the Treatment Effects of Reducing Cholesterol (ARBITER) 2: a double-blind, placebo-controlled study of extended-release niacin on atherosclerosis progression in secondary prevention patients treated with statins. Circulation 2004; 110(23):3512–7.
91. Goldberg RB, Jacobson TA. Effects of niacin on glucose control in patients with dyslipidemia. Mayo Clin Proc 2008;83(4):470–8.
92. Bays HE. Safety considerations with omega-3 fatty acid therapy. Am J Cardiol 2007;99(6A):35C–43C.
93. Davidson MH, Stein EA, Bays HE, et al. Efficacy and tolerability of adding prescription omega-3 fatty acids 4 g/d to simvastatin 40 mg/d in hypertriglyceridemic patients: an 8-week, randomized, double-blind, placebo-controlled study. Clin Ther 2007;29(7):1354–67.
94. Nambi V, Ballantyne CM. Combination therapy with statins and omega-3 fatty acids. Am J Cardiol 2006;98(4A):34i–8i.
95. Gruppo Italiano per lo Studio della Sporavvivenza nell'Infarto Miocardico - Prevenzione Investigators. Dietary supplementation with n-3 polyunsaturated fatty acids and vitamin E after myocardial infarction: results of the GISSI-Prevenzione trial. Lancet 1999;354:447–55.
96. Marchioli R, Barzi F, Bomba E, et al. Early protection against sudden death by n-3 polyunsaturated fatty acids after myocardial infarction: time-course analysis of the results of the Gruppo Italiano per lo Studio della Sporavvivenza nell'Infarto Miocardico (GISSI)-prevenzione. Circulation 2002;105:1897–903.
97. Freund-Levi Y, Eriksdotter-Jonhagen M, Cederholm T, et al. Omega-3 fatty acid treatment in 174 patients with mild to moderate Alzheimer disease: OmegAD study: a randomized double-blind trial. Arch Neurol 2006;63(10):1402–8.
98. Harris WS. Expert opinion: omega-3 fatty acids and bleeding-cause for concern? Am J Cardiol 2007;99(6A):44C–6C.
99. Benner JS, Glynn RJ, Mogun H, et al. Long-term persistence in use of statin therapy in elderly patients. JAMA 2002;288(4):455–61.
100. Nichols GA, Nag S, Chan W. Intensity of lipid-lowering therapy and low-density lipoprotein cholesterol goal attainment among the elderly before and after the 2004 National Cholesterol Education Program Adult Treatment Panel III update. Am Heart J 2007;154(3):554–60.

Lipid Management in Patients Who Have HIV and Are Receiving HIV Therapy

Judith A. Aberg, MD

KEYWORDS

- HIV-related dyslipidemia • Hypertriglyceridemia
- Drug interactions • Statins • Fibrates

HIV-infected persons may be at increased risk for the development of coronary heart disease because of the chronic inflammatory state associated with the virus itself and the metabolic side effects of the antiretroviral therapies in addition to the known traditional and genetic host factors.[1–7] Current guidelines support managing dyslipidemia in HIV-infected persons as in the general population, per the National Cholesterol Education Program (NCEP).[8–10] Investigators of the Data Collection on Adverse Events of Anti-HIV Drugs (D:A:D) observational cohort applied the Framingham equation to individual study participants receiving combination antiretroviral therapy and found that their observed rates of myocardial infarction correlated with the Framingham predicted rates.[11] Therefore it has been recommended that HIV-infected patients who have two or more of the traditional cardiac risk factors should have their cardiac risk score calculated by the Framingham equation. Lipid goals should be assessed for every individual. Lifestyle modifications such as smoking cessation, diet, and exercise should be prescribed. If further intervention is needed to achieve lipid goals, lipid-lowering therapy should be initiated, or a switch in antiretroviral therapy should be made (**Fig. 1**). Special considerations for the HIV-infected person include whether the patient had existing lipid abnormalities before the initiation of antiretroviral therapy, whether specific antiretroviral therapy might contribute to lipid disturbances, and whether there might be drug interactions between antiretroviral therapy and lipid-lowering therapy.

This work was supported in part by National Institute of Allergy and Infectious Diseases grant AI-068636 to the AIDS Clinical Trials Group and grant AI-069532 to the New York University AIDS Clinical Trials Unit.

Bellevue Hospital Center, AIDS Clinical Trials Unit, New York University School of Medicine, 550 First Avenue, BCD 5 (Room 558), NY 10016, USA

E-mail address: judith.aberg@nyumc.org

Endocrinol Metab Clin N Am 38 (2009) 207–222
doi:10.1016/j.ecl.2008.11.009
0889-8529/08/$ – see front matter

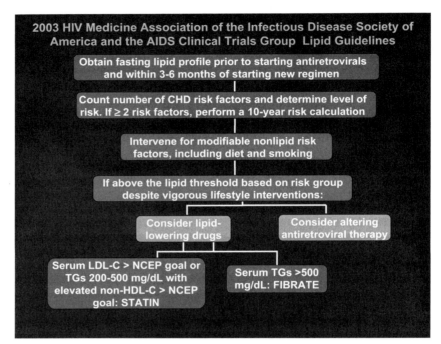

Fig. 1. Guidelines for managing lipid disorders and risk of cardiovascular disease in patients receiving antiretroviral therapy. (*Modified from* Dube MP, Stein JH, Aberg JA, et al. Guidelines for the evaluation and management of dyslipidemia in human immunodeficiency virus (HIV)-infected adults receiving antiretroviral therapy: recommendations of the HIV Medical Association of the Infectious Disease Society of America and the Adult AIDS Clinical Trials Group. Clin Infect Dis 2003;37:614; with permission.)

DRUG INTERACTIONS BETWEEN ANTIRETROVIRAL AGENTS AND LIPID-LOWERING THERAPY

The Food and Drug Administration (FDA) has approved 25 agents among five classes of antiretroviral therapy for the treatment of HIV (**Table 1**). Drug–drug interactions between lipid-lowering agents and antiretroviral agents may influence the selection of therapy (**Table 2**). Not all medications in the statin class can be used safely in the HIV-infected population receiving antiretroviral therapy. The protease inhibitors (PIs) and non-nucleoside reverse transcriptase inhibitors (NNRTIs) and many of the statins are metabolized by the cytochrome P450 isoenzyme CYP3A4. For example, significant interactions of 30-fold increases in simvastatin area under the curve (AUC) have been demonstrated when given with ritonavir-boosted saquinavir.[12] These interactions suggest that simvastatin is contraindicated in the presence of PIs, especially because excessively elevated levels may place patients at risk for rhabdomyolysis.[13] Lovastatin would be expected to behave in the same way. In the presence of PIs, moderate increases occur in the levels of atorvastatin; it can be prescribed, but at lower doses than in the general population.[12,14] Because pravastatin is eliminated by multiple pathways that do not include CYP3A4, it can be used safely in patients receiving PIs other than darunavir; in the presence of darunavir, pravastatin levels increase by up to fivefold in some subjects through a mechanism that has not yet been described.[12,15,16] Hence, the package insert recommends that the lowest

Table 1
FDA-approved antiretroviral therapies

Generic Name	Trade Name
Nucleoside reverse transcriptase inhibitors	
Abacavir (ABC)	Ziagen
Didanosine (ddl)	Videx
Emtricitabine (FTC)	Emtriva
Lamivudine (3TC)	Epivir
Stavudine (d4T)	Zerit
Tenofovir (TDF)	Viread
Zalcitabine (ddC) *withdrawn 2005*	Hivid
Zidovudine (ZDV or AZT)	Retrovir
3TC/ABC	Epzicom
3TC/ABC/ZDV	Trizivir
3TC/ZDV	Combivir
FTC/TDF	Truvada
Non-nucleoside reverse transcriptase inhibitors	
Delavirdine (DLV)	Rescriptor
Efavirenz (EFV)	Sustiva
Nevirapine (NVP)	Viramune
Etravirine (ETV)	Intelence
Multiple Class Fixed Dose Combination	
Tenofovir/Emtricitabine/Efavirenz (TDF/FTC/EFV) Atripla	
Protease inhibitors	
Amprenavir (APV) *discontinued 2004*	Agenerase
Atazanavir (ATV)	Reyataz
Darunavir (DRV)	Prezista
Fosamprenavir (FPV)	Lexiva
Indinavir (IDV)	Crixivan
Lopinavir/ritonavir (LPV/RTV)	Kaletra
Nelfinavir (NFV)	Viracept
Ritonavir (RTV)	Norvir
Saquinavir (SQV hgc)	Invirase
Tipranavir (TPV)	Aptivus
Fusion inhibitors	
Enfuvirtide (ENF or T-20)	Fuzeon
CCR5 antagonists	
Maraviroc (MRV)	Selzentry
Integrase inhibitors	
Raltegravir (RAL)	Isentress

possible dose of pravastatin, atorvastatin, or rosuvastatin be prescribed in patients taking darunavir.[16] Except in patients taking darunavir, pravastatin may be less effective in lipid lowering in patients receiving PIs, because the induction of enzymes responsible for the metabolism of pravastatin results in decreased levels of pravastatin. Because no information regarding pharmacokinetic interactions with antiretroviral

Table 2
Dosing recommendations based on drug–drug interactions between commonly used lipid-lowering agents and antiretroviral agents

Lipid-Lowering Drug	Protease Inhibitors	Efavirenz	Nevirapine
Simvastatin	↑ AUC 506%–3059%: do not coadminister[12]	↓ AUC 58%: may need increased dose simvastatin[19]	No data
Atorvastatin	↑ AUC 71%–488%: use lowest starting dose atorvastatin[12,14]	↓ AUC 43%: may need increased dose atorvastatin[19]	No data
Pravastatin	Minimal change: no dose adjustment[12,14,15] except use lowest dose with darunavir[16]	—	No data
Rosuvastatin	↑ AUC 210%–470%: use lowest starting dose[17,18]	No data	No data
Fibrates	No dose adjustment	No dose adjustment	No dose adjustment
Bile acid sequestrants	May interfere with absorption of antiretroviral therapy: do not co-administer	May interfere with absorption of antiretroviral therapy: do not co-administer	May interfere with absorption of antiretroviral therapy: do not co-administer
Niacin	No dose adjustment	No dose adjustment	No dose adjustment
Ezetimibe	No dose adjustment	No dose adjustment	No dose adjustment
Fish Oil	No dose adjustment	No dose adjustment	No dose adjustment

agents was available, the HIV Medicine Association/AIDS Clinical Trials Group guidelines do not include rosuvastatin, a lipid-lowering medication that was approved by the FDA after the publication of those guidelines. Subsequently, two pharmacokinetic studies have suggested that rosuvastatin levels increase similarly to atorvastatin levels in the presence of ritonavir-boosted lopinavir.[17,18]

Drug–drug interactions also occur between statins and the antiretroviral class of NNRTIs. Efavirenz has been shown to decrease the AUC of atorvastatin by 43% and of simvastatin by 58%, suggesting that higher doses of atorvastatin and simvastatin may be needed to reduce low-density lipoprotein (LDL) cholesterol effectively in patients taking efavirenz.[19] Raltegravir, an integrase inhibitor, is eliminated mainly by UGT1A1 glucouronidation and not by a substrate of cytochrome P450 enzymes.[20] Although significant interactions with lipid-lowering drugs would not be expected, there are no published data regarding interactions between raltegravir and the lipid-lowering agents. Alternatively, elvitegravir, an integrase inhibitor in development, is a moderate inducer of CYP3A; drug interaction studies have not been reported as of the time of this publication.[21] Maraviroc, a CCR5 entry inhibitor, is a substrate of the cytochrome P450 enzyme system (CYP3A) and p-glycoprotein and as such may have significant interactions with lipid-lowering therapies.[21] Caution always should be used in the absence of data regarding drug interactions between lipid-lowering drugs and the newer classes of antiretroviral therapy. Patients should be monitored for any signs or symptoms of toxicity or less-than-expected responses.

DATA FROM INTERVENTIONAL STUDIES OF LIPID-LOWERING DRUGS

In accordance with the guidelines, the type of lipid abnormality should be determined first to guide the choice of lipid-lowering therapy. Some of studies of the lipid-management therapy in HIV-infection persons included all types of dyslipidemias within the trial, and this practice may have affected outcomes of these trials. A common belief among providers is that lipid-lowering therapy may not work as well among persons who have HIV infection, but the percent reductions in lipids achieved by the individual agents are similar to those reported in the general population. Given the safety of pravastatin with most PIs and NNRTIs, pravastatin was the statin most often studied in clinical trials.

Moyle and colleagues[22] conducted a randomized, open-label comparative 24-week trial of dietary advice alone or dietary modification plus pravastatin in 31 male patients taking PIs who had total cholesterol levels greater than 252 mg/dL (6.5 mmol/L). The mean total cholesterol level at baseline was 286 mg/dL (7.4 mmol/L) in the dietary advice arm and 290 mg/dL (7.5 mmol/L) in the pravastatin arm. At week 24, total cholesterol fell significantly in the pravastatin arm (46 mg/dL; 1.2 mmol/L; 17.3%; $P < .05$) but not in the dietary advice arm (12 mg/dL; 0.3 mmol/L; 4%). The difference between the two groups approached significance at week 24 ($P = .051$). The reduction in LDL cholesterol was 48 mg/dL (1.24 mmol/L; 19%) in the pravastatin arm and 3 mg/dL (0.07 mmol/L; 5.5%) in the dietary advice arm. The high-density lipoprotein (HDL) cholesterol level rose nonsignificantly by 23 mg/dL (0.6 mmol/L) in both groups. As expected, there was no significant change in triglycerides (TG).

Calza and colleagues[23] conducted an open-label, randomized, prospective study of the efficacy and safety of bezafibrate, gemfibrozil, fenofibrate, pravastatin, and fluvastatin as pharmacologic treatment for PI-related dyslipidemia. Of the 106 evaluable subjects, bezafibrate was used in 25 cases, gemfibrozil in 22, fenofibrate in 22, pravastatin in 19, and fluvastatin in 18. The investigators reported that the use of fibrates (n = 69) resulted in reductions in TG of 41% and of 23% for LDL cholesterol while increasing HDL cholesterol by 20%. Statins (n = 37) reduced TG by 35% and LDL cholesterol levels by 26%, and the HDL cholesterol level increased by 24%.

The AIDS Clinical Trials Group (ACTG) A5087[24] was a randomized, open-label trial for subjects who had mixed dyslipidemia as defined by elevated LDL cholesterol, elevated TG, and low HDL cholesterol by NCEP criteria. Subjects were assigned to fenofibrate, 200 mg/d (n = 88), or pravastatin, 40 mg/d (n = 86). Subjects who did not reach the NCEP composite goal on monotherapy by week 12 received both drugs. Although the composite goal at week 12 was achieved by only 1% of fenofibrate and 5% of pravastatin subjects, 36% of the randomly assigned subjects achieved LDL cholesterol goals, 49% achieved HDL cholesterol goals, and 18% achieved TG goals with pravastatin monotherapy. Treatment with fenofibrate monotherapy led to 9%, 66%, and 48% of subjects achieving LDL, HDL, and TG goals, respectively. The percent reductions in lipid parameters were similar to the expected results in the general population. Furthermore, combination therapy with fenofibrate and pravastatin for HIV-related dyslipidemia provided substantial improvements in all lipid parameters and seemed to be safe, even if it was unlikely to achieve all NCEP targets for lipid levels.

In a pharmacokinetic study of healthy, HIV-seronegative subjects, the rosuvastatin AUC and maximal drug concentration were increased 2.1- and 4.7-fold, respectively, in combination with lopinavir/ritonavir, but the LDL reduction was attenuated when the subjects were given both drugs. This finding led to questions about the clinical utility of rosuvastatin in HIV-infected persons taking PIs.[18] Van der Lee and colleagues[17] also explored the lipid-lowering effect of rosuvastatin and assessed the effect of lopinavir/ritonavir on the pharmacokinetics of rosuvastatin in a small (n = 22) HIV-infected population. They found that the minimal dosage levels of rosuvastatin were about 1.6-fold higher than the levels reported among the general population. The mean reductions in total cholesterol and LDL cholesterol from baseline to week 4 in subjects taking rosuvastatin, 10 mg once daily, were 27.6% and 31.8%, respectively.

The French Agence Nationale de Recherche sur le Sida[25] conducted ANRS 126, a randomized, open-label trial comparing pravastatin, 40 mg/d (n = 42), with rosuvastatin, 10 mg/d (n = 42). The median baseline total cholesterol level was 292 mg/dL (7.48 mmol/L), the median baseline LDL cholesterol level was 192 mg/dL (4.93 mmol/L), the median baseline TG level was 204 mg/dL (2.29 mmol/L), and the median baseline HDL level was 50 mg/dL (1.27 mmol/L). Rosuvastatin reduced LDL cholesterol by 37%, compared with a 19% reduction by pravastatin ($P < .001$). TG levels were reduced by 19% in persons taking rosuvastatin and by 7% in persons taking pravastatin ($P = .035$). HDL levels did not differ between arms. This study suggests that rosuvastatin may be superior to pravastatin for the management of elevated LDL in HIV-infected persons taking PIs.

No studies have been conducted evaluating long-term cardiac outcomes of different statins prescribed to HIV-infected persons, so statin preference usually is based on safety and tolerability as well as on inferences from data from the general population. Similarly, the use of ezetimibe either alone or in combination is based largely on its benefits reported in the general population. The results of the simvastatin/ezetimibe combination in the Ezetimibe and Simvastatin in Hypercholesterolemia Enhances Atherosclerosis Regression (ENHANCE) study[26] were disappointing, because the study failed to show an additive effect on the surrogate clinical marker, carotid intima media thickness (IMT), even after producing a further lowering of LDL cholesterol of approximately 50 mg/dL. Eighty percent of the subjects had been treated with statins and had very thin baseline carotid IMT, suggesting that previous treatment already may have lowered the risk and thinned the intima media and may have precluded finding differential IMT changes in just 2 years. Therefore this study should not be used to preclude the use of ezetimibe in who have HIV, because the combination of ezetimibe with any statin is less likely to produce significant drug interactions with HIV therapy than the use of very high-dose statins alone. Nevertheless, maximizing statin therapy should be the first goal in all situations.

Negredo and colleagues[27] reported the first prospective, open-label study evaluating the addition of ezetimibe, 10 mg/d, in 19 HIV-infected subjects who had LDL levels higher than 130 mg/dL and who were taking pravastatin, 20 mg/d. At week 24, 61.5% of patients achieved the end point of the study (LDL cholesterol level < 130 mg/dL). Significant declines in mean total and LDL cholesterol levels were observed between baseline and weeks 6, 12, and 24, irrespective of the type of anti-retroviral agent (PI or NNRTI). Also of importance, no differences were observed in the minimal drug levels of lopinavir or nevirapine levels measured just before and 12 weeks after ezetimibe introduction.

Bennett and colleagues[28] retrospectively analyzed lipid parameters in 33 HIV-infected patients who were prescribed ezetimibe, 10 mg/d. The mean total cholesterol level was reduced from 269 mg/dL (6.95 mmol/L) to 213 mg/dL (5.51 mmol/L; 21% reduction; $P < .001$). The mean LDL cholesterol level was reduced from 157 mg/dL (4.05 mmol/L) to 102 mg/dL (2.63 mmol/L; 35% reduction; $P < .001$), and the mean TG level was reduced from 551 mg/dL (6.22 mmol/L) to 341 mg/dL (3.85 mmol/L; 34% reduction; $P = .006$). The mean HDL level increased from 41 mg/dL (1.07 mmol/L) to 45 mg/dL (1.16 mmol/L; 8% increase; $P = .038$).

Furthermore a double-blind, placebo-controlled, crossover design study evaluated ezetimibe, 10 mg/d, on the lipid levels of 48 HIV-infected subjects not taking any other lipid-lowering therapy.[29] The investigators reported a small but significant change in the LDL cholesterol level (mean baseline level, 128 mg/dL), with 35% of subjects having at least a 17% reduction in LDL cholesterol, as has been reported in the general population. Unlike the previously mentioned studies, there were no significant changes in TG or HDL cholesterol levels.

Hypertriglyceridemia remains the most common lipid abnormality among patients who have HIV. Although controversy still exists, many experts believe hypertriglyceridemia is an independent risk for coronary heart disease.[30–32] Although statins have mild or moderate effects on TG, the first-line therapy for hypertriglyceride-mia is a fibric acid followed by fish oil and niacin in no particular order. Lipid guidelines recommend administration of gemfibrozil or fenofibrate for patients who have hypertriglyceridemia.[8–10] Some fibrates (eg, gemfibrozil) are metabolized in the liver via uridine 5'-diphosphate-glucuronosyl transferase enzymes, which are induced by most PIs. Therefore one would expect a decrease in their plasma concentrations, and this decrease might explain the low efficacy reported with the use of gemfibrozil. Miller and colleagues[33] conducted a 16-week, randomized, double-blind, comparative study of a low-saturated-fat diet versus a low-saturated-fat diet with gemfibrozil, 600 mg twice daily, in patients who had TG levels of 3 mmol/L ($\geq$266 mg/dL) or higher and who were taking PIs. Subjects were assigned randomly to gemfibrozil or matching placebo following a 4-week period of dietary intervention alone. The primary outcome was the difference between the two groups in mean change in fasting TG at week 16. Seventeen men were assigned to the gemfibrozil arm, and 20 were assigned to the placebo arm; the median fasting TG level was 496 mg/dL (5.6 mmol/L). Mean changes in the TG level from week 4 to week 16 were -108 mg/dL (-1.22 mmol/L) for the gem-fibrozil group and $+31$ mg/dL ($+0.35$ mmol/L) for placebo groups. The between-group mean difference was 139 mg/dL (1.57 mmol/L) (95% confidence interval, -594–310 mg/dL [-6.7–3.5 mmol/L]; $P = 0.08$). Only one patient treated met the TG goal of

2.00 mmol/L ($\leq$177 mg/dL) or lower. No significant changes in the other metabolic parameters were observed. The investigators concluded that gemfibrozil is safe and demonstrated, at most, modest efficacy for hypertriglyceridemia in HIV-infected patients taking PIs. They also stated that, given the level of response, it is unclear whether these reductions will confer clinical benefit, at least in the presence of continued PI use.

Because drug–drug interactions between fenofibrate and antiretroviral therapy are unlikely and because data suggest that fenofibrate improves cardiovascular outcomes, fenofibrate has become the fibrate most commonly prescribed for HIV-infected patients who have hypertriglyceridemia. Thomas and colleagues[34] initially reported two case reports of significant TG-lowering activity. TG levels decreased from 1450 to 337 mg/dL (76.8%) in one patient and from 1985 to 322 mg/dL (83.8%) in another with the use of fenofibrate. A subsequent case report by de Luis[35] reiterated the lipid-lowering benefit and safety among nine patients. In the study described earlier in this article, Calza and colleagues[23,36] further demonstrated safety and efficacy in 60 cases. Caramelli and colleagues[37] then reported a 45.7% reduction in TG levels (mean baseline, 486 mg/dL) in 13 patients treated with fenofibrate. Palacios and colleagues[38] conducted a prospective study of 20 subjects taking antiretroviral therapy who had baseline TG levels higher than 400 mg/dL, with or without high total cholesterol, despite adherence to fitness and dietary measures. The mean TG level of 812 mg/dL at baseline was reduced to 376.6 mg/dL (54% reduction; $P = .0001$) after 24 weeks of treatment with micronized fenofibrate, 200 mg/d.

Badiou and colleagues[39] conducted an open-label, randomized study of the effects of fenofibrate and/or vitamin E on the lipoprotein profile in 36 HIV-infected adults taking antiretroviral therapy who had fasting TG levels of 2 mmol/L (177 mg/dL) or higher. Subjects were assigned randomly to receive either micronized fenofibrate (200 mg/d) or vitamin E (500 mg/d) for 3 months and then to take both for an additional 3-month period. Total cholesterol, HDL cholesterol, LDL cholesterol, TG, apolipoprotein (apo)A1, apoB, apoCIII, lipoprotein composition, LDL particle size, and LDL resistance to copper-induced oxidation were determined before the initiation of fenofibrate or vitamin E and 3 and 6 months thereafter. The mean baseline TG level was 309 mg/dL (3.49 mmol/L). Three months of fenofibrate treatment resulted in a significant decrease in TG (-40%), apoCIII (-21%), total cholesterol (-14%), apoB (-17%), and non-HDL cholesterol levels (-17%) levels and in the TG to apoA1 ratio in HDL cholesterol (-27%) and was associated with an increase in HDL cholesterol ($+15\%$) and apoA1 ($+11\%$) levels. In addition, fenofibrate increased LDL particle size and enhanced LDL resistance to oxidation. The investigators concluded that fenofibrate therapy improves the atherogenic lipid profile in HIV-positive adults who have hypertriglyceridemia. Rao and colleagues[40] reported similar reductions in TG levels among 55 patients receiving fenofibrate.

Dual therapy with a statin and a fibrate may be the best approach for achieving NCEP Adult Treatment Panel III lipid targets in patients who have HIV infection; the results of the ACTG 5087 study[24] described earlier have demonstrated the effectiveness of this approach. As A5087 and other studies have shown, however, it remains unlikely that HIV-infected patients who have hypertriglyceridemia will reach NCEP goals with fibrate therapy alone, and further intervention is needed. Fish oil is an attractive supplement because of its desirable anti-inflammatory properties, reduction of cardiovascular atherogenic effects, and lack of drug interactions with antiretroviral therapy. The American Heart Association' dietary guidelines recommend that healthy adults eat at least two servings of fish per week and that people who have elevated TG levels need 2 to 4 g/d of eicosapentaenoic acid (EPA) and docosahexaenoic acid

(DHA) as a dietary supplement.[41] A few studies evaluating the TG-lowering effects of fish oil have been conducted in HIV-infected subjects.

In a randomized, double-blind, placebo-controlled study by DeTruchis and colleagues,[42] administration of fish oil supplement (EPA + DHA, 1.8 g/d) three times daily for 8 weeks to 60 HIV-infected subjects receiving antiretroviral therapy who had a mean baseline TG level of 450 mg/dL resulted in a median 25.5% decrease in TG level, compared with a decrease of only 1% among 62 control subjects receiving a paraffin oil. In the open-label phase of the study, subjects who switched from placebo to fish oil supplement demonstrated a 21.2% decrease in serum TG levels. Wohl and colleagues[43] administered EPA plus DHA, 2.9 g/d, to HIV-infected subjects receiving antiretroviral therapy who had a mean baseline TG level of 461 mg/dL and demonstrated a mean decrease in fasting TG levels of 25%.

In the ACTG A5186[44] phase II open-label study of 100 patients, twice-daily administration of 3 g fish oil supplement (EPA + DHA, 4.86 g/d) or once-daily administration of fenofibrate, 160 mg, reduced median TG levels by 283 mg/dL (46%) and 367 mg/dL (58%), respectively. Patients not achieving the NCEP goal of a TG level below 200 mg/dL on either medication alone and subsequently treated with both agents demonstrated a 65.5% reduction in TG level from baseline. Although this combination therapy achieved TG levels of 200 mg/dL or lower in only 22.7% of study subjects, the median TG level at baseline was 667 mg/dL.

Baril and colleagues[45] conducted a study with an open-label, parallel and crossover design to evaluate the effects of 1 g salmon oil (EPA + DHA, 0.9 g/d) administered three times daily. The salmon oil group (n = 26) received treatment for 24 weeks, and the no-intervention arm (n = 32) received salmon oil during weeks 12 through 24. At week 12, the salmon oil group experienced a nonsignificant decrease in TG level of 97 mg/dL (1.1 mmol/L), and the no-intervention arm had a nonsignificant increase in TG level of 27 mg/dL (0.3 mmol/L). The limitations of this study were the absence of a dietary intervention before the study, the low dose of EPA plus DHA prescribed, and concomitant lipid-lowering therapies taken by 58.6% of the subjects.

Bile acid sequestrants and niacin are alternative therapies recommended in the lipid guidelines. There are no published studies regarding bile sequestrants, probably reflecting the concern that these drugs may decrease the absorption and therefore the virologic efficacy of antiretroviral therapy. Investigators at Washington University[46] conducted an open-label pilot study evaluating the safety of extended-release niacin in 14 HIV-infected subjects taking antiretroviral therapy who had TG levels higher than 200 mg/dL at baseline. Niacin was initiated at a dose of 500 mg/d and was increased to a maximum of 2000 mg/d. Although the investigators reported that the median TG level decreased by 34%, 7 of 11 evaluable subjects were glucose intolerant (3 of these subjects developed glucose intolerance during the study).

ACTG 5148 was a similar study evaluating extended-release niacin in 33 HIV-infected subjects taking antiretroviral therapy who had TG levels of 200 mg/dL or higher and non-HDL levels of 180 mg/dL or higher.[47] Forty-two percent of the subjects had prediabetes at entry. Overall niacin was well tolerated, with only four subjects discontinuing therapy. Twenty-three subjects (70%) received the full 2000-mg dose of niacin. At 48 weeks, the median percent reduction in TG level was 38% and in non-HDL level was 8%. Although no subjects developed diabetes by fasting glucose definition, one subject did meet criteria by 2-hour glucose tolerance testing, and other subjects had mild glucose elevations, as anticipated with niacin.

Although there are limited data regarding the effect of lipid-lowering therapies on the long-term cardiovascular outcomes, the HIV Outpatient Study,[48] composed of more than 8000 patients followed since 1993, reported that the incidence of myocardial infarction has been decreasing since a peak in the year 2000. Investigators attribute the decrease to the increasing use of lipid-lowering therapy. They reported hazard ratios of 2.38 for being over the age 40 years, 2.45 for having diabetes, 2.22 for smoking, and 0.34 for the use of lipid-lowering therapy.

SWITCHING ANTIRETROVIRAL THERAPIES

Given the extent and severity of lipid abnormalities reported among persons who have HIV, it is not surprising that single- or dual-agent lipid-lowering therapies may not meet the NCEP goal. Another strategy that has been considered is changing specific antiretroviral agents. Readers are referred to an extensive review by Barragan and colleagues.[49] The HIV Medicine Association/AIDS Clinical Trials Group guidelines emphasize that altering a treatment regimen to improve the lipid profile may not produce the anticipated result because of the multifactorial nature of dyslipidemia in patients receiving treatment for HIV infection.[9] The dyslipidemia that is labeled "HIV related" is complex. The lipid abnormalities may be caused by HIV itself, by antiretroviral therapy, or by host factors. Results of the Strategies for Management of Antiretroviral Therapy study[5] demonstrated that discontinuation of antiretroviral therapy resulted in increased cardiovascular deaths compared with continued antiretroviral therapy. The D:A:D observational cohort study[4] suggests that long-term exposure to PIs is associated with an increased risk for myocardial infarction but that the risk is not as high as that of traditional risk factors such as male gender, advanced age, and smoking. An analysis of the D:A:D cohort[50] suggested that recent use didanosine and abacavir was associated with the risk of coronary heart disease, but in the past the thymidine analogues (zidovudine and stavudine) were associated with mitochondrial toxicity and alterations in the sterol regulatory–binding proteins leading to permutations of metabolic pathways and resulting in insulin resistance and dyslipidemia.[51] The association of didanosine and abacavir with coronary heart disease has not been confirmed by prospective, randomized studies, and no mechanism for such an association has been elucidated.

One cannot attribute an abnormal lipid parameter simply to one specific agent, because studies now show that these abnormalities may not be the effect of an individual drug or even a class effect. Instead, the abnormalities may be caused by a particular drug or by combinations of antiretroviral therapy in specific individuals who have particular drug metabolism polymorphisms or genetic predispositions toward the development of dyslipidemia.[52,53] Not everyone given a specific agent develops abnormal lipid values, suggesting that genomics do in fact play a role. Also, there never has been a study demonstrating that pre-existing lipid abnormalities before HIV infection and antiretroviral therapy that worsen on antiretroviral therapy will normalize after a switch. Switching medications should be reserved for those who have developed lipid abnormalities on a specific regimen and for whom such a switch will not adversely affect virologic or immunologic control. Also, results from clinical studies suggest that a change in antiretroviral therapy may have only limited effects on overall cardiovascular risk.

Although the PIs were the class of antiretroviral therapy most commonly associated with the development of dyslipidemia, combination studies demonstrated that certain combinations of drugs were most often associated with lipid abnormalities. The PI ritonavir and the nucleoside reverse transcriptase inhibitor stavudine (d4T) are more commonly associated with elevated total cholesterol, LDL cholesterol, and TG levels than other agents. The ESS40002 study[54] comparing zidovudine/lamivudine/abacavir, zidovudine/lamivudine/nelfinavir, and stavudine/lamivudine/nelfinavir highlighted the varying effects of combinations and suggested that race/ethnicity and gender also play important roles. The investigators noted that among nelfinavir recipients, women were more likely than men to develop increased LDL cholesterol levels, and the association between female sex and LDL elevations was even stronger in the stavudine-containing arm than in the zidovudine-containing arm. Also, blacks were more likely than whites and Hispanics to develop increased LDL levels. Overall, subjects in the three-nucleoside arm had the most favorable lipid parameters, but this combination has lower virologic efficacy than the efavirenz-containing regimens and no longer is listed as a preferred regimen by national guidelines. Tenofovir (TDF), a nucleotide, seems to be one of the more "lipid-friendly" of the nucleoside reverse transcriptase inhibitors.[55,56] At week 24 in the TDF intensification study, there was a decrease in total cholesterol and TG levels of 17.5 mg/dL and 24 mg/dL, respectively, in the TDF group compared with a decrease in 3.8 mg/dL and 3.4 mg/dL in the placebo group.[56] When this placebo group was rolled over to receive TDF from weeks 24 to 48, the total cholesterol level decreased by 12.1 mg/dL, and the TG level decreased by 22.0 mg/dL. In the Gilead 903 extension study[57] comparing TDF with d4T on an efavirenz-containing regimen, subjects taking d4T experienced a mean increase in fasting TG level of 102 mg/dL and a mean increase in fasting total cholesterol level of 59 mg/dL by year 3 in the original study; after switching from d4T to tenofovir, TG levels decreased by a mean of 61 mg/dL, and total cholesterol levels declined by a mean 21 mg/dL by the end of year 5 (both, $P < .001$).

A study of 88 HIV-infected patients assessed the metabolic effects of switching from a ritonavir-boosted, lopinavir-containing regimen to ritonavir-boosted atazanavir.[58] This switch resulted in a 13% decrease in total cholesterol levels and a 30% decrease in TG levels but resulted in only slight reductions, from 12% to 10%, in the Framingham-calculated 10-year risk of coronary heart disease. The Switching to Atazanavir study (n = 419) was a 2:1 randomization of subjects taking a PI-based regimen to switch to atazanavir or continue the current PI-containing regimen.[59] Of note, only 9% of subjects who switched to atazanavir took ritonavir for boosting. Significant decreases in total cholesterol levels (15% versus 3%) and TG levels (33% versus an increase of 9%) were reported upon switching to primarily unboosted atazanavir compared with staying on the current PI regimen. There were no significant changes in HDL cholesterol or LDL cholesterol levels, however, and the impact of the switch on Framingham risk was not assessed.

Another important aspect of switching antiretroviral therapy is that one may be able to discontinue lipid-lowering therapies after the switch and subsequent improvements in lipid parameters. Martinez and colleagues[60] reported 162 subjects who switched to ritonavir-boosted atazanavir as part of the Bristol Myers Squibb early access program. Thirty-four percent of subjects were taking boosted lopinavir at time of the switch. Six months after the switch they reported mean decreases of 12%, 10%, and 18% in total cholesterol, LDL cholesterol, and TG levels, respectively. Almost one third of the subjects were able to discontinue lipid-lowering therapy.

Switching Antiretroviral Therapy Versus Lipid-Lowering Therapy

There are limited data comparing the benefits and risks of switching or modifying antiretroviral therapy compared with lipid-lowering therapy. One randomized, prospective study[61] in HIV-infected patients who had mixed hyperlipidemia and who were being treated with their first antiretroviral therapy regimen compared the lipid-lowering effects of switching from a PI to a NNRTI (either nevirapine or efavirenz) or of treatment with either pravastatin or bezafibrate added to the current unchanged antiretroviral therapy regimen for up to 12 months. These treatment strategies resulted in reductions in mean TG levels of 25.2%, 9.4%, 41.2%, and 46.6%, respectively, with statistically significant differences noted between the NNRTI arms and the lipid-lowering agents ($P < .01$). In addition, treatment with pravastatin or bezafibrate resulted in significantly greater decreases in mean plasma total and LDL cholesterol than in the nevirapine- and efavirenz -treated patients. This study was powered to compare the strategies of switching versus lipid-lowering therapy and could not detect differences among the four arms. Although this strategy was commonly used at the time the study was conducted, data today suggest that efavirenz is associated with lipid abnormalities more commonly than nevirapine, so it is not surprising that the switch to efavirenz was suboptimal compared with lipid-lowering agents.

Another analysis from the D:A:D cohort[62] compared the effects of lipid-lowering treatments with switching from PI- to NNRTI-based antiretroviral therapy. The results showed significant reductions in total cholesterol with both lipid-lowering treatments and antiretroviral therapy switching, compared the absence of either intervention. Intervention with lipid-lowering treatments resulted in greater mean reductions in total and LDL cholesterol levels (P = not significant), whereas switching to NNRTI-based antiretroviral therapy resulted in a greater mean reduction in the HDL cholesterol level. Both strategies had similar reductions in serum TG levels and total cholesterol to HDL ratios.

SUMMARY

HIV-infected patients may have lipid abnormalities caused by the HIV infection itself, by antiretroviral therapy, or by host factors (genetic and lifestyle). The current management guidelines recommend that patients who have HIV infection be managed similarly to the general population with the exception that drug-induced hyperlipidemia may be modifiable by a switch in antiretroviral therapy. Switching should be done only when there are antiretroviral therapy options that may result in a more favorable lipid profile and will maintain virologic suppression. Patients who already are taking antiretroviral therapy should not discontinue it except under the guidance of an HIV expert, because as discontinuation of antiretroviral therapy may lead to increased risk of coronary heart disease. Patients who have two or more cardiovascular risk factors should have their absolute risk of coronary heart disease assessed with the Framingham score calculations used to provide guidance for management and treatment. The HIV-infected population may have other characteristics dissimilar to the general population that warrant additional strategies. For instance, the HIV-infected community is reported to have higher rates of smoking. Smoking cessation programs should be readily available. HIV-infected patients also may have other comorbidities such as wasting, and the typical American Heart Association diet may be contraindicated. It is strongly encouraged that patients who have HIV be referred to a nutritionist who is knowledgeable about HIV disease. Finally, the drug interactions between lipid-lowering agents and antiretroviral therapy pose additional challenges, and caution should be used whenever prescribing additional medications to an already complex disease and its therapies. Future studies probably will explore the strategy of switching from current PIs and NNRTIs to the newly approved classes of integrase inhibitors and entry inhibitors as a means for improving lipid parameters and reducing cardiovascular risk.

REFERENCES

1. Grinspoon S, Carr A. Cardiovascular risk and body-fat abnormalities in HIV-infected adults. N Engl J Med 2005;352:48–62.
2. Riddler SA, Smit E, Cole SR, et al. Impact of HIV infection and HAART on serum lipids in men. JAMA 2003;289:2978–82.

3. Friis-Moller N, Sabin CA, Weber R, et al. Combination antiretroviral therapy and the risk of myocardial infarction. N Engl J Med 2003;349:1993–2003.
4. DAD Study Group, Friis-Moller N, Reiss P, et al. Class of antiretroviral drugs and the risk of myocardial infarction. N Engl J Med 2007;356:1723–35.
5. El-Sadr WM, Lundgren JD, Neaton JD, et al. CD4+ count-guided interruption of antiretroviral treatment. N Engl J Med 2006;355:2283–96.
6. Cespedes MS, Aberg JA. Cardiovascular and endothelial disease in HIV infection. Curr Infect Dis Rep 2005;7(4):309–15.
7. Lichtenstein K, Armon C, Buchacz K. Analysis of cardiovascular risk factors in the HIV outpatient study (HOPS) cohort. Presented at the Thirteenth Conference on Retroviruses and Opportunistic Infections (CROI); February 5–8, 2006, Denver, Colorado.
8. National Cholesterol Education Program N. Third report of the Expert Panel on Detection, Evaluation and Treatment of High Blood Cholesterol in Adults (Adult Treatment Panel III). Available at: http://www.nhlbi.nih.gov/guidelines/cholesterol/atp3_rpt.htm. Accessed May 23, 2008.
9. Dube MP, Stein JH, Aberg JA, et al. Guidelines for the evaluation and management of dyslipidemia in human immunodeficiency virus (HIV)-infected adults receiving antiretroviral therapy: recommendations of the HIV Medical Association of the Infectious Disease Society of America and the Adult AIDS Clinical Trials Group. Clin Infect Dis 2003;37:613–27.
10. Lundgren JD, Battegay M, Behrens G, et al. European AIDS Clinical Society (EACS) guidelines on the prevention and management of metabolic diseases in HIV. HIV Med 2008 Feb;9(2):72–81. Available at: http://www.eacs.eu/guide/index.htm. Accessed May 23, 2008.
11. Law MG, Friis-Moller N, El-Sadr WM, et al. The use of the Framingham equation to predict myocardial infarctions in HIV-infected patients: comparison with observed events in the D:A:D study. HIV Med 2006;7(4):218–30.
12. Fichtenbaum CJ, Gerber JG, Rosenkranz SL, et al. Pharmacokinetic interactions between protease inhibitors and statins in HIV seronegative volunteers: ACTG study A5047. AIDS 2002;16:569–77.
13. Aboulafia DM, Johnston R. Simvastatin-induced rhabdomyolysis in an HIV-infected patient with coronary artery disease. AIDS Patient Care STDS 2000;14:13–8.
14. Carr R, Andre A, Bertz R. Concomitant administration of ABT-378/ritonavir (ABT-378/r). Results in a clinically important pharmacokinetic (PK) interaction with atorvastatin but not pravastatin [abstract 1644]. 40th Interscience Conference on Antimicrobial Agents and Chemotherapy. Toronto, September 17–20, 2000.
15. Aberg JA, Rosenkranz S, Fichtenbaum CJ, et al. Pharmacokinetic interaction between nelfinavir and pravastatin in HIV-seronegative volunteers: ACTG study A5108. AIDS 2006;20:725–9.
16. Raritan NJ. Prezista (Darunavir) package insert. Tibotec Theraputics February 2008. Available at: http://www.tibotectherapeutics.com/tibotectherapeutics/documents/us_package_insert.pdf. Accessed April 27, 2008.
17. van der Lee M, Sankatsing R, Schippers E, et al. Pharmacokinetics and pharmacodynamics of combined use of lopinavir/ritonavir and rosuvastatin in HIV-infected patients. Antivir Ther 2007;12(7):1127–32.
18. Kiser JJ, Gerber JG, Predhomme JA, et al. Drug/drug interaction between lopinavir/ritonavir and rosuvastatin in healthy volunteers. J Acquir Immune Defic Syndr 2008;47(5):570–8.
19. Gerber JG, Rosenkranz S, Fichtenbaum CJ, et al. The effect of efavirenz on the pharmacokinetics of simvastatin, atorvastatin, and pravastatin: results of ACTG 5108 study. J Acquir Immune Defic Syndr 2005;39:307–12.

20. Croxtall JD, Lyseng-Williamson KA, Perry CM. Raltegravir. Drugs 2008;68(1):131–8.

21. Kiser JJ. Pharmacologic characteristics of investigational and recently approved agents for the treatment of HIV. Curr Opin HIV AIDS 2008;3(3):330–41.

22. Moyle GJ, Lloyd M, Reynolds B, et al. Dietary advice with or without pravastatin for the management of hypercholesterolaemia associated with protease inhibitor therapy. AIDS 2005;15(12):1503–8.

23. Calza L, Manfredi R, Chiodo F. Statins and fibrates for the treatment of hyperlipidaemia in HIV-infected patients receiving HAART. AIDS 2003;17(6):851–9.

24. Aberg JA, Zackin RA, Brobst SW, et al. A randomized trial of the efficacy and safety of fenofibrate versus pravastatin in HIV-infected subjects with lipid abnormalities: AIDS Clinical Trials Group Study 5087. AIDS Res Hum Retroviruses 2005;21:757–67.

25. Aslangul E, Assoumou L, Bittar R, et al. ANRS 126, a prospective, randomized, open label trial comparing the efficacy and safety of rosuvastatin versus pravastatin in HIV-infected subjects receiving ritonavir boosted PI with lipid abnormalities [abstract LBPS7/2]. Eleventh European AIDS Conference. Madrid, October 24–27, 2007.

26. Kastelein JJ, Akdim F, Stroes ES, et al. Simvastatin with or without ezetimibe in familial hypercholesterolemia. N Engl J Med 2008;358:1431–43.

27. Negredo E, Molto J, Puig J, et al. Ezetimibe, a promising lipid-lowering agent for the treatment of dyslipidaemia in HIV-infected patients with poor response to statins. AIDS 2006;20:2159–64.

28. Bennett MT, Johns KW, Bondy GP. Ezetimibe is effective when added to maximally tolerated lipid lowering therapy in patients with HIV. Lipids Health Dis 2007;6:15.

29. Wohl D, Hsue P, Richard S, et al. Ezetimibe' effects on the LDL cholesterol levels of HIV-infected patients receiving HAART [abstract 39]. 14th Conference on Retroviruses and Opportunistic Infections. Los Angeles, February 25–28, 2007.

30. Hokanson JE, Austin MA. Plasma triglyceride level is a risk factor for cardiovascular disease independent of high-density cholesterol level: a meta-analysis of population-based prospective studies. J Cardiovasc Risk 1996;3:213–9.

31. Cullen P. Evidence that triglycerides are an independent coronary artery disease risk factor. Am J Cardiol 2000;86:943–9.

32. McBride PE. Triglycerides and risk factors for coronary heart disease: editorial. JAMA 2007;298:236–8.

33. Miller J, Brown D, Amin J, et al. A randomized, double-blind study of gemfibrozil for the treatment of protease inhibitor-associated hypertriglyceridaemia. AIDS 2002;16:2195–200.

34. Thomas JC, Lopes-Virella MF, Del Bene VE, et al. Use of fenofibrate in the management of protease inhibitor-associated lipid abnormalities. Pharmacotherapy 2000;20(6):727–34.

35. de Luis DA, Bachiller P, Aller R. Fenofibrate in hyperlipidaemia secondary to HIV protease inhibitors. Fenofibrate and HIV protease inhibitor. Nutrition 2001;17(5):414–5.

36. Calza L, Manfredi R, Chiodo F. Use of fibrates in the management of hyperlipidemia in HIV-infected patients receiving HAART. Infection 2002;30(1):26–31.

37. Caramelli B, de Bernoche CY, Sartori AM, et al. Hyperlipidemia related to the use of HIV-protease inhibitors: natural history and results of treatment with fenofibrate. Braz J Infect Dis 2001;5(6):332–8.

38. Palacios R. Efficacy and safety of fenofibrate for the treatment of hypertriglyceridemia associated with antiretroviral therapy. J Acquir Immune Defic Syndr 2002;31(2):251–3.

39. Badiou S. Fenofibrate improves the atherogenic lipid profile and enhances LDL resistance to oxidation in HIV-positive adults. Atherosclerosis 2004;172(2):273–9.

40. Rao A, D'Amico S, Balasubramanyam A, et al. Fenofibrate is effective in treating hypertriglyceridemia associated with HIV lipodystrophy. Am J Med Sci 2004; 327(6):315–8.

41. Kris-Etherton PM, Harris WS, Appel LJ, for the AHA Nutrition Committee. Omega-3 fatty acids and cardiovascular disease: new recommendations from the American Heart Association. Arterioscler Thromb Vasc Biol 2003;23:151–2.

42. De Truchis P, Kirstetter M, Perier A, et al. Reduction in triglyceride levels with N-3 polyunsaturated fatty acids in HIV-infected patients taking potent antiretroviral therapy: a randomized prospective study. J Acquir Immune Defic Syndr 2007; 44:278–85, for the VIH Study Group.

43. Wohl DA, Tien H-C, Busby M, et al. Randomized study of the safety and efficacy of fish oil (omega-3 fatty acids) supplementation with dietary and exercise counseling for the treatment of antiretroviral therapy-associated hypertriglyceridemia. Clin Infect Dis 2005;41:1498–504.

44. Gerber JG, Kitch DW, Fichtenbaum CJ, et al. Fish oil and fenofibrate for the treatment of hypertriglyceridemia in HIV-infected subjects on antiretroviral therapy: results of ACTG A5186. J Acquir Immune Defic Syndr 2008;47(4):459–66.

45. Baril JG, Kovacs CM, Trottier S, et al. Effectiveness and tolerability of oral administration of low-dose salmon oil to HIV patients with HAART-associated dyslipidemia. HIV Clin Trials 2007;8(6):400–11.

46. Gerber MY, Mondy KE, Yarasheski KE, et al. Niacin in HIV-infected individuals with hyperlipidemia receiving potent antiretroviral therapy. Clin Infect Dis 2004; 39(3):419–25.

47. Dubé MP, Wu JW, Aberg JA, et al. for the AIDS Clinical Trials Group Study A5148. Safety and efficacy of extended-release niacin for the treatment of dyslipidemia in patients with HIV infection: AIDS Clinical Trials Group study A5148. Antivir Ther 2006;11:1081–9.

48. Lichtenstein K, Armon C, Buchacz K, et al. Analysis of cardiovascular risk factors in the HIV outpatient study cohort [abstract 735]. In: Program and abstracts of the 13th conference on retroviruses and opportunistic infections. 2006; Denver, February 5–8, 2006.

49. Barragan P, Fisac C, Podzamczer D. Switching strategies to improve lipid profile and morphologic changes. AIDS Rev 2006;8(4):191–203.

50. D:A:D Study Group. Use of nucleoside reverse transcriptase inhibitors and risk of myocardial infarction in HIV-infected patients enrolled in the D:A:D study: a multi-cohort collaboration. Lancet 2008;371:1417–26.

51. Jones SP, Qazi N, Morelese J, et al. Assessment of adipokine expression and mitochondrial toxicity in HIV patients with lipoatrophy on stavudine- and zidovudine-containing regimens. J Acquir Immune Defic Syndr 2005;40(5):565–72.

52. Tarr PE, Taffe P, Bleiber G, et al. Modeling the influence of APOC3, APOE, and TNF polymorphisms on the risk of antiretroviral therapy–associated lipid disorders. J Infect Dis 2005;191:1419–26.

53. Foulkes AS, Wohl DA, Frank I, et al. Associations among race/ethnicity, ApoC-III genotypes, and lipids in HIV-1-infected individuals on antiretroviral therapy. PLoS Med 2006;3(3):e52.

54. Kumar PN, Rodriguez-French A, Thompson MA, et al. A prospective, 96-week study of the impact of Trizivir, Combivir/nelfinavir, and lamivudine/stavudine/nelfinavir on lipids, metabolic parameters and efficacy in antiretroviral-naive patients: effect of sex and ethnicity. HIV Med 2006;7:85–98.

55. Gallant JE, Staszewski S, Pozniak AL, et al. Efficacy and safety of tenofovir DF vs stavudine in combination therapy in antiretroviral-naive patients: a 3-year randomized trial. JAMA 2004;292:191–201.

56. Squires K, Pozniak AL, Pierone G Jr, et al. Tenofovir disoproxil fumarate in nucleoside-resistant HIV-1 infection: a randomized trial. Ann Intern Med 2003;139: 313–20.

57. Madruga JR, Cassetti I, Suleiman JMAH, et al. [903E Study Team]. The safety and efficacy of switching stavudine to tenofovir df in combination with lamivudine and efavirenz in HIV-1-infected patients: three-year follow-up after switching therapy. HIV Clin Trials 2007;8(6):381–90.

58. Guillemi S, Toulson A, Joy R. Changes in lipid profile upon switching from lopinavir/ritonavir (LPV/r) to atazanavir + ritonavir (ATZ + RTV) based HAART. Paper presented at the XVI International AIDS Conference. Toronto, August 13–18, 2006.

59. Gatell J, Salmon-Ceron D, Lazzaria A. Efficacy and safety of atazanavir-based highly active antiretroviral therapy in patients with virologic suppression switched from a stable, boosted or unboosted protease inhibitor treatment regimen: the SWAN study (AI424-097) 48-week results. Clin Infect Dis 2007;44(11):1484–92.

60. Martinez E, Azuaje C, Antela A. Effects of switching to ritonavir-boosted atazanavir on HIV-infected patients receiving antiretroviral therapy with hyperlipidemia [abstract # 850]. 12th Conference on Retroviruses and Opportunistic Infections. Boston, February 22–25, 2005.

61. Calza L, Manfredi R, Colangeli V, et al. Substitution of nevirapine or efavirenz for protease inhibitor versus lipid-lowering therapy for the management of dyslipidaemia. AIDS 2005;19:1051–8.

62. Van Der Valk M, Friis-Møller N, Sabin C. Effect of interventions to improve dyslipidaemia. Paper presented at the 8th International Congress on Drug Therapy in HIV Infection. Glasgow, United Kingdom, November 12–16, 2006.

Lipid Management in Chronic Kidney Disease, Hemodialysis, and Transplantation

Terri Montague, MD[a],*, Barbara Murphy, MD[b]

KEYWORDS

- Chronic kidney disease • Hyperlipidemia • Statin
- Hemodialysis • Renal transplantation

The optimal management of lipid abnormalities in patients who have chronic kidney disease (CKD) remains controversial. There are limited data to guide the use of lipid-lowering drugs in this population, because most of the landmark trials that showed benefits of lipid-lowering therapy on cardiovascular mortality in the general population included few patients who had CKD.[1–3] This issue is important, because cardiovascular morbidity and mortality are high in the CKD population. If pharmacologic therapy lowers the risk of cardiovascular events even modestly, the impact in this high-risk group is substantial. The high rates of cardiovascular disease in the CKD, end-stage renal disease (ESRD), and renal transplant population are multifactorial; risk factors include general risk factors, such as diabetes, hypertension, and smoking, and also factors unique to renal disease, such as vascular calcification and chronic low-grade inflammation. The impact of dyslipidemia and lipid-lowering therapy in this population is unclear.

Recent studies have shown the spectrum of dyslipidemia in patients who have CKD or ESRD to be different from that of the general population. There seems to be a shift to a uremic profile as the renal function deteriorates.[4,5] The magnitude of the abnormalities is not disclosed fully by routine laboratory chemistries that test only total cholesterol, LDL cholesterol, HDL cholesterol, and triglyceride levels. Other modifications such as oxidation and glycation of lipoproteins may promote further atherosclerosis.[6] The few trials aimed at studying dyslipidemia in the ESRD and renal transplant population have shown mixed benefits from lipid-lowering therapy.[7,8] This article discusses the pathophysiology of dyslipidemia in CKD, dialysis, and renal transplant patients, the therapeutic options, and their association with clinical

[a] Division of Kidney Disease and Hypertension, 593 Eddy Street, APC 9, Brown Medical School, Providence, RI 02903, USA
[b] Division of Nephrology, Mount Sinai School of Medicine, 1468 Madison Avenue, Annenberg Building, New York, NY 10029, USA
* Corresponding author.
E-mail address: tmontague@lifespan.org (T. Montague).

Endocrinol Metab Clin N Am 38 (2009) 223–234
doi:10.1016/j.ecl.2008.11.004
0889-8529/08/$ – see front matter © 2009 Published by Elsevier Inc.

endo.theclinics.com

outcomes. Whenever possible, comparisons are made to outcomes in the general population.

PATHOPHYSIOLOGY AND PREVALENCE OF DYSLIPIDEMIA IN CHRONIC KIDNEY DISEASE, DIALYSIS, AND TRANSPLANTATION

Lipids are insoluble in plasma and thus require association with proteins (apolipoproteins) to form dissolvable particles called "lipoproteins." These lipoproteins function mainly in transporting cholesterol or triglycerides from sites of absorption (gut) or synthesis (liver) to sites of use (peripheral tissues) or metabolism. Lipoprotein profiles seem to be affected by the severity of renal dysfunction and proteinuria.[9] High-density lipoprotein (HDL), total cholesterol, and low-density lipoprotein (LDL) levels tend to decrease with declining renal function and on average are lower in patients who have stage 3 to stage 5 CKD than in the general population.[10]

As CKD advances to renal failure and dialysis, the levels of total cholesterol and LDL cholesterol tend to decrease. Despite this decrease, more than 50% of dialysis patients have LDL cholesterol levels greater than 100 mg/dL or non–high-density (non-HDL) lipoprotein cholesterol levels greater than 130 mg/dL.[11] The prevalence of LDL cholesterol levels greater than 100 mg/dL is 85%, 70%, and 90%, respectively, in patients who have nephrotic syndrome, patients who are being treated with peritoneal dialysis, and renal transplant patients.[12] In general, patients treated with peritoneal dialysis tend to have a more atherogenic lipid profile, with increased LDL cholesterol and oxidized LDL levels, than patients treated with hemodialysis.[12] This difference may result in part from the use of dextrose-containing peritoneal dialysate and glucose absorption across the peritoneal membrane.[13]

Measurements of serum LDL cholesterol in patients who have kidney disease also may underestimate the atherogenic potential if it does not measure the LDL subfractions, such as small, dense LDL particles and lipoprotein (a), which are increased in these patients.[14] Small, dense LDL particles tend to penetrate the vascular endothelium, become oxidized, and be taken up by scavenger receptors on macrophages and vascular smooth muscle cells. Once overloaded with cholesterol esters, these macrophages transform into foam cells, further accelerating atherosclerosis.[15] The increased levels of oxidative stress and inflammation in CKD may promote the conversion of LDL to this more atherogenic form.[16]

Lipoprotein (a), a modified form of LDL that exists in different isoforms, has been found to be a risk factor for cardiovascular disease (CVD) in the general population and is highly atherogenic.[17] Structurally it resembles plasminogen and interferes with fibrinolysis,[18] and it also binds to macrophages, promoting foam cell formation. Plasma lipoprotein (a) levels are affected by renal function. In patients who have large lipoprotein (a) isoforms, levels have been found to increase as the glomerular filtration rate (GFR) decreases.[19] After successful kidney transplantation, a decrease in large isoforms of plasma lipoprotein (a) is noted in patients previously treated with hemodialysis, and a decrease in all isoforms is seen in patients previously treated with peritoneal dialysis.[20,21] Elevated lipoprotein (a) is an independent risk factor for CVD in patients treated with hemodialysis and has been associated with vascular events.[22,23]

Triglyceride levels tend to increase early in CKD and are particularly high in patients who have nephrotic syndrome and patients treated with dialysis.[14] In the plasma, triglycerides are found predominantly in chylomicrons and in very-low-density lipoproteins (VLDLs). Chylomicrons are assembled in the intestine and transport dietary fatty acids, whereas VLDLs are produced in the live rand transport endogenous fatty acids. The increase in triglycerides is caused partly by the decreased catabolic rate of these lipoproteins resulting from the decreased activity of vascular endothelium-associated lipases such as lipoprotein lipase and hepatic triglyceride lipase.[24] Impaired lipase activity may be caused by an inhibitor effect of hyperparathyroidism, calcium accumulation in islet cells leading to impaired insulin secretion, or depletion of the enzyme pool by frequent heparinization during hemodialysis.[25,26] This decreased catabolism leads to prolonged exposure of the arterial vasculature to triglyceride-rich lipoprotein remnants that are atherogenic.[18] Studies in the general population have shown elevated triglyceride levels to be an independent risk factor for CVD.[27]

Patients who have CKD and patients treated with dialysis tend to have lower plasma HDL cholesterol levels than common in the general population.[28] HDL plays a role in the reverse cholesterol transport, moving cholesterol from peripheral cells to the liver. This decrease leads to increased cholesterol levels peripherally and in the vasculature, thereby promoting atherosclerosis.

These relative differences in the lipid profiles of uremic patients render questionable the extrapolation of data on the benefits of lipid-lowering therapy derived from the general population. In addition, given the relatively lower levels of total cholesterol and LDL cholesterol on standard lipid profile measurements that do not measure small, dense LDL particles, lipoprotein (a), VLDL, and chylomicron, potentially beneficial therapy may be withheld if guidelines for initiation are not met (ie, LDL cholesterol level >100 mg/dL).

DYSLIPIDEMIA AND CARDIOVASCULAR MORTALITY IN CHRONIC KIDNEY DISEASE, DIALYSIS, AND TRANSPLANTATION

In the general population, clinical trials have demonstrated that cardiovascular mortality decreases proportionally with the rate of LDL cholesterol reduction.[3,29,30] There are few data on the contribution of dyslipidemia toward cardiovascular morbidity and mortality in the CKD population. It is possible that in the setting of CKD with contributing factors such as anemia, inflammation, and proteinuria, dyslipidemia may contribute differently to the overall risk. In a prospective cohort study, Muntner and colleagues[31] evaluated the contribution of different risk factors to cardiovascular mortality in the nondialysis CKD population. The study involved 14,856 participants with a mean follow-up period of 10.5 years. The association between the severity of dyslipidemia and future cardiovascular events was similar to that in patients who had normal renal function. The study included patients who had mild (GFR 60–90 mL/min/1.73 m^2 body surface area [bsa]) and moderate to severe CKD (GFR 15–59 mL/min/1.73 m^2 bsa). Based on their data, the authors predicted that for every 42-mg/dL (1.1-mmol/L) reduction in total cholesterol, there would be a 19.7% reduction in cardiovascular events. This study, however, did not show that treatment of dyslipidemia actually decreases cardiovascular mortality in the CKD population.

The data in the dialysis population are conflicting. Two prospective studies in patients treated with hemodialysis showed no relationship between total cholesterol, triglyceride, LDL cholesterol, or HDL cholesterol levels and future cardiovascular events, but a cross-sectional and a prospective study showed a positive association.[19,22,32–35] In 1995, Lowrie and colleagues,[36] in a retrospective study involving 12,000 patients undergoing hemodialysis, found a U-shaped relationship between cholesterol levels and mortality. Patients who had low total cholesterol levels (<100 mg/dL) had more than four times the mortality risk of patients who had total cholesterol levels between 200 and 250 mg/dL. Once adjusted for albumin, the relationship became more linear, suggesting a potential role of malnutrition. In a 10-year prospective study of 1167 Japanese patients undergoing hemodialysis, low cholesterol was associated independently with higher C-reactive protein levels and mortality in patients who had low albumin levels.[37] In a subgroup of patients who had albumin levels higher than 4.5 mg/dL, however, higher levels of cholesterol were associated with increased mortality. Liu and colleagues,[38] in a prospective study of 823 patients starting hemodialysis or peritoneal dialysis in the United States, found that an increase in total cholesterol levels in the setting of inflammation and malnutrition decreased all-cause mortality. In the absence of inflammation and malnutrition, however, higher total cholesterol levels were associated positively with all-cause mortality. Both these studies show hypercholesterolemia to be a risk factor for all-cause mortality in the dialysis population, which is modified in the presence of inflammation and malnutrition.

In the renal transplant population, the incidence of both hyperlipidemia and CVD is high. The hyperlipidemia is multifactorial, and causes include previously discussed factors such as renal dysfunction, proteinuria, obesity, and diabetes as well as risk factors unique to transplant recipients, including immunosuppressive medications. In this population studies have not demonstrated conclusively a causal relationship between hyperlipidemia and CVD. Several small studies, however, have shown that treatment leads to decreased rates of mortality, rejection, and chronic allograft nephropathy.[39,40]

CURRENT TREATMENT GUIDELINES

The National Kidney Foundation has established guidelines that recommend aggressive therapy of dyslipidemia in patients who have kidney disease.[41] These guidelines are based on the risk reductions achieved in the general population in patients who have or are at high risk for CVD, on the high risk of CVD in patients who have kidney disease, and on the overall safety of most pharmacologic therapies. These guidelines, however, also acknowledge the paucity of data in this population.

In keeping with the National Cholesterol Education Program (NCEP) guidelines for hyperlipidemia in the general population, the National Kidney Foundation guidelines recommend lifestyle modifications with diet and exercise.[42] Both sets of guidelines endorse therapeutic lifestyle changes including reduced intake of saturated fat, trans fats, and cholesterol, increased intake of fiber, weight loss, increased exercise, avoidance of (or moderation in the use of) alcohol, and treatment of high blood glucoses. The work group also concluded that, with a few notable differences, many of the NCEP guidelines are applicable to stage 1 to stage 5 CKD, including patients who have received a renal transplant (regardless of whether the GFR is >90 mL/min/1.73 m^2 bsa). One guideline places all patients who have renal insufficiency, including renal transplant recipients, in the highest category of cardiovascular risk. As a result, a target LDL cholesterol level of less than 100 mg/dL is recommended for all renal patients. Furthermore, for renal patients who have an LDL cholesterol level between 100 and 129 mg/dL, pharmacologic therapy should be used after only 3 months of lifestyle changes, although this guideline is considered optional in the general population. For renal patients whose LDL cholesterol is greater than 120 mg/dL, lifestyle changes should be initiated concurrently with pharmacologic therapy. The National Kidney Foundation guidelines also suggest that fibrates may be used in stage 5 CKD for patients who have triglyceride levels higher than 500 mg/dL or patients who have triglyceride levels higher than 200 mg/dL, non-HDL cholesterol levels greater than 130 mg/dL, and who cannot tolerate statins. This guideline is in contrast to the NCEP Adult Treatment Panel guidelines, in which fibrates are contraindicated in stage 5 CKD.

PHARMACOLOGIC MANAGEMENT OF DYSLIPIDEMIA IN CHRONIC KIDNEY DISEASE, DIALYSIS, AND TRANSPLANTATION
Antioxidants

Oxidative stress, as discussed previously, plays a role in promoting atherosclerosis in patients who have CKD. As a result, antioxidants such as vitamin E have been used in attempts to decrease atherogenic oxidized lipid levels. Randomized trials in the general population did not demonstrate any cardiovascular benefits.[43,44] Boaz and colleagues,[45] however, in a trial of 196 patients treated with hemodialysis who had pre-existing cardiovascular disease, found that vitamin E given for median time of 519 days resulted in a 54% reduction in the composite end point of myocardial infarction, peripheral vascular disease, and ischemic stroke as compared with placebo. In another study, vitamin E was found to increase HDL cholesterol levels in patients treated with dialysis.[46] Larger randomized studies are needed to validate these results.

3-Hydroxy-3-Methylglutaryl Coenzyme A Reductase Inhibitors (Statins)

In the general population, studies have shown a direct correlation between increasing levels of total and LDL cholesterol and cardiovascular mortality.[47,48] Treatment with lipid-lowering therapy has shown clear benefits in cardiac outcomes in both primary and secondary prevention studies.[1,49,50] Studies of statin use in patients treated with peritoneal dialysis or hemodialysis and in renal transplant recipients have shown that statins are effective in reducing LDL cholesterol levels, but few studies have evaluated the correlation between statin use and a reduction in cardiovascular mortality.[7,8,51,52]

Stage 2 through stage 4 chronic kidney disease
In large, randomized trials in the general population, there have been several post hoc analyses of subgroups with impaired renal function. The Pravastatin Pooling Project combined patient results of three randomized trials of pravastatin versus placebo in the general population.[53] The three trials were the West of Scotland Coronary Prevention Study, the Cholesterol and Recurrent Events study, and the Long-term Intervention with Pravastatin in Ischemic Disease study.[2,3,54] The primary outcome studied was time to myocardial infarction, coronary death, or cardiac intervention. Of the 19,700 patients included, 4491 had moderate CKD defined by a GFR between 30 and 60 mL/min/1.73 m^2 bsa. CKD was associated with increased risk for the primary outcome with a hazard ratio of 1.26 (95% confidence interval, 1.07–1.49). In the patients who had CKD, 40 mg of pravastatin was associated with a 23% reduction in the composite outcome over 5 years. This result was similar to those obtained in patients who did not have CKD. In the Anglo-Scandinavian Cardiac Outcomes Trial, subgroup analysis of 6517 patients who had kidney dysfunction followed for a median of 3.3 years revealed that 10 mg of atorvastatin led to a significant (39%) reduction in nonfatal myocardial infarction and cardiac death.[55] Both these studies included patients who had or who were at high risk for coronary artery disease. It is unknown whether there is a benefit to patients who have moderate CKD without coronary artery disease.

Dialysis

In patients treated with dialysis, Seliger and colleagues,[56] in the Dialysis Morbidity and Mortality wave 2 study, studied the effect on mortality of starting statins at the initiation of dialysis. The cohort of 3716 prospective study participants included patients treated with peritoneal dialysis and a random sample of 20% of the patients treated with hemodialysis from the US Renal Data System. The rate of statin use at the initiation of dialysis was low, at 9.7%, and recipients tended to have pre-existing coronary artery disease and diabetes. In this study cardiovascular mortality decreased by 37% in the statin recipients. This trial was not a randomized, controlled study, however, and it is uncertain if the results are generalizable to the entire dialysis population. These findings were not confirmed by the Die Deutsche Diabetes-Dialyse (4D) study.[8] This controlled trial randomly assigned 1255 diabetic patients treated with hemodialysis to atorvastatin, 20 mg, or placebo. Despite a 42% reduction in the LDL cholesterol level in the atorvastatin group, the rate of the composite end point of death from cardiac causes, fatal stroke, nonfatal myocardial infarction, and nonfatal stroke was similar in the two groups at 3 years. The rate of coronary interventions was 18% lower in the atorvastatin group, but the risk of fatal stroke was doubled. Statin drugs may have limited benefit in advanced CVD, but further studies are needed to establish this benefit firmly.

Renal transplantation

To date, only one trial has examined the mortality benefits of statin treatment in renal transplant recipients. The Assessment of Fluvastatin in Renal Transplantation study evaluated the effect of fluvastatin, 40 mg, compared with placebo on the cardiac outcomes of renal transplant recipients.[7] This study, which enrolled 2102 stable transplant recipients 6 months after transplantation, is notable for its size. The follow-up duration was 5 to 6 years. Fluvastatin lowered LDL cholesterol levels by 32%, but no significant reduction was seen in the combined primary end points of cardiac death, definite or probable myocardial infarction, or coronary intervention. A post hoc analysis examining the effect of fluvastatin on definite myocardial infarction or cardiac death (omitting the end point of coronary intervention) showed that fluvastatin was associated with a statistically significant risk reduction of 35%.[57]

Overall there may be a benefit of statin use in early CKD that decreases as renal failure advances. Two ongoing randomized trials are evaluating statin use in patients who have CKD. The Study of Heart and Renal Protection (SHARP) will evaluate the combined effect of simvastatin and ezetimibe versus placebo in the primary prevention of heart disease and stroke.[58] Six thousand patients who have CKD with plasma creatinine levels greater than 1.7 mg/dL in men and greater than 1.5 mg/dL in women and 3000 patients being treated with dialysis will be recruited. A second trial, the Study to Evaluate the Use of Rosuvastatin in Subjects on Regular Hemodialysis: an Assessment of Survival and Cardiovascular Events (AURORA), will evaluate the effect of rosuvastatin on the incidence of cardiovascular deaths, heart attacks, and strokes in patients with and without diabetes who are being treated with hemodialysis.[59,60] Neither study has lipid inclusion criteria.

A serious and common complication of statin therapy is myositis, the importance of which was emphasized by the recall of cerivastatin in 2001. This concern was not recognized in either the 4D study or the other large studies. Most statins are metabolized by the cytochrome P450 (CYP) 3A4, and myotoxicity is increased if they are taken with medications that inhibit this metabolism (eg, immunosuppressive medications such as cyclosporine, tacrolimus, and sirolimus and other medications such as verapamil, diltizaem, erythromycin, and several antidepressants).[61] Exceptions among statins include fluvastatin, which is metabolized by CYP2C9, and pravastatin and rosuvastatin, which are metabolized by a non–cytochrome-dependent mechanism. The potential for drug–drug interactions are substantial, and thus caution and close monitoring are recommended. Current recommendations are that, except for atorvastatin and pravastatin, the statin dose be reduced by 50% in patients being treated with dialysis.[62,63] In transplant recipients, the current recommendations are that a lower initial dose of statin be used, particularly with concomitant use of cyclosporine.[41] Studies involving rosuvastatin in patients who had severe renal insufficiency noted higher rosuvastatin levels than seen in patients who had normal renal function, and thus a lower starting dose of 5 mg is recommended.[64]

Statin and additional effects

Statins may exert additional effects independent of the effect on LDL cholesterol. The results of one small observational study in patients treated with hemodialysis suggest that statins may have anti-inflammatory properties, because significant decreases were seen in C-reactive protein levels after 8 weeks of simvastatin treatment.[65] Other small, randomized trials suggest that statins also may help slow the decline in GFR.[66,67] Bianchi and colleagues[66] studied the effect of atorvastatin, 10 to 40 mg/d, versus placebo in 56 patients who had CKD. They found that after 1 year the rate of proteinuria decreased significantly with atorvastatin compared with placebo. In a post hoc analysis of a subgroup of 690 patients who had moderate CKD (GFR < 60 mL/min/1.73 m^2 bsa), statin therapy slowed the decline in GFR, especially in patients who had proteinuria.[67]

Fibrates

In the general population, fibrates reduce plasma triglyceride levels and modestly increase HDL cholesterol concentrations. They are indicated when a triglyceride level greater than 500 mg/dL is the primary lipid abnormality and may reduce these levels by up to 50%.[11] Gemfibrozil was associated with 20% reduction in cardiovascular events in patients who had mild to moderate renal insufficiency (GFR 30–75 mL/min/1.73 m^2 bsa).[68] In patients who had dyslipidemia who were treated with continuous ambulatory peritoneal dialysis, gemfibrozil led to significant reductions in triglyceride levels without myositis or liver toxicity.[69,70] The dose used in these studies was less than that used in the general population (600 mg/d or 600 mg every other day). There have been case reports of rhabdomyolysis associated with use of fibrates in ESRD and hypothyroidism, however.[71,72] There also have been reports of worsening kidney function associated with the use of clofibrate, bezafibrate, and fenofibrate in patients who had mild to moderate CKD.[73] Recent guidelines discourage the use of fibrates in patients who have a GFR of less than 15 mL/min/1.73m^2 bsa.[11]

Bile Acid Sequestrants

Treatment with cholestyramine in asymptomatic individuals who had normal kidney function reduced cardiovascular mortality by 19%.[29] In the general population, bile acid sequestrants used in combination with statins lower LDL cholesterol levels by up to 20%. Because these drugs are not absorbed in the gastrointestinal tract, in theory no dose adjustments are needed for patients who have reduced kidney function. Bile acid sequestrants do interfere with cyclosporine absorption, however, and also may cause increases in triglyceride levels. There are few data on the safety and cardiac outcomes of these agents in the CKD population.

Nicotinic Acid

Nicotinic acid reduces the secretion of VLDL by the liver.[74] The National Kidney Foundation guidelines recommend nicotinic acid as an alternative second agent for LDL cholesterol reduction in combination with a statin.[11] The side effects associated with the administration of niacin, such as flushing, hyperglycemia, and hepatoxicity, decrease its tolerability, leading to high rates of noncompliance. One study compared the results of nicotinic acid, clofibrate, and pravastatin on LDL cholesterol levels in patients treated with continuous ambulatory peritoneal dialysis or hemodialysis.[75] There were no adverse effects with any of the treatments, but statins were superior in reducing LDL cholesterol levels.

Sevelamer Hydrochloride

Sevelamer is a cationic polymer that binds phosphates via ion exchange. It also has been found to reduce plasma total cholesterol levels by 18% to 22% and plasma LDL cholesterol levels by 30% to 37% by binding bile acids in the intestine.[76] An open-label study involving 192 patients treated by hemodialysis who used sevelamer for 46 weeks showed a 36% reduction in LDL cholesterol level and an 18% increase in HDL cholesterol level.[77] In the Treat to Goal Study, patients receiving sevelamer were found to have significantly lower rates of coronary artery calcification and an associated decrease in LDL cholesterol levels.[78] There have been no long-term outcome studies of the cardiovascular benefits of sevelamer.

SUMMARY

Commonly used clinical assays that measure only triglyceride, LDL cholesterol, HDL cholesterol, and total cholesterol levels may not measure the additional lipid abnormalities prevalent in uremia. Post hoc analysis of large clinical trials in the general population seems to support the beneficial effects of statins in renal transplant recipients and patients in the early stages of CKD, but the evidence is unclear in the latter stages of CKD. Data on the use of statins in the ESRD population are sparse, and the results have been discouraging in the one completed study, the 4D trial. Patients who have CKD, in particular the subset treated by dialysis, are at high risk for cardiovascular morbidity and mortality, and thus this lack of data represents a significant gap in knowledge. It is hoped that the results of the ongoing SHARP and AURORA trials will help guide the use of statins in this population.

REFERENCES

1. MRC/BHF heart protection study of cholesterol lowering with simvastatin in 20,536 high-risk individuals: a randomised placebo-controlled trial. Lancet 2002;360: 7–22.
2. Sacks FM, Pfeffer MA, Moye LA, et al. The effect of pravastatin on coronary events after myocardial infarction in patients with average cholesterol levels. Cholesterol and Recurrent Events trial investigators. N Engl J Med 1996; 335(14):1001–9.
3. Shepherd J, Cobbe SM, Ford I, et al. Prevention of coronary heart disease with pravastatin in men with hypercholesterolemia. West of Scotland Coronary Prevention Study Group. N Engl J Med 1995;333(20):1301–7.
4. Kronenberg F, Kuen E, Ritz E, et al. Lipoprotein(a) serum concentrations and apolipoprotein(a) phenotypes in mild and moderate renal failure. J Am Soc Nephrol 2000;11(1):105–15.

5. Weintraub M, Burstein A, Rassin T, et al. Severe defect in clearing postprandial chylomicron remnants in dialysis patients. Kidney Int 1992;42(5):1247–52.
6. Galle J, Wanner C. Modification of lipoproteins in uremia: oxidation, glycation and carbamoylation. Miner Electrolyte Metab 1999;25(4–6):263–8.
7. Holdaas H, Fellstrom B, Jardine AG, et al. Effect of fluvastatin on cardiac outcomes in renal transplant recipients: a multicentre, randomised, placebo-controlled trial. Lancet 2003;361(9374):2024–31.
8. Wanner C, Krane V, Marz W, et al. Atorvastatin in patients with type 2 diabetes mellitus undergoing hemodialysis. N Engl J Med 2005;353(3):238–48.
9. Molitch ME. Management of dyslipidemias in patients with diabetes and chronic kidney disease. Clin J Am Soc Nephrol 2006;1(5):1090–9.
10. Kasiske BL. Hyperlipidemia in patients with chronic renal disease. Am J Kidney Dis 1998;32(Suppl 3):S142–56.
11. K/DOQI clinical practice guidelines for management of dyslipidemias in patients with kidney disease. Am J Kidney Dis 2003;41(Suppl 3):S1–91.
12. Weiner DE, Sarnak MJ. Managing dyslipidemia in chronic kidney disease. J Gen Intern Med 2004;19(10):1045–52.
13. Attman PO, Samuelsson O, Johansson AC, et al. Dialysis modalities and dyslipidemia. Kidney Int 2003;84:S110–2.
14. Kwan BC, Kronenberg F, Beddhu S, et al. Lipoprotein metabolism and lipid management in chronic kidney disease. J Am Soc Nephrol 2007;18(4):1246–61.
15. Zioncheck TF, Powell LM, Rice GC, et al. Interaction of recombinant apolipoprotein (a) and lipoprotein (a) with macrophages. J Clin Invest 1991;87(3):767–71.
16. Maggi E, Bellazzi R, Falaschi F, et al. Enhanced LDL oxidation in uremic patients: an additional mechanism for accelerated atherosclerosis? Kidney Int 1994;45(3):876–83.
17. Craig WY, Neveux LM, Palomaki GE, et al. Lipoprotein (a) as a risk factor for ischemic heart disease: metaanalysis of prospective studies. Clin Chem 1998;44(11):2301–6.
18. Nogueira J, Weir M. The unique character of cardiovascular disease in chronic kidney disease and its implications for treatment with lipid-lowering drugs. Clin J Am Soc Nephrol 2007;2(4):766–85.
19. Kronenberg F, Neyer U, Lhotta K, et al. The low molecular weight apo(a) phenotype is an independent predictor for coronary artery disease in hemodialysis patients: a prospective follow-up. J Am Soc Nephrol 1999;10(5):1027–36.
20. Kerschdorfer L, Konig P, Neyer U, et al. Lipoprotein(a) plasma concentrations after renal transplantation: a prospective evaluation after 4 years of follow-up. Atherosclerosis 1999;144(2):381–91.
21. Kronenberg F, Konig P, Lhotta K, et al. Apolipoprotein(a) phenotype-associated decrease in lipoprotein(a) plasma concentrations after renal transplantation. Arterioscler Thromb 1994;14(9):1399–404.
22. Cressman MD, Heyka RJ, Paganini EP, et al. Lipoprotein(a) is an independent risk factor for cardiovascular disease in hemodialysis patients. Circulation 1992;86(2):475–82.
23. Longenecker JC, Klag MJ, Marcovina SM, et al. High lipoprotein(a) levels and small apolipoprotein(a) size prospectively predict cardiovascular events in dialysis patients. J Am Soc Nephrol 2005;16(6):1794–802.
24. Arnadottir M. Pathogenesis of dyslipoproteinemia in renal insufficiency: the role of lipoprotein lipase and hepatic lipase. Scand J Clin Lab Invest 1997;57(1):1–11.
25. Arnadottir M, Nilsson-Ehle P. Has parathyroid hormone any influence on lipid metabolism in chronic renal failure? Nephrol Dial Transplant 1995;10(12):2381–2.

26. Nishizawa Y, Shoji T, Kawagishi T, et al. Atherosclerosis in uremia: possible roles of hyperparathyroidism and intermediate density lipoprotein accumulation. Kidney Int Suppl 1997;62:S90–2.

27. Assmann G, Schulte H, Funke H, et al. The emergence of triglycerides as a significant independent risk factor in coronary artery disease. Eur Heart J 1998; 19(Suppl M):M8–14.

28. Farbakhsh K, Kasiske BL. Dyslipidemias in patients who have chronic kidney disease. Med Clin North Am 2005;89(3):689–99.

29. The Lipid Research Clinics Coronary Primary Prevention Trial results. II. The relationship of reduction in incidence of coronary heart disease to cholesterol lowering. JAMA 1984;251(3):365–74.

30. Sever PS, Dahlof B, Poulter NR, et al. Prevention of coronary and stroke events with atorvastatin in hypertensive patients who have average or lower-than-average cholesterol concentrations, in the Anglo-Scandinavian Cardiac Outcomes Trial–Lipid Lowering Arm (ASCOT-LLA): a multicentre randomised controlled trial. Drugs 2004;64(Suppl 2):43–60.

31. Muntner P, He J, Astor BC, et al. Traditional and nontraditional risk factors predict coronary heart disease in chronic kidney disease: results from the atherosclerosis risk in communities study. J Am Soc Nephrol 2005;16(2):529–38.

32. Cheung AK, Sarnak MJ, Yan G, et al. Atherosclerotic cardiovascular disease risks in chronic hemodialysis patients. Kidney Int 2000;58(1):353–62.

33. Hahn R, Oette K, Mondorf H, et al. Analysis of cardiovascular risk factors in chronic hemodialysis patients with special attention to the hyperlipoproteinemias. Atherosclerosis 1983;48(3):279–88.

34. Koch M, Kutkuhn B, Grabensee B, et al. Apolipoprotein A, fibrinogen, age, and history of stroke are predictors of death in dialysed diabetic patients: a prospective study in 412 subjects. Nephrol Dial Transplant 1997;12(12):2603–11.

35. Stack AG, Bloembergen WE. Prevalence and clinical correlates of coronary artery disease among new dialysis patients in the United States: a cross-sectional study. J Am Soc Nephrol 2001;12(7):1516–23.

36. Lowrie EG, Lew NL. Death risk in hemodialysis patients: the predictive value of commonly measured variables and an evaluation of death rate differences between facilities. Am J Kidney Dis 1990;15(5):458–82.

37. Iseki K, Yamazato M, Tozawa M, et al. Hypocholesterolemia is a significant predictor of death in a cohort of chronic hemodialysis patients. Kidney Int 2002;61(5):1887–93.

38. Liu Y, Coresh J, Eustace JA, et al. Association between cholesterol level and mortality in dialysis patients: role of inflammation and malnutrition. JAMA 2004; 291(4):451–9.

39. Kobashigawa JA, Katznelson S, Laks H, et al. Effect of pravastatin on outcomes after cardiac transplantation. N Engl J Med 1995;333(10):621–7.

40. Wenke K, Meiser B, Thiery J, et al. Simvastatin reduces graft vessel disease and mortality after heart transplantation: a four-year randomized trial. Circulation 1997;96(5):1398–402.

41. Kasiske B, Cosio FG, Beto J, et al. Clinical practice guidelines for managing dyslipidemias in kidney transplant patients: a report from the Managing Dyslipidemias in Chronic Kidney Disease Work Group of the National Kidney Foundation Kidney Disease Outcomes Quality Initiative. Am J Transplant 2004;4(Suppl 7):13–53.

42. Third report of the National Cholesterol Education Program (NCEP) Expert Panel on Detection, Evaluation, and Treatment of High Blood Cholesterol in Adults (Adult Treatment Panel III) final report. Circulation 2002;106(25):3143–421.

43. Stephens NG, Parsons A, Schofield PM, et al. Randomised controlled trial of vitamin E in patients with coronary disease: Cambridge Heart Antioxidant Study (CHAOS). Lancet 1996;347(9004):781.

44. Yusuf S, Dagenais G, Pogue J, et al. Vitamin E supplementation and cardiovascular events in high-risk patients. The Heart Outcomes Prevention Evaluation Study investigators. N Engl J Med 2000;342(3):154–60.

45. Boaz M, Smetana S, Weinstein T, et al. Secondary Prevention with Antioxidants of Cardiovascular Disease in Endstage Renal Disease (SPACE): randomised placebo-controlled trial. Lancet 2000;356(9237):1213–8.

46. Khajehdehi P. Effect of vitamins on the lipid profile of patients on regular hemodialysis. Scand J Urol Nephrol 2000;34(1):62–6.

47. Pekkanen J, Linn S, Heiss G, et al. Ten-year mortality from cardiovascular disease in relation to cholesterol level among men with and without preexisting cardiovascular disease. N Engl J Med 1990;322(24):1700–7.

48. Stamler J, Wentworth D, Neaton JD. Is relationship between serum cholesterol and risk of premature death from coronary heart disease continuous and graded? Findings in 356,222 primary screenees of the Multiple Risk Factor Intervention Trial (MRFIT). JAMA 1986;256(20):2823–8.

49. Cannon CP, Braunwald E, McCabe CH, et al. Intensive versus moderate lipid lowering with statins after acute coronary syndromes. N Engl J Med 2004; 350(15):1495–504.

50. Downs JR, Clearfield M, Weis S, et al. Primary prevention of acute coronary events with lovastatin in men and women with average cholesterol levels: results of AFCAPS/TexCAPS. Air Force/Texas Coronary Atherosclerosis Prevention Study. JAMA 1998;279(20):1615–22.

51. Harris KP, Wheeler DC, Chong CC. A placebo-controlled trial examining atorvastatin in dyslipidemic patients undergoing CAPD. Kidney Int 2002;61(4):1469–74.

52. Saltissi D, Morgan C, Rigby RJ, et al. Safety and efficacy of simvastatin in hypercholesterolemic patients undergoing chronic renal dialysis. Am J Kidney Dis 2002;39(2):283–90.

53. Tonelli M, Isles C, Curhan GC, et al. Effect of pravastatin on cardiovascular events in people with chronic kidney disease. Circulation 2004;110(12):1557–60.

54. Prevention of cardiovascular events and death with pravastatin in patients with coronary heart disease and a broad range of initial cholesterol levels. The Long-Term Intervention with Pravastatin in Ischaemic Disease (LIPID) Study Group. N Engl J Med 1998;339(19):1349–57.

55. Sever PS, Dahlof B, Poulter NR, et al. Prevention of coronary and stroke events with atorvastatin in hypertensive patients who have average or lower-than-average cholesterol concentrations, in the Anglo-Scandinavian Cardiac Outcomes Trial–Lipid Lowering Arm (ASCOT-LLA): a multicentre randomised controlled trial. Lancet 2003;361(9364):1149–58.

56. Seliger SL, Weiss NS, Gillen DL, et al. HMG-CoA reductase inhibitors are associated with reduced mortality in ESRD patients. Kidney Int 2002;61(1):297–304.

57. Jardine AG, Holdaas H, Fellstrom B, et al. Fluvastatin prevents cardiac death and myocardial infarction in renal transplant recipients: post-hoc subgroup analyses of the ALERT study. Am J Transplant 2004;4(6):988–95.

58. Baigent C, Landry M. Study of Heart and Renal Protection (SHARP). Kidney Int Suppl 2003;84:S207–10.

59. Fellstrom B, Holdaas H, Jardine AG, et al. Effect of rosuvastatin on outcomes in chronic haemodialysis patients: baseline data from the AURORA study. Kidney Blood Press Res 2007;30(1):314–22.

60. Fellstrom B, Zannad F, Schmieder R, et al. Effect of rosuvastatin on outcomes in chronic haemodialysis patients—design and rationale of the AURORA study. Curr Control Trials Cardiovasc Med 2005;6(5):9.
61. Bilchick KC, Henrikson CA, Skojec D, et al. Treatment of hyperlipidemia in cardiac transplant recipients. Am Heart J 2004;148(2):200–10.
62. Grundy SM, Cleeman JI, Merz CN, et al. Implications of recent clinical trials for the National Cholesterol Education Program Adult Treatment Panel III guidelines. J Am Coll Cardiol 2004;44(3):720–32.
63. Stern RH, Yang BB, Horton M, et al. Renal dysfunction does not alter the pharmacokinetics or LDL-cholesterol reduction of atorvastatin. J Clin Pharmacol 1997;37(9):816–9.
64. Launay-Vacher V, Izzedine H, Deray G. Statins' dosage in patients with renal failure and cyclosporine drug-drug interactions in transplant recipient patients. Int J Cardiol 2005;101(1):9–17.
65. Chang JW, Yang WS, Min WK, et al. Effects of simvastatin on high-sensitivity C-reactive protein and serum albumin in hemodialysis patients. Am J Kidney Dis 2002;39(6):1213–7.
66. Bianchi S, Bigazzi R, Caiazza A, et al. A controlled, prospective study of the effects of atorvastatin on proteinuria and progression of kidney disease. Am J Kidney Dis 2003;41(3):565–70.
67. Tonelli M, Moye L, Sacks FM, et al. Pravastatin for secondary prevention of cardiovascular events in persons with mild chronic renal insufficiency. Ann Intern Med 2003;138(2):98–104.
68. Tonelli M, Collins D, Robins S, et al. Gemfibrozil for secondary prevention of cardiovascular events in mild to moderate chronic renal insufficiency. Kidney Int 2004;66(3):1123–30.
69. Lee MS, Kim SM, Kim SB, et al. Effects of gemfibrozil on lipid and hemostatic factors in CAPD patients. Perit Dial Int 1999;19(3):280–3.
70. Lucatello A, Sturani A, Di Nardo AM, et al. Safe use of gemfibrozil in uremic patients on continuous ambulatory peritoneal dialysis. Nephron 1998;78(3):338.
71. Clouatre Y, Leblanc M, Ouimet D, et al. Fenofibrate-induced rhabdomyolysis in two dialysis patients with hypothyroidism. Nephrol Dial Transplant 1999;14(4):1047–8.
72. Schonfeld G. The effects of fibrates on lipoprotein and hemostatic coronary risk factors. Atherosclerosis 1994;111(2):161–74.
73. Broeders N, Knoop C, Antoine M, et al. Fibrate-induced increase in blood urea and creatinine: is gemfibrozil the only innocuous agent? Nephrol Dial Transplant 2000;15(12):1993–9.
74. Kamionna VS, Kashyap ML. Mechanism of action of niacin. Am J Cardiol 2008;101(8A):20B–6B.
75. Nishizawa Y, Shoji T, Tabata T, et al. Effects of lipid-lowering drugs on intermediate-density lipoprotein in uremic patients. Kidney Int Suppl 1999;71:S134–6.
76. Chertow GM, Burke SK, Raggi P. Sevelamer attenuates the progression of coronary and aortic calcification in hemodialysis patients. Kidney Int 2002;62(1):245–52.
77. Chertow GM, Burke SK, Dillon MA, et al. Long-term effects of sevelamer hydrochloride on the calcium × phosphate product and lipid profile of haemodialysis patients. Nephrol Dial Transplant 1999;14(12):2907–14.
78. Block GA, Spiegel DM, Ehrlich J, et al. Effects of sevelamer and calcium on coronary artery calcification in patients new to hemodialysis. Kidney Int 2005;68(5):1815–24.

Index

Note: Page numbers of article titles are in **boldface** type.

A

Abacavir, interactions with lipid-lowering agents, 209, 216
ACCORD trial, on fibrates, for geriatric patient, 199
Acyl cholesterol acyl transferase, cholesterol absorption inhibitors impact on, 114
Adenosine triphosphate binding membrane cassette transport protein A1 (ABCA1),
    in high-density lipoprotein function, 159–160
    in reverse cholesterol transport, 154–157
Adhesion molecules, expression of, high-density lipoproteins effect on, 155
Adipose triglyceride lipase, in chylomicron metabolism, 138, 145
Advanced lipoprotein testing, **1–31**
    apolipoprotein B in, 3
    evidence as coronary heart disease predictor, 6–24
        all variables compared in one population, 17–22
        ApoB vs. LDL-C results, 12–14
            less favorable, 14
        in diabetic patients, 22–24
        LDL-C particle number vs. LDL-C results, 15–16
        non-HDL-C, LDL-C, and ApoB results, 22–24
        non-HDL-C vs. LDL-C results, 6–7
            less favorable, 7, 12
            trial comparisons of, 6, 8–11
        summary of all studies, 24
    laboratories for, 2, 4
    low-density lipoprotein levels in, 2–3
    measures of, 2, 4
    non–high-density lipoprotein levels in, 2–3
    nuclear magnetic resonance spectroscopy in, 5–6
    recommendations for, 24–26
    segmented gradient gel electrophoresis in, 5
    summary of, 1–2, 26–27
    vertical density gradient ultracentrifugation in, 4–5
Aegerion, as systemic microsomal triglyceride transfer protein inhibitor, 109
AEGR-733, as systemic microsomal triglyceride transfer protein inhibitor, 109
Aerobic exercise, for lipid management, 56–57, 61–62
African Americans, risk score prediction of coronary heart disease in, 36
Age, in risk score prediction, of coronary heart disease, 35–36, 40–41
AIDS patients. See *HIV patients.*
Air Force/Texas Coronary Atherosclerosis Prevention Study (AFCAPS/TEXCAPS),
    on statins, advanced lipoprotein testing in, 10, 13
        for geriatric patient, 190–192
Alanine aminotransferase (ALT), mipomersen impact on, 105, 107
    squalene synthase inhibitors impact on, 112

Endocrinol Metab Clin N Am 38 (2009) 235–264
doi:10.1016/S0889-8529(09)00024-3
0889-8529/09/$ – see front matter © 2009 Elsevier Inc. All rights reserved.

endo.theclinics.com